T0296525

The scientific revolution of the sixteenth and seventeenth centuries is usually characterized in terms of astronomy and the physics of motion. In *The French Paracelsians* Allen Debus narrates an important episode whose contribution to the scientific revolution has been largely ignored: the long-standing contention between Paracelsians and Galenists.

Shortly after the medical authority of Galen had been reestablished during the Renaissance, Paracelsus, a Swiss-German firebrand, proposed a new approach to natural philosophy and medicine – through chemistry. The resulting debate between Paracelsians and Galenists lasted more than a century, embroiling medical establishments across Europe. In France the debate was particularly bitter, with the Medical Faculty of Paris determined to block the introduction of chemistry to medicine in any field. Debus elucidates this important polemic, not only in regard to Paracelsian pharmaceutical chemistry and clinical cosmology, but also in regard to the development of chemical physiology and its struggle with seventeenth-century medicine dominated by mechanical philosophy. Debus shows how the purported triumph of the mechanists in the scientific academies was partial at best, recounting the osmotic acceptance of chemistry by the academies. This persistent influence of medical chemistry, which was significant for the chemical revolution as well as being one of the driving forces behind the scientific revolution, deserves greater recognition by historians.

The French Paracelsians

THE FRENCH PARACELSIANS

*The Chemical Challenge to Medical and
Scientific Tradition in Early Modern France*

ALLEN G. DEBUS

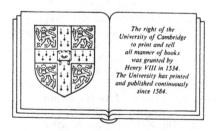

The right of the
University of Cambridge
to print and sell
all manner of books
was granted by
Henry VIII in 1534.
The University has printed
and published continuously
since 1584.

CAMBRIDGE UNIVERSITY PRESS

CAMBRIDGE

NEW YORK   PORT CHESTER   MELBOURNE   SYDNEY

PUBLISHED BY THE PRESS SYNDICATE OF THE UNIVERSITY OF CAMBRIDGE
The Pitt Building, Trumpington Street, Cambridge, United Kingdom

CAMBRIDGE UNIVERSITY PRESS
The Edinburgh Building, Cambridge CB2 2RU, UK
40 West 20th Street, New York NY 10011–4211, USA
477 Williamstown Road, Port Melbourne, VIC 3207, Australia
Ruiz de Alarcón 13, 28014 Madrid, Spain
Dock House, The Waterfront, Cape Town 8001, South Africa

http://www.cambridge.org

© Cambridge University Press 1991

First published 1991
First paperback edition 2002

A catalogue record for this book is available from the British Library

Library of Congress Cataloguing in Publication data
Debus, Allen G.
The French Paracelsians: the chemical challenge to medical and
scientific tradition in early modern France / by Allen G. Debus.
p.   cm.
Includes bibliographical references.
ISBN 0 521 40049 X
1. Chemistry – France – History.   2. Paracelsus, 1493–1541.
3. Medicine – France – 15th–18th centuries.   I. Title.
QD18.F8D43   1991
540′.944′0903–dc20   90-26163

ISBN 0 521 40049 X hardback
ISBN 0 521 89444 1 paperback

This book is dedicated to
John J. Murray
and to the late
A. Haire Forster,
both true educators, without
whose advice and encouragement
many years ago this book would
never have been written.

Contents

Contents

Illustrations

Preface

The present book has resulted from a long-time interest in the relationship of chemistry and medicine during the early modern period that began when I was a graduate student at Indiana University more than forty years ago. It continued through the years I worked as a research chemist at Abbott Laboratories and finally resulted in my decision to leave my position there to enter the then small graduate program in the History of Science at Harvard University in 1956. There, in the Tudor and Stuart seminars of Professor W. K. Jordan I prepared papers on the English followers of the Swiss-German reformer, Paracelsus. In the year 1959–60, with the aid of a Fulbright Award and a Fellowship from the Social Sciences Research Council, I was able to spend a year devoted to research in England where I became acquainted with Walter Pagel, surely this century's greatest authority on the Paracelsians. I will always be indebted to him and to his wife, Magda, for the interest they took in my work.

My doctoral dissertation on the English Paracelsians was completed in 1961 under the direction of Professor I. B. Cohen and published with few changes four years later. This early work resulted in a series of related studies, but my interests were never centered on English science and medicine alone. Rather, my primary concern has always been to broaden our understanding of the scientific revolution of the sixteenth and seventeenth centuries. Thirty years ago this term referred almost exclusively to the progression from Copernicus to Galileo to Newton and, with the exception of the Harveyan circulation, was confined to problems of astronomy and the physics of motion. My own background and interests led me to another area, to the relationship of chemistry and medicine in the period of the scientific revolution.

Following my work on the English Paracelsians I turned to a more general study of the followers of Paracelsus, which was completed in the early 1970s but not published until 1977 as *The Chemical Philosophy: Paracelsian Science and Medicine in the Sixteenth and Seventeenth Centuries*. The following year my book *Man and Nature in the Renaissance* was published by Cambridge University Press. In this I attempted to show the impor-

tance of the Paracelsian chemical debates and their relation to better
known developments of the science of the sixteenth and early seventeenth centuries. Over the next few years I published papers on Spanish
and Portuguese Paracelsism, and even the introduction of Paracelsian
thought in the Ottoman Empire. Separate studies such as these led to an
interest in comparing the reception of Paracelsian thought in the different countries of Europe. A paper devoted to this topic titled "The Chemical Philosophy and the Scientific Revolution" was presented at the
meeting on "Revolutions in Science" sponsored by the University of
Coimbra and the International Union of the History and Philosophy of
Science (1988).

However, throughout these years I have always had a special interest
in the work of the French Paracelsists. I had first become aware of the
importance of Joseph Duchesne and Theodore Turquet de Mayerne during my years as a student at Harvard. I expanded the work in my
dissertation when writing *The Chemical Philosophy* and decided then that
I would eventually prepare a book on the challenge that chemistry
posed to the French medical establishment in the early modern period.
My first essay specifically on the French scene was written for the
Festschrift in honor of Professor I. B. Cohen, but due to long delays in the
completion of that volume the essay appeared first in *Ambix* in 1981 as
"The Paracelsians in Eighteenth Century France: A Renaissance Tradition in the Age of the Enlightenment." This research led me to take a
special interest in the Paracelsian influence in France throughout the
eighteenth century. With the aid of a Fellowship at the Institute for
Research in the Humanities at the University of Wisconsin I was able to
continue my research using the rich resources of the Duveen Collection
at the Memorial Library in Madison during the year 1981–2. At that time
I also prepared a paper on the opening decades of the century, "Alchemy in the Age of Reason: The Chemical Philosophers in Early Eighteenth Century France," for an international meeting on Hermeticism
held at the Folger Shakespeare Library in March 1982. It was eventually
to appear in the proceedings of that conference, *Hermeticism and the
Renaissance: Intellectual History and the Occult in Early Modern Europe*,
edited by Professor Ingrid Merkel and myself. Although this paper was
intended to be the second chapter of a book on eighteenth-century
French Paracelsism, it was actually to form the basis of the fifth chapter
of the present work.

A fellowship from The Folger Shakespeare Library made it possible for
me to spend the first six months of 1987 in Washington where I had
access to the Folger collections as well as the more specialized holdings
of the National Library of Medicine in Bethesda. Because I was able to
spend much of my time writing, it was then that this book took its
present organization. My first thought was to write a book largely confined to the eighteenth century with an introductory chapter on the

period before 1700. However, I soon found that there was so much untouched material from the sixteenth and seventeenth centuries that the manuscript took a new form, beginning with the Galenic world of the early sixteenth century and then going on to the debates resulting from the introduction of chemistry to medicine over the next two centuries.

The picture that emerges from this study is of a Galenic medical establishment challenged by a group of chemical physicians who saw their new preparations as the basis for a sweeping program of chemical reform. Many, if not all, of these Paracelsians added to this a world system founded on the supposed interrelation between the microcosm of man and the great world of the macrocosm. The story of this conflict between tradition and reform took place at the same time as the more familiar debate over the new and the old astronomy and the resultant search for a new physics of motion. Both should form integral parts of any discussion of the scientific revolution. And surely, the significance of medical history for the understanding of the period is nowhere more evident.

The reader should be advised from the start that this work is not meant to be exhaustive. It should be looked upon rather as a preliminary study of a very complex period. I have tried to explain in the prefatory comments to the bibliography that the identification of the works was not always an easy task, and there was often little or no biographical information to rely on. As in my earlier work I found here as well that the authors writing on chemical medicine most frequently presented their work in the vernacular. There are notable exceptions to this rule, but it would seem that the chemists throughout Europe tried to appeal to a larger audience by writing in their native languages. Although Latin was more common among the members of the Medical Faculty of Paris, even they frequently used French in their polemical attacks on the chemists.

I should add that this book does not pretend to be a sociological study. My primary aim has been to identify the major issues dividing the Galenists and the chemists on the basis of the printed sources. To be sure, religious issues are evident, and in the case of Théophraste Renaudot the debate involves politics at a high level; but I have been interested primarily in the intellectual history of this debate. I gladly leave the sociological aspects to others.

As mentioned earlier, this work has evolved from earlier studies. I have used this earlier work here, but generally I have added much new material. The end product shows a far more complex, and far more bitter, confrontation in France than that which existed in the other European countries I have studied. This was surely due in large measure to the importance of and the conservative nature of the Parisian Medical Faculty. Although this debate did not result in a key figure of the stature of Newton, this could not have been foreseeable to scholars of the late sixteenth century. They would only have seen a debate being argued as fiercely as any aspect of the new astronomy. I am convinced that any comprehensive study of the scientific revolution, viewed in historical context, must include the medicochemical debates of the period as a major component.

As always I am indebted to the Morris Fishbein Center for the Study of the History of Science and Medicine and the University of Chicago for support and for a willingness to let me pursue my research elsewhere on occasion. I am also grateful to the National Science Foundation for a research grant during the year 1980–1 which was helpful during the early stages of this research. A year spent at the Institute for Research in the Humanities (1981–2) made it possible to become thoroughly acquainted with the rich holdings of the Duveen and Cole Collections of the Memorial Library at the University of Wisconsin. My work there was made much easier by the aid and interest of John Neu whose knowledge of these collections, and of the bibliography of the history of science, is second to no one's. His friendship and that of the late William Coleman and his wife, Louise, made our year in Madison truly memorable. The fellowship at the Institute at the University of Wisconsin as well as that at the Folger Shakespeare Library in Washington during the first half of 1987 was funded by the National Endowment for the Humanities. Without this support the manuscript would not now be finished.

In addition to the Folger Shakespeare Library and the Memorial Library at the University of Wisconsin my research has been carried out largely at the National Library of Medicine in Bethesda, the Wellcome Historical Medical Library and the British Library in London, and the University of Chicago Library.

I wish to thank Dr. Elsa González and Mr. Michael Kugler, the former for finding numerous articles and references pertinent to my work and the latter for working with me during the final stages of proofreading and indexing.

Finally, at the Morris Fishbein Center, I must give a special note of thanks to Mrs. Elizabeth Bitoy for typing the manuscript not only in its final form, but several times over in earlier forms and in derivative papers. At home, my wife, Bruni, has never ceased to encourage me to complete my work even if it meant that she had to pack and leave home with me for long periods in the pursuance of my research.

Deerfield, Illinois
August 1989

1

Paracelsism and medical tradition

The Galenic revival

At the time, early in the sixteenth century, few people recognized that the medical and scientific communities were on the threshold of a fundamental change. Revered texts by ancient and medieval authorities were soon to be replaced by a wave of new translations as the spirit of fourteenth- and fifteenth-century humanism passed from literary texts to the sciences and to medicine.[1] In 1417, Poggio Bracciolini (1380–1459) found a copy of the *De rerum natura* of Lucretius (ca. 99–55 B.C.), a work that was eventually to spur a new interest in atomic explanations of natural phenomena. Georg von Peuerbach (1423–1461) and his disciple Johann Müller (Regiomontanus) (1436–1476) sought to reform astronomy in their quest for an accurate manuscript of Ptolemy's *Almagest* (second century A.D.). This quest led first to Peuerbach's textbook, the *Theoricae novae planetarum* (published ca. 1473) and then to Müller's *Epitome* of the *Almagest* (1496). The new emphasis on Ptolemy influenced the young Copernicus (1473–1543) whose own work was to be essentially a sun-centered restatement of Ptolemaic astronomy.

In 1428, Guarino da Verona (1370–1460) discovered the long lost encyclopedic treatise on medicine by Celsus (second century A.D.), and by the end of the fifteenth century, prominent medical humanists such as Thomas Linacre (ca. 1460–1524) were planning extensive new translations of ancient medical authors.[2] This intense activity emphasized the primacy of Galen as a medical authority, one of whose major works, *De usu partium*, appeared in several new translations by 1500. Linacre added his own translations, among them the important *De naturalibus facultatibus* (1523). The first edition of the collected works of Galen in Greek appeared in 1525, and the medical humanist, Jacques Du Bois (Iacobus Sylvius) (1478–1555), wrote that "After Apollo and Aesculapius they [Hippocrates and Galen] were the greatest powers in medicine, most

---

[1] On humanism in the sciences, see A. C. Crombie (1953), pp. 267–70; Lynn Thorndike (1941), vol. 4, passim; Allen G. Debus (1978), passim; and the papers by A. Buck (1973).

[2] The most valuable volume on Linacre is the collection of essays edited by Francis Maddison, Margaret Pelling, and Charles Webster (1977), which includes Walter Pagel's essential paper on "Medical Humanism – A Historical Necessity in the Era of the Renaissance," pp. 375–86.

1

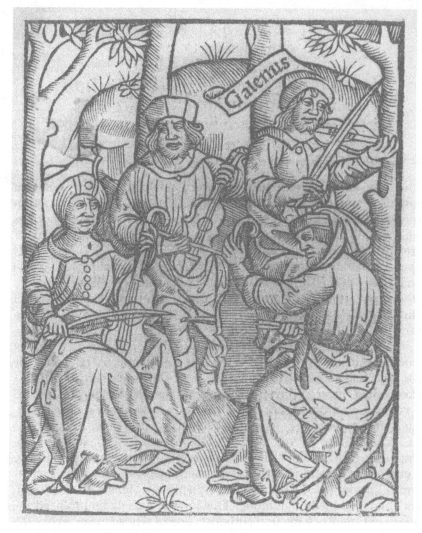

The harmony of Galen, Hippocrates, Plato, and Aristotle. From Symphorien Champier, *Symphonia Platonis cum Aristotle, et Galeni cum Hyppocrate* (1516). Courtesy of the National Library of Medicine, Bethesda.

perfect in every respect, and they had never written anything in physiology or other parts of medicine that was not entirely true."[3]

Even more important was the work of Johannes Guinter of Andernach

---

[3] Owsei Temkin (1973), p. 126, quote from "Vaesani cuiusdam calumniarum in Hippocratis Galenique rem anatomicam depulsio," *Opera medica* (1680), p. 135. The work of Sylvius has recently been discussed by G. Baader in Wear, French and Lonie (1985). The papers in this volume are an excellent source for studying the impact of the ancient classics on medicine in the sixteenth century.

(ca. 1497–1574),[4] who not only prepared new editions and translations of the medical works of Paul of Aegina (late seventh century), Caelius Aurelianus (seventh century), Oribasius (ca. 325–400), and Alexander of Tralles (sixth century), but also wrote new texts himself. Andernach translated much of Galen into Latin, including the work *De anatomicis administrationibus* (1531), which was strongly to influence his own *Institutionum anatomicarum secundum Galeni sententiam ad candidatos medicinae* (1536). Andernach's assistant during the preparation of this work was a young medical student, Andreas Vesalius (1514–1564). Vesalius's anatomical masterwork, the *De humani corporis fabrica* (1543), was to be as important to the development of anatomy as the *De revolutionibus* of Copernicus was to be for astronomy, and his debt to the new Galenic studies was as great as Copernicus's debt to the corrected Greek text of Ptolemy.

Andernach had a second assistant among his students, Michael Servetus (ca. 1511–1553), who was to be the first author to describe the lesser circulation of the blood from the right ventricle through the lungs to the left ventricle. His interest in the passage of the blood stemmed from a religious concern, the assimilation of the Heavenly Spirit in the body through respiration; he published these thoughts in his *Christianismi Restitutio* (1553). But Servetus was also a Galenist. In his discussion of syrups (1536) he openly praised the work of the Greek physician as the basis of true medicine in contrast to the outmoded works of the Arabs and the medical translators:

> In our happy age [Galen] once shamefully misunderstood is reborn and reestablishes himself to shine in his former lustre; so that like one returning home he has delivered the citadel which had been held by the forces of the Arabs, and he has cleansed those things which had been bespattered by the sordid corruptions of the barbarians.[5]

The medical humanists of the early decades of the sixteenth century presented physicians with a flood of new translations of texts, some unknown earlier and others known imperfectly. It was a labor performed by recognized scholars. In the case of Linacre we recognize the founder of the London College of Physicians (1518) whereas with Sylvius and Guinter we are in the presence of leading figures of the Parisian medical establishment. These men accepted Galen as the "Prince of Physicians" and sought medical truth through accurate translations of the best manuscripts they could locate. It was a period when scholars in all fields were judged through the now traditional academic disputation; in the case of medical texts, this meant that specific theses were discussed and defended by the author before a panel of medical experts.

---

[4] For Guinter as a medical humanist, see C. D. O'Malley (1964); for Guinter as a proponent of chemical medicine, see Allen G. Debus (1972), vol. 1. See also Georges Schaff (1976).
[5] Michael Servetus (1953), p. 60.

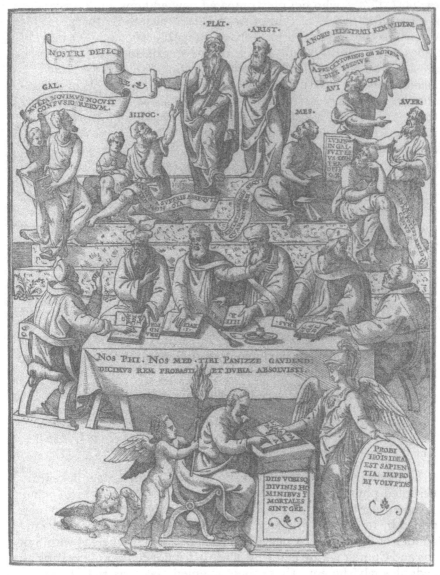

A sixteenth-century academic disputation from Ludovico Panizza, *De venae sectione in inflammationibus quibuscunque fluxione genitis, per sanguinis missionem curandis . . . disputatio ac decisio* (Venice: Ex Officina Farrea, 1544). Courtesy of the National Library of Medicine, Bethesda.

The touchstone of truth was to be found in the work of the ancient and medieval authorities whose work their texts reflected. Tradition rather than innovation was emphasized. When these medical humanists disagreed with the ancients, they followed in the steps of their literary forebears; corrections were welcomed, but the original was not to be discarded.

With little controversy these new translations and texts gradually superseded the Arabic medical texts and the "barbarous" translations made during the twelfth and thirteenth centuries. In essence this medical reform was accomplished through an extension of the spirit of literary humanism to the sciences, an early, but essential, phase of the scientific revolution, which was welcomed by most members of the medical community. The stamp of Galen shone brightly on this "new" establishment medicine of the sixteenth century, both in medical education and among the growing number of associations of prominent physicians.[6]

Hermeticism and natural magic

The Galenic revival was only one of the medical results of humanism. The search for ancient texts had also yielded the Greek text of the *Corpus Hermeticum* (ca. 1460). Cosimo d'Medici (1389–1464) had instructed Marsilio Ficino (1433–1499) to turn from his translation of Plato to these treatises, which were ascribed to Hermes, a legendary figure who was thought to have lived at the time of Moses or Abraham. The *Corpus Hermeticum* had been known to St. Augustine and other Fathers of the Church, and these tracts seemed to offer Renaissance scholars a gentile revelation contemporary with the books of Moses.[7] In the *Pymander* was a description of the creation and the fall of man that paralleled the account in Genesis. However, the *Pymander* account left man with the power to act in nature on his own. Had not the Creator concealed treasures in the earth for the health and wealth of mankind? He had identified these with signs, which the seeker – when informed by Grace – might discover and learn to use for the benefit of his fellow man. This was the proper role of the physician, but at the same time it was a doctrine similar to the role of the natural magician in the Hermetic tradition. Man could be a natural magician capable of learning of the wonders of the Lord while examining His Book of Nature. In this sense magic was seen as a religious quest.

For these Hermeticists, these natural magicians, the universe was a unified whole, interconnected in all of its parts. This unity was ex-

---

[6] Dr. John Geynes, a member of the London College of Physicians, was forced to recant after suggesting that Galen was not infallible (1559). W. S. C. Copeman (1960), p. 36.

[7] Dame Frances A. Yates was largely responsible for the current interest in the Hermetic revival and its relation to the scientific revolution. She developed this theme in *Giordano Bruno and the Hermetic Tradition* (1964) and in a number of volumes over the next seventeen years. A conference on Renaissance Hermeticism at The Folger Shakespeare Library in 1982 permitted scholars to reassess this influence in many areas: Ingrid Merkel and Allen G. Debus, eds. (1988). See also Allen G. Debus (1977), vol. 1, pp. 30–4 on "The Hermetic Revival and the Study of Nature."

pressed in the duality of the macrocosm and the microcosm: All things
in the great world were also to be found in the small world of man.
These two worlds were connected by astral influences and the Holy
Spirit, though much on the motion and action we perceive was explained in terms of sympathetic or antipathetic influences. Because of
the role that man could play in this view of the cosmos, Hermeticism
and natural magic were to have a profound effect on medicine and the
sciences.

Paracelsus

Perhaps the chief beneficiaries of this more mystical hermetic view of the
world in the sixteenth century were Philippus Aureolus Theophrastus
Bombastus von Hohenheim, called Paracelsus (1493–1541), and his followers.[8] A lifelong rebel, Paracelsus was exposed as a boy to practical
medicine by his father, who served as a country doctor in several Swiss
towns, among them Eins. .deln where Paracc¹sus was born. His father
also carried out alc' ,cmic.ı experiments at the hearth whenever he had
time. Tradition has it that Paracelsus was taught by the Abbott Johannes
Trithemius of Sponheim, also known for his esoteric interests, including
alchemy. The family moved to the mining town of Villach in 1502 where
the boy worked as an apprentice in the mines owned by the wealthy
Fugger family. Here he surely became acquainted with mining lore and
metallurgical practices and with the diseases associated with this profession, which were to become the subject of one of his books.

In 1507, at the age of fourteen, Paracelsus left home as a wandering
scholar, visiting many universities and taking employment of various
kinds. Whether or not he took a medicine degree is in doubt, but he did
work as a surgeon in the mercenary armies of the period. Although he
referred to many towns and countries in writing of these years of travel,
we cannot be certain that he actually went to all of them. We can only
speak with confidence of his travels in the last fifteen years of his life
when he confined himself to the cities and villages of Switzerland and
southern Germany. We need not recount his well-known difficulties in
Basel in 1527 or his final call to Salzburg in 1541. It suffices to say that he
died at the rather early age of forty-eight after more than thirty years of
almost constant travel and conflict with local authorities. At the time of
his death, few of his more important works had been published, but this
was to change in the decades afterward.

Paracelsus became famous after his death, primarily because he was
thought to have accomplished wondrous cures. As a result, his manuscripts – many had been left behind as he moved from town to town –

---

[8] Of the numerous studies of Paracelsus, I have relied primarily on those of Walter Pagel,
particularly Pagel (1982, 1962). See also Debus (1977), vol. 1, pp. 45–61.

were sought out, published, and commented on by physicians who may never have heard of him during his lifetime. Beginning about 1550 a trickle of Paracelsian publications grew into a flood in the closing decades of the century. Paracelsians called for a new medicine – their own medicine – to supersede that of the schools. It is not hard to understand why most Galenists demanded the suppression of this medical heresy, though some were more open minded, such as the long-lived medical humanist Guinter von Andernach who recommended (1571) that physicians take whatever they found useful from the works of either camp. In his own case, Guinter meant by this the theoretical medicine of the ancients plus the revolutionary metal-based remedies of the Paracelsians.

By the early years of the seventeenth century, the Paracelsian–Galenist debate had reached a fever pitch, not only among physicians but among everyone concerned with the question of a new philosophy. John Cotta (ca. 1575–ca. 1650), a Northampton physician, wrote in 1612 that

> The innumer*.ble* 'issen*.ions* amongst the learned concerning the Arabicke and Chymicke remedies at this day infinitely, with opposite and contradictorie writings, and inuectives, burthen the whole world. Some learned Phisitions and writers extoll and magnifie them as of incomparable vse and diuine efficacie. Some with execration accuse and curse them as damned and hellish poysons. Some because they find not these remedies in the common & vulgar readings of the Antients (the famous and learned Grecians) with feare and horror endure their very mention, farre therein vnlike and differing from that ingenuous spirit of the thrise worthy and renowned Pergamene Claudius Galen who . . . did . . . with humble and daigning desire search & entertaine from any sort of people, yea from the most unlearned Empiricke himselfe, any their particular remedies or medicines, which after by his purer and more eminent iudgement, and clearer light of understanding, refining, he reduced to more proper worth, and thereby gave admired presidents of their wondered ods in his learned prescription and accomodation. Some contrarily contemning the learning and knowledge of the Grecian, and with horrid superstition, deifying an absolute sufficiencie in Chymicke remedies, reiect the care or respect of discreet and prudent dispensation. A third and more commendable sort differeth from both these, and leaving in the one his learned morositie and disdainfull impatience of different hearing, and in the other his ignorant and peruerse Hermeticall monopoly, with impartiall and ingenuous desire free from sectarie affectation, doth from both draw whatsoeuer may in either seem good or profitable vnto health or physicke vse: from the Grecian deriving the sound & ancient truth, & from both Greeke, Chymicke, or Arabian, borrowing with thankfull diligence any helpfull good to needfull vse.[9]

[9] John Cotta of Northampton, Doctor in Phisicke (1612), pp. 82–3.

The chemical philosophy

This passage by Cotta is testimony of the intensity of the medical debate in the early years of the seventeenth century.[10] But what had the Paracelsians proposed that was so objectionable to the Galenists? Certainly the Paracelsians were opposed to the educational establishment, believing that Aristotle, Galen, and their followers and commentators must be discarded as the ultimate authorities in philosophy and medicine. They had been heathens. Galen had attacked the Christians in his works, and the philosophy of Aristotle had been condemned by the Church time and time again.[11] In short, the Galenic medical humanists sought to magnify the authority of the ancients whereas the Paracelsians, whom we might call "Hermetic humanists," sought to destroy the authority of the ancients and replace it with a more Christian system of learning.

Paracelsian medicine and philosophy were to be based on the two books of divine revelation, Holy Scripture and God's Book of Creation. It was quite clear to Thomas Tymme (1605): "The Almighty Creatour of the Heauvens and the Earth, (Christian Reader), hath set before our eyes two most principall Bookes: the one of Nature, the other of his written Word . . ."[12] Clearly the biblical books were incontrovertible, but nature was no less so if read correctly. Finding the myriad treasures that God had hidden in the earth and heavens for the benefit of man was hopeless for those who thought the answer was to be found in reading the books of the ancients or studying at the universities. In 1571 Peter Severinus (1540–1602) encouraged seekers of truth to

> sell your lands, your houses, your clothes and your jewelry; burn up your books. On the other hand, buy yourselves stout shoes, travel to the mountains, search the valleys, the deserts, the shores of the sea, and the deepest depressions of the earth; note with care the distinctions between animals, the differences of plants, the various kinds of minerals, the properties and mode of origin of everything that exists. Be not ashamed to study diligently the astronomy and terrestrial philosophy of the peasantry. Lastly, purchase coal, build furnaces, watch and operate with the fire without wearying. In this way and no other, you will arrive at a knowledge of things and their properties.[13]

10 See my chapter on "The Paracelsian Debates" in Debus (1977), vol. 1, pp. 127–204.

11 Much of the work of Pierre Duhem and subsequent writers on the history of physics in the Middle Ages has dealt with the significance of the condemnation of Aristotelian philosophy by Church councils in the thirteenth century. For a discussion of Galen's references to the Christians, see R. Walzer (1949). The attack on Aristotle and Galen as heathens by the Paracelsians is a common theme. R. Bostocke (1585) refers to Galen as "that heathen and professed enemy of Christ" (sig. H^{v-r}) and "The heathnish Phisicke of *Galen* doth depend uppon that heathnish Philosophie of Aristotle" (sig. Av^{v}).

12 Thomas Tymme (1612), sig. A3.

13 Petrus Severinus (1660), p. 39.

Like Severinus, Joseph Duchesne (ca. 1544–1609) wrote of the need of the physician to travel in order to learn of local diseases that had not yet reached his own country. He wrote of the strange sweating sickness in England, scorbitum (scurvy) in Germany, colic in Alsatia, a new fever in Hungary, and a disease called plica in Poland. None of these were known to the ancients.[14] Paracelsus himself had traveled constantly and believed that the physicians should "learn of old Women, Egyptians, and such-like persons; for they have greater experiences in such things than all the Academians."[15]

The Paracelsians called for a new study of nature that went far beyond the debate over the use of chemical medicines referred to by John Cotta. Man as the microcosm contained within him all things that were to be found in the great world surrounding him. Paracelsus, in one of his earliest works, the *Volumen medicinae paramirum* (ca. 1520), had written that all things in heaven and earth exist in man.

> All this you should know exists in man and realize that the firmament is within man, the firmament with its great movements of bodily planets and stars which result in exaltations, conjunctions, oppositions and the like, as you call these phenomena as you understand them. Everything which astronomical theory has searched deeply and gravely by aspects, astronomical tables and so forth, – this self-same knowledge should be a lesson and teaching to you concerning the bodily firmament. For, none among you who is devoid of astronomical knowledge may be filled with medical knowledge.[16]

The Paracelsians certainly wanted a new understanding of nature, but their concept of science was quite different from ours. Not only did they insist on the validity of the macrocosm–microcosm analogy, they also found little value in mathematics as an interpreter of natural phenomena. Mathematics was thought to be a form of logic (as exemplified by geometry), a link with the Greek past and the establishment educational system, which they rejected. Peter Severinus wrote that the source of Galen's failure had been his fascination with the beauty of mathematical proofs and his desire to base medicine on a foundation as firm as geometry is.[17] Galenic medicine had failed in the treatment of the diseases that were the scourge of sixteenth-century Europe. The mathematics of Paracelsus was a cosmic "sidereal" mathematics, more

---

[14] Joseph Duchesne (1618), pp. 151–4. "Plica polonica" was a disease endemic in sixteenth-century Poland. It was a disorder of the hair in which it became twisted, matted, and crusted as a result of filth, neglect, and infestation by vermin.

[15] Paracelsus (1656), p. 88. For the original text, see Paracelsus, *Sämtliche Werke*, ed. Karl Sudhoff and Wilhelm Mathiessen, 15 vols. (Munich: R. Oldenbourg [vols. 6–9: O. W. Barth], 1922–33), vol. 14, p. 541.

[16] Paracelsus (1949), p. 36.   [17] Severinus (1660), pp. 2, 3, 21.

akin to Pythagorean and Cabalistic number mysticism than to logic.[18] Other practitioners with more practical needs turned to Wisdom 11:17 (Douay version 11:21) to show that God had created "all things in number, weight and measure." This statement fitted the experience of the chemist, the pharmacist, and even the alchemist, all of whom weighed and measured their reagents in the laboratory.

This new philosophy of nature was to be founded on chemistry rather than mathematical abstraction and the study of motion. Although the Creation had been a mathematical process, it had been no less a chemical separation. In his *Phisophiae* [sic] *ad Athenienses* (published 1564), Paracelsus had written of a chemical unfolding of nature; and Thomas Tymme (1605) described the Creation as a divine "Halchymicall Extraction, Seperation, Sublimation, and Coniunction" of the "original indigested Chaos or masse."[19] Gerhard Dorn prepared a Paracelsian commentary on the six days of Creation in which he insisted that the division of the waters (second day) was the familiar alchemical separation of pure essence – or spirit – from the impure residue, the *caput mortuum*.[20]

Surely this emphasis on the Creation led to the problem of the elements, which were a necessary first product of the process. Paracelsus himself frequently used the four Aristotelian elements (earth, water, air, and fire) in his work, as he had in his *Philosophy to the Athenians*. But he also used a second set of elementary substances, the *tria prima* or three principles: mercury, sulfur, and salt. These were clearly derived from and were an extension of the traditional alchemical mercury and sulfur, which had been introduced in the eighth or ninth centuries by Arabic chemists to account for the metals. It was understood that the three principles were not the common substances met in the laboratory but were their essences, or even "souls," and were frequently termed "the sulfur and mercury of the philosophers."

The relationship of the material elements to their principles was not clear to Paracelsus because any tangible substance might be composed of material elements that could be made of the spiritual principles, or the reverse.[21] Whatever his real thought might have been, element theory was thrown into confusion until well into the eighteenth century. This confusion had far-flung consequences because the cosmology, the physics, and the medicine of the European universities were all based on the

---

[18] I have written at greater length on the mathematics of the Paracelsians in my "Mathematics and Nature in the Chemical Texts of the Renaissance," Debus (1968). The subject is discussed by Paracelsus in his *Astronomia magna*.

[19] From the dedication to Sir Charles Blunt in Joseph Duchesne (Quercitanus) (1605), sig. A³ʳ.

[20] Dorn's *Liber de natura luce physica, ex Genesi desumpta* (1583) was assured a wide audience by being included in the first volume of the *Theatrum Chemicum* published by Lazarus Zetzner, which went through three editions between 1602 and 1659–61.

[21] Walter Pagel discussed the relationship of the elements and the principles in the Paracelsian texts in his *Paracelsus*, (1958), pp. 100–4.

traditional Aristotelian elements. The Paracelsian attack on these elements, no less than their rejection of formal deductive logic in favor of fresh observations, were potentially serious challenges to the educational establishment.

Although there was little initial agreement on the natures of the elements and their principles, chemists gradually placed increasing emphasis on the principles, which seemed to conform to the products of their distillations: spiritous liquors (mercury), inflammable oils (sulfur), and residue (salt). By the mid-seventeenth century these three elements plus water (phlegm) and earth had become commonly accepted as a five-element–principle system, which was incorporated in the most successful of the many seventeenth-century chemical textbooks.[22]

Interest in the chemical Creation spread beyond the subject of the elements to that of the earth and man. In the possibly apocryphal *Liber Azoth* (1591) Paracelsus wrote of the similarity between life and combustion and pointed to the fact that air was essential for both.[23] More specifically, the Paracelsians argued that a part of air was the essential ingredient: an aerial niter or salt-peter.[24] This was practically equated with the Heavenly Spirit and was required for life of all kinds: mineral as well as animal and vegetable.

The earth itself was pictured as a vast distillation flask with an enormous central fire. This fire was the cause of volcanoes and of mountain streams, which derived from underground waters that were distilled in the alembiclike mountains. The internal fire also produced a radical moisture required by vegetation, and it distilled other subterranean substances, readying them for accepting the needed celestial virtues requisite for developing into metals.[25]

The Paracelsian chemical philosophy was meant to replace the cosmology and natural philosophy of the ancients, and in this sense it can rightly be compared with the mechanical philosophy of the seventeenth century. However, the chemical philosophy was always of special interest to physicians who opposed the medicine of the Galenists. The Paracelsian physicians thought of themselves as natural magicians, able to effect cures because they had been touched by Divine Grace. They repeatedly referred to Ecclesiasticus 38:1, "Honor the physician for the need thou hast of him: for the most high hath created him."

Belief in the macrocosm–microcosm analogy solidified the connection between nature and man, and the acceptance of a chemical Creation led naturally to a willingness to explain natural phenomena by chemical analogies. If chemical analogy held for the macrocosm, it should also be valid for the microcosm.

[22] This development is discussed in Debus (1977), vol. 1, pp. 78–84.
[23] Paracelsus, *Liber Azoth* in the *Opera Bücher und Schrifften* (1616), vol. 2, p. 520.
[24] See Debus (1964), 43–61.
[25] Examples are given in Debus (1977), vol. 1, pp. 84–96.

In their opposition to ancient philosophy, the Paracelsians turned to sympathetic action in nature and argued that magnetic action was accomplished not by contact, as in Aristotelian physics, but at a distance. The most famous medical example of sympathetic action was in the use of weapon-salve: The weapon that caused the wound, rather than the victim, was treated with the salve, which included blood from the victim.[26] Sympathy among the weapon, the salve, and the wound assured medical success. This is hardly a chemical cure by our definition of the word, but cure by weapon-salve, frequently referred to as the "powder of sympathy," was generally considered part of the chemical philosophy by seventeenth-century savants.

And what of disease theory? Galenic medicine was grounded on the four humors – blood, phlegm, yellow bile, and black bile – which were an extension of Greek element theory. Humoral balance fostered health whereas imbalance resulted in illness.[27] Paracelsians who rejected the Aristotelian elements rejected the humors as well. Rather than seek an explanation of disease in terms of fluid imbalance, these chemists sought the origin of disease in external factors that entered the body through food or respiration and became localized in body organs.[28] The various organs had within them certain forces or *archei*, which separated pure essences from waste. The essence was distributed where needed and the waste eliminated through the pores, the digestive tract, and the lungs. If the archeus of any organ did not function properly, the waste might not be completely eliminated, and disease or even death could result.

Seeds of disease that did become lodged in the body grew in a fashion similar to the growth of metals in the earth; that is, in the earth, metalline seeds were thought to grow into a metal or metallic ore when introduced into a proper earthly matrix whereas in the human body, a disease seed would grow if lodged in an appropriate organ.[29] Microcosmic chemical analogies were also found in the common cold, which was viewed as a distillation process within the body that caused phlegm in the nose.[30] This explanation was similar to that for the origin of mountain streams. Hot and burning diseases were explained as the result of the reaction of an aerial sulfur and an aerial niter after inhalation in the respiration process.[31] The same reaction occurring in the atmosphere resulted in thunder and lightning, which seemed much like the explosion of gunpowder.[32]

26 On the weapon-salve and sympathetic action, see Debus (1964), 389–417.
27 On the humoral pathology and Galenic medical philosophy, see Temkin (1973), pp. 10–50.
28 For Paracelsian disease theory, see Walter Pagel (1982), pp. 134–44.
29 On the similarities between diseases and minerals, see ibid., p. 136. At one point Paracelsus compares man with a mine, ibid, p. 134.
30 Here see Joseph Duchesne (1626), p. 183.
31 Paracelsus, *Bertheonae* (1618), p. 354.
32 Paracelsus, ibid., *Grossen Wundarznei*, p. 52.

The Paracelsian chemical philosophy thus openly rejected the ancients and called for a new, Christian approach to nature founded on fresh observations, which were best interpreted through chemistry or chemical analogies. The debate over the new chemical remedies highlighted by John Cotta was at most only one aspect in a much larger conflict. Still, the acceptance or rejection of the new remedies was to be the single most difficult problem to resolve. Paracelsian physicians, obsessed with their chemical explanations, sought a chemical approach to the virulence of new diseases – particularly the venereal diseases – which were then ravaging the Continent. They were convinced that new medicines were required to replace the relatively mild herbal remedies that formed the bulk of the Galenic *materia medica*. John Hester (d. 1593), one of the earliest of the English Paracelsians, argued (1590) that neither Galen nor Hippocrates could be used as a guide to diseases that did not exist in ancient times.

> Now that the diseases of the French Pockes was neyther knowne to them, nor to theyr successors for many yeeres . . . is a matter so far out of question, that it refuseth all shew of disputation, and therefore as this latter age of ours sustaineth the scourge thereof, a iust whyp of our lycentiousnesse, so let it (if ther be any to be had) carry the credite of the cure, as some rewarde of some mens industries.[33]

These cures were to be found in chemical remedies made from metals and minerals. Here, too, the Paracelsians drew from their medieval alchemical heritage. Roger Bacon (ca. 1214–ca. 1294), Arnald of Villanova (1235–1311), and John of Rupescissa (mid-fourteenth century) had all found the greatest value of chemistry to be in the preparation of medicines rather than in the quixotic quest for the precious metals.[34] This tradition remained influential during the lifetime of Paracelsus through the works of Hieronymus Brunschwig (ca. 1440–ca. 1512), Philip Ulstadius (fl. first half of the sixteenth century), Conrad Gesner (1516–1565), and many others who urged the chemical distillation of herbs for the production of the most efficacious medicinal oils and waters.[35] Even

[33] See the preface to Philip Herman (1590), p. 31.
[34] Robert P. Multhauf has studied the medieval medical applications of distilled substances in his "John of Rupescissa and the Origin of Medical Chemistry" (1954), 359–67, and "The Significance of Distillation in Renaissance Medical Chemistry" (1956), 329–46. A study of the continuation of distillation methods in the sixteenth and seventeenth centuries is much to be desired.
[35] *The Book of Distillation*, Brunschwig (1971), is conveniently available with an authoritative introduction by Harold J. Abrahams. Conrad Gesner, *Thesaurus Euonymi* (Part 1), translated in the sixteenth century as *The Treasure of Euonymus: Conteyninge the wonderfull hid secretes of nature* (1559). The second part appeared in English as *The New Jewell of Health* (1576). The rapid translation of these texts testifies to the intense contemporary interest in distillation. Also of interest was the addition of short distillation texts to other medical works. Ambroise Paré included a section on distillation at the end of his surgical works, and later editions of Petrus Andreas Mattioli's famed edition of *Dioscorides* included an appendix on distillation, which was updated during the course of the next century.

Jean Fernel (ca. 1497–1558), professor of medicine at Paris, thought chemistry should be of interest to the physician. His *Universa Medicina* (1567) was one of the most successful medical texts of the sixteenth and seventeenth centuries, and in it he maintained a traditional Galenic physiology.[36] However, in his *De abditis rerum causis* (1548, and included in the *Universa Medicina*) Fernel wrote of the sympathetic action of medicines which he compared to magnetic attraction and repulsion.[37] He proceeded then to discuss chemistry, noting that fire separated substances to the original four elements before he went on to take up the philosopher's stone and the process of transmutation.[38] Brunschwig, Gesner, Fernel, and many others who were interested in chemistry sought primarily to add useful new remedies to traditional ones, but many Paracelsians sought much more. They argued for a total break with tradition, hoping to replace Galenic herbal remedies with their own chemical preparations derived from metals.

Here again was a direct challenge to the medical establishment. Galenists charged their adversaries with indiscriminate prescription of poisons. Not so, countered the chemical physicians; not only did they remove the poisonous qualities of metals by chemical preparation, but they also gave careful attention to proper dosage with their stronger substances.[39] But they could not deny that they used reagents that were originally poisons.

Galenic medical cure was dominated by the belief that contraries cure: A disease characterized as hot and of a given degree must be cured by an opposed medicine, one that was cold and of the same degree;[40] in this fashion humoral balance might be achieved. Paracelsians turned to folk tradition and insisted on cure by similitude, arguing that a poisonous disease had to be cured by a like poison. For this reason we find that the Paracelsians had a great interest in drugs compounded from mercury, arsenic, antimony, and a host of other metals and minerals.[41] These substances were frequently used as purges, to the anger and despair of the Galenists. The most debatable substance of all was antimony (prepared in many forms and prescribed frequently as the sulfide). It was the subject of numerous texts, the most important of which was the *Currus triumphalis antimonii* (1604), ascribed to Basil Valentine, who supposedly had lived in the fifteenth century.[42]

---

36 On Fernel, see C. S. Sherrington (1946).
37 Jean Fernel, *De abditis rerum causis*, in *Universa Medicina* (1656), p. 526.
38 Ibid., p. 531.   39 Bostocke (1585), sig. Ev^v.
40 Pagel (1982), pp. 243–7.
41 Robert P. Multhauf (1954) points to the fact that a very high percentage of Paracelsus' chemical preparations were based on distillation and that the interest in residues developed primarily later in the century. Although this may be true in general, a number of important salts are discussed in the works of Paracelsus. See Debus (1977), vol. 1, pp. 115–17.
42 Although the present work does not deal with the actual chemistry of the early modern

Educational reform and the growth of iatrochemistry

The sixteenth-century Paracelsians did borrow from Aristotle and Galen, to the extent that Walter Pagel emphasized their similarities to the ancients. However, they saw themselves primarily as proponents of a reformed medicine and natural philosophy and were convinced that their view of nature, as well as their medical philosophy, must replace the old curricula at the schools and universities of Europe. R. Bostocke (1585) complained bitterly that

> in the scholes nothing may be receiued nor allowed that sauoreth not of *Aristotle, Gallen, Auicen,* and other Ethnikes, whereby the yong beginners are either not acquainted with this doctrine, or els it is brought into hatred with them. And abrode likewise the *Galenists* be so armed and defended by the protection, priuiledges and authoritie of Princes, that nothing can be allowed that they disalowe, and nothing may bee receiued that agreeth not with their pleasures and doctrine.[43]

These Paracelsists called openly for educational reform so that their message might be heard. And they had some success. Although no European university ever embraced their demand for a total overhaul of the educational curriculum, chemistry was gradually accepted in the course of the late sixteenth and seventeenth centuries for its practical pharmaceutical value. When the College of Physicians in London considered issuing an official pharmacopoeia in 1585, a committee on chemical medicines was appointed that included Thomas Moffett (1553–1604), perhaps the most distinguished of the early English Paracelsians.[44] The project was long delayed, but the *Pharmacopoeia Londinensis* finally appeared in 1618, due largely to the efforts of Theofore Turquet de Mayerne (1573–1655), a chemical physician who had weathered the then recent Parisian confrontation between the Galenists and the Paracelsians.

An increasing number of chemical physicians were finding positions at European courts in the early years of the seventeenth century. In

pharmaceutical products, it is interesting to note that antimony compounds are still found in pharmacopoeias. The 1980 British *Pharmacopoeia* lists antimony sodium tartrate, antimony standard solution, antimony trichloride in 1,2-dichloroethane solution, and antimony trichloride reagent. The 1985 U.S. *Pharmacopoeia* lists antimony pentachloride, antimony potassium tartrate, and antimony trichloride. The tartrate is used against an infection caused by schistosoma japonicum. *Remington's Pharmaceutical Sciences* (1980) notes that antimony continues to be used as an emetic because of its expectorant action. Reference is also made to the fact that it occasionally causes diarrhea and may cause sudden death, although rarely (p. 1180). A concise overview of seventeenth-century medicinal antimony preparations will be found in Daems (1976), pp. 26–33.

[43] Bostocke (1585), sig. F ii^v.
[44] Debus (1977), vol. 1, pp. 182–91.

England, Mayerne was appointed chief physician to James I. Previously he had been médecin ordinaire to Henry IV of France, a post obtained for him by another proponent of chemical medicine, Ribit de la Rivière, the premier médecin to the king. In Denmark, Peter Severinus was physician to the king, and Paracelsians filled many posts in the smaller political entities of central Europe. Oswald Crollius (1560–1609), the famed author of the *Basilica Chymica* (1609), was the chief physician to Prince Christian I of Anhalt-Bernberg, and Johann Hartmann (1568–1631) became the first professor of chemistry (chymiatria or chemical medicine) in Europe at the University of Marburg. Hartmann, a Paracelsist, was appointed to a medical faculty to teach the preparation of chemical medicines. It was in this fashion that chemistry entered the existing medical curricula of European universities.[45] By the close of the seventeenth century professors of chemistry were associated with most medical faculties in Europe.

[45] Allen G. Debus (1986).

2

Chemistry and medicine in France: the early years

Quãt aux Paracelsistes, où autres plus subtils inuẽteurs de leur secte, ils ne me ferõt quiter les bons, & approuuez autheurs pour suivre leurs nouuelles inventions: par lesquelles ils peruertissent tout ordre diuin & humain, de tout temps, & ancienneté, & par toutes nations, iusques icy tenu, gardé & obserué en la Medecine, ny moins d'approuuer leurs nouueaux secrets où entrent toute sortes de mortiferes poisons: l'experience desquels a faict mourir vne infinité de peuple, comme ils continuent chacun iour.[1]

André du Breil (1580)

Setting the stage

Early in the sixteenth century the Parisian Medical Faculty was a center of medical humanism that was reestablishing Galen as the touchstone of medical authority. To be sure, the use of chemistry was approved by some physicians, even then, for the distillation of herbs and the preparation of a limited number of remedies. The fourteenth-century works of Arnald of Villanova, which emphasized chemical methods, were frequently reprinted in the early sixteenth century and even recommended to medical students. Because respected herbalists were familiar with the advantages of distillation, many tracts on the benefits of spa waters included chemical methods for the analysis of those waters.[2] But this type of chemistry had not posed a threat to the medical establishment; thus, in France as in Germany, little attention was paid to Paracelsus during his lifetime or in the years immediately after his death.

After 1560, as the texts of Paracelsus began to be collected and published in quantity, the implications of the new medicine became better understood. Then, because these works posed specific threats to traditional medicine, physicians began to choose sides in the inevitable medi-

[1] André du Breil (1586), sig. a vi^v–a vii^r. This work was published first in 1580.
[2] Allen G. Debus (1962).

17

cal debate.[3] Perhaps the most distinguished early defender of the Paracelsian system was Peter Severinus (1542–1602), physician to Frederick II of Denmark.[4] In 1571 Severinus published his *Idea medicinae philosophicae*, an attack on the insufficiency of Galenic medicine and also an attempt to present the Paracelsian doctrine in a short and orderly form. His attempt was successful and was frequently referred to by continental savants. It was reprinted in 1616, and again in 1660 with a very long commentary by William Davisson.

The *Idea* opens by complaining that Galenic medicine had failed to suppress the new diseases that were ravaging Europe. If physicians would discard the works of the ancients and turn to their own observations in nature, they would find that a proper understanding of the relation of man and nature is expressed clearly in the analogy of the macrocosm and the microcosm.[5] Severinus accepted the doctrine of signatures and, as a follower of Paracelsus, rejected the traditional doctrine of the humors and the belief that contraries cure.[6]

Like Paracelsus he used both the four elements (earth, water, air, and fire) and the three principles (mercury, sulfur, and salt) on different levels (material and philosophical), but the three principles seemed the most important concepts to him because they corresponded to the threefold classification of substances obtained by distillation: liquors, oils, and solids. "Haec vera est corporum Analysis. In hac Anatomia exercitatum oportet esse Medicum."[7]

Severinus presented a theoretical defense of Paracelsian medicine that spread the concept of a chemical medicine far beyond the confines of central Europe, but it was in Germany that the new medical system was first criticized in detail. Thomas Erastus (Liebler) (1524–1583), professor of medicine at Heidelberg, prepared his four-part *Disputationes de medicina nova Paracelsi*, which appeared between 1572 and 1574.[8] Renowned as a theologian and as a physician (he was to become professor of theology and moral philosophy in 1580), Erastus wrote at length against witchcraft, astrology, and the use of amulets. It is understandable, then, that he should have looked at Paracelsus as something more than a medical heretic. Indeed, he accused Paracelsus of magic and of having been informed by the devil.[9] He was a dangerous charlatan who had dared to describe the divine Creation in terms of chemical separation and then

---

3 The following discussion of Severinus, Erastus, Wimpenaeus, and Andernach is derived from Allen G. Debus (1977), vol. 1, pp. 128–45.

4 See Allen G. Debus, "Peter Severinus," in *Dictionary of Scientific Biography*, vol. 12 (New York: Scribner's, 1975), pp. 334–6.

5 Peter Severinus (1660), pp. 19–21 (from chap. 3: Universalis totius medicinae adumbratio).

6 Ibid., pp. 186–8.   7 Ibid., pp. 36–40.

8 On Erastus, see Walter Pagel's biography (1971), pp. 386–8; and see Pagel (1958), pp. 311–22. I have discussed his work in Debus (1965), pp. 37–9.

9 Thomas Erastus (1572), p. 2.

had proceeded to describe the universe in terms of the macrocosm and the microcosm.[10] But man could not fly or lay eggs like a bird, and he could not live in the water like a fish.[11] Indeed, he should be able to do all of these things if all of the virtues seen in other beings existed in his own body. Surely this analogy was untrue.

As for medicine, the humoral medicine of Galen and the other ancient medical authorities was one of the glories of antiquity.[12] To scrap this in favor of a new medicine based on poisonous metals and minerals was unthinkable. And why turn to a new set of principles when earth, air, fire, and water were clearly the elements of all things?[13] Chemistry might well have a limited use in the preparation of some medicines, but it was certainly not the proper basis for either medicine or natural philosophy.

The works of Severinus and Erastus reflect the increasing sharpness of the differences between the Paracelsians and the Galenists in the third quarter of the sixteenth century, but notice should also be taken of more moderate authors. At Munich, Johannes Albertus Wimpenaeus (von Wimpfen) published his *De concordia Hippocraticorum et Paracelsistarum* (1569), in which he tried to show that both medicines could be used together. True wisdom could be found in the works of all the great physicians of the past;[14] and although the followers of Paracelsus might use different terms, their views were in most cases compatible with those of the ancients. Thus, the four elements are really the same as the three principles,[15] and the Paracelsian view that man is a small copy of the macrocosm is not so very different from the ancient belief that man is made of the four elements.[16] Indeed, we need the works of the Paracelsians because we now know more about the relation of the macrocosm and the microcosm than the ancients did. At the same time we also know more about diseases and have developed more effective medicines for their cure.

This work of conciliation was to be supplemented two years later by the *De medicina veteri et noua tum cognoscenda tum faciunda commentarij duo* (1571) of Johannes Guinter of Andernach, the great Parisian medical humanist of the 1530s. Probably born in 1497, Guinter attended Louvain in 1523, and then moved to Paris three years later where he took his medical degree (1526). Although he is best known for his work on the classical medical texts, Guinter read widely in the Paracelsian texts when they began issuing from the presses of Europe. Far from being willing to discard the Galenist foundation of medicine, Guinter nevertheless found himself strongly attracted to the reports of cures accomplished by

10 Ibid., (Pars prima), p. 3.
11 Pagel (1958), pp. 323–4.   12 Ibid., pp. 324–26.
13 Erastus (1572), pp. 37–9.
14 Johannes Albertus Wimpenaeus (1569), sig. A6ᵛ.
15 Ibid., sig. Glʳ–Glᵛ.   16 Ibid., sig. G3ʳ.

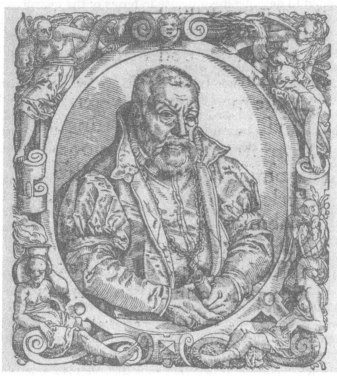

Johannes Guinter of Andernach (1497–1574). From his *De medicina veteri et noua tum cognoscenda, tum faciunda commentarij duo* (1571). Courtesy of the Wellcome Institute Library, London.

the new chemical medicines. He did condemn the magic found in the Paracelsian texts, as well as the arrogance of his followers,[17] but like Wimpenaeus, Guinter found the Paracelsian principles similar to the Aristotelian elements[18] and saw also that the ancients had used the macrocosm–microcosm analogy.[19]

This being the case, the establishment physicians could hardly reject this view of man and the cosmos outright. Nor need there be such a storm of protest over the Paracelsian dictum, *similia similibus*. Surely the poisons of the Paracelsian metals might be altered in the process of chemical change in such a way that in final form they cause action, as the Galenists wish, by contrary qualities.[20] As for the new chemical medicines, he thought their value had clearly been shown. Guinter devoted a large portion of his section on *materia medica* to chemical preparations. Iron, antimony, and mercury compounds are described, and the

[17] J. Guintherius (Guinter) von Andernach (1571), vol. 2, pp. 11, 651.
[18] Ibid., p. 39.
[19] Ibid., pp. 28–31.   [20] Ibid., pp. 25–6.

preparation of *turpeth minerale* (mercury base) is presented as a true cure for the French disease. Above all, *aurum potabile* is lauded as the most valuable of the chemicals because it seemed to cure most diseases.[21]

In short, for Wimpenaeus and Guinter of Andernach it was not a case of using the old medicine or the new but of using both in concert. Guinter wrote that "the ancients on account of time-honored authority are to be given first place," but there is much of great value in the work of the more recent chemists. There seemed to him to be faults and virtues in the work of both factions, and physicians must choose the best from each.[22]

Paracelsism in France: the opening debate

Although Severinus had taken his medical degree in France,[23] and Guinter had been one of the two professors of medicine at Paris as well as one of the royal physicians (1534–8), neither was to affect the development of chemical medicine during his years in France. Severinus returned to Denmark, and Andernach does not seem to have become aware of the Paracelsian works until after he left Paris, first for Metz (1538) and later for Strasbourg (ca. 1540).

The earliest significant notice of Paracelsus in France occurred in the exchange between Loys de Launay (M.D., Montpellier, 1557) and Jacques Grévin (1538–1570) concerning the medical use of antimony.[24] De Launay, a physician at La Rochelle, had learned of the virtues of antimony from the 1561 French translation of the *Commentaries* on Dioscorides by Pietro Andrea Mattioli (1500–1577), which was first published in 1544. The fifth book of this work dealt with stones, minerals, and metals.[25] In the chapter on antimony Mattioli claimed that this substance was a valuable cure for the plague, melancholic humors, persistent fevers, asthma, spasms, paralysis, and colic. He referred to numerous authors, both ancient and modern. As far as he could determine, Paracelsus was the first to describe the internal use of antimony as a strong laxative, though several more recent authors including George Handsch and André Gallus, physician to Emperor Ferdinand, had described its strong purgative action. Handsch gave an account of his personal experience. Suffering from nausea, he had taken three grains of antimony mixed with "Succre rosat" [conserve of roses], after which he had vomited in less than half an hour, and his stomach upset had disap-

21 Ibid., pp. 192–8, 650–1, 673.   22 Ibid., pp. 31–2.
23 A useful guide to the French language medical literature of the sixteenth century is to be found in Howard Stone (1963), 315–46.
24 On the "antimony war," see Pascal Pilpoul (1928); A. G. Chevalier (1940), pp. 418–23.
25 M. Pierre Andre Matthioli (1561); the chapter on antimony is on pp. 444–5. My citations are from the similarly paginated edition of 1566.

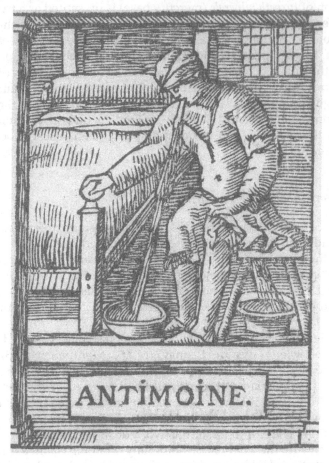

ANTiMOiNE.

The action of antimony on the body. From H. Barlet, *Le vray et methodique cours de
la physique resolutive, vulgairement dite chymie* (1657). Courtesy of the Wellcome
Institute Library, London.

peared. Further evacuations improved his condition. He soon regained
his appetite and gave thanks to God for his recovery from a dangerous
illness by means of antimony.[26]

---

[26] Ibid., p. 445. Mattioli states that George Handsch took antimony that had been pul-
   verized and mixed with conserve of roses (3 grains):
   Peu d'heure aprés il sent que ceste medecine luy renuersoit l'estomac, luy causant
   quelque petite chaleur: & soudain cõmença à vomir quelques morceaux de viande
   comment il l'auoit prinse, encores qu'il n'eust souppé le iour precedent. Après ce
   vomissent ensuyuit vn autre semblable au precedent: & pour le tiers vomissement il
   ietta plus de quatre onces d'humeurs coleriques: & le tout en moins de demye heure.
   Dés lors il perdit toute la douleur qu'il auoit en l'estomac. Vne heure aprés cela, il fit
   trois selles toutes d'humeurs coleriques, amassees auec quelques peu d'humeurs
   grosses & visqueuses: & pouoit peser son operatiõ, enuiron trois liures. Dés la il perdit

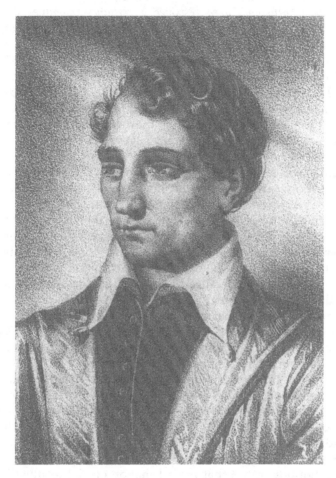

Jacques Grévin (1540–1570). Courtesy of the National Library of Medicine, Bethesda.

But why should antimony act in this fashion? Mattioli explained that the alchemists affirmed that gold was freed of its impurities when heated with antimony, and since gold was the perfect metal in the mineral kingdom as man is the perfect being among animals, it seemed reasonable that antimony should purge man of his impurities (and illnesses).

De Launay credited Mattioli with reviving the medical use of antimony, knowledge that had long been lost.[27] In his *De la Facvlté & vertue*

le bat de coeur, & furent arrestees les fluxiõs du cerueau: ioint q̃ la lãguette du col du poulmõ se desenfla soudain: & par ce moyẽ se trouua desalteré, & recouura l'appetit. Et du depuis se porta tres bien: rẽdant graces à Dieu de l'auoir retiré de ceste dangereuse maladie par le moyen de l'Antimoine.

27 Loys de Launay (1564), sig. Aivʳ.

admirable de l'Antimoine, avec responce à certaines calomnies (1564) de Launay referred to earlier accounts of Dioscorides, Paul Aegineta, Actuarius, Avicenna, Aliabbas, and others.[28] In their references to metallic poisons these authors had not mentioned antimony. Indeed, although some physicians insisted that antimony's purgative action was poisonous, de Launay could not agree. He asserted that he and two or three friends had taken antimony, which he had prepared, both through the nose and by mouth. Neither he nor they had suffered headaches or upset stomachs.[29] However, de Launay gave credit primarily to Mattioli, not to Paracelsus.

De Launay was answered by Jacques Grévin, a Parisian physician and dramatist who was well known for his comedies and tragedies.[30] His *Discovrs . . . sur les vertus & facultez de l'Antimoine* (1566) is a short text, but clear and to the point. Grévin pointed to the growing use of this drug, which was being prescribed by theologians, nobles, merchants, and peasants, all of whom were ignorant of medicine.[31] They should be warned that antimony can be dangerous. He himself was not opposed to alchemy (chemistry) "because I know well that in alchemy there are many valuable secrets: and I approve of the extracts of oils and the quintessences provided that they are made by good masters who are learned in the art. . . ."[32] And regarding the account of Mattioli's edition of Dioscorides, he noted that the ancient author had recognized that lead and antimony had similar effects.[33] Have not Pliny, Dioscorides, and Albertus Magnus written "that the fumes of calcined lead are deathly dangerous – would they wish to understand anything else of antimony."[34] Because antimony was considered to be a fourth type of lead and more impure, "it follows then that Antimony is more dangerous than lead."[35]

The method of preparation was also a matter of concern because accepted authorities agreed that the calcination of lead resulted in a poison. But "the artificial preparation of Antimony is done by dry roasting and burning called calcination."[36] Even Paracelsus in his *De gradibus* had noted that antimony was reduced to a chalklike powder, cinders, and glass at the fourth degree of fire.[37]

In short, for Grévin, antimony was not the harmless purgative that de Launay and others had claimed it to be. Like de Launay he had tried it himself, with very different results. It was indeed a purgative, but a violent one that left him weakened for eight days. He had little doubt

---

[28] Ibid., sig. Cii[v].   [29] Ibid., sig. Di[r].
[30] On the multifaceted career of Grévin, see Lucien Pinvert (1899). Here the exchange with de Launay is discussed on pp. 91–7.
[31] Jacques Grévin (1566), fol. 3[v].   [32] Ibid., fol. 4[r].
[33] Ibid., fol. 7[v].   [34] Ibid., fol. 27[r].
[35] Ibid.   [36] Ibid., fol. 22[v].
[37] Ibid., fol. 24[r].

that "Antimony is a poison; not a medicine."[38] Whether one should accept Grévin's account or that of de Launay involves the relation among science, observation, and experience.

> Experience, according to Aristotle and Galen, is a recollection of things which have happened many times the same way so that many examples having the same results engender an experience upon which one can base some rules on which to erect an art or a science. Such rules cover in general form that which experience has found only in particular.[39]
> . . . Even Paracelsus, one of the first authors to discuss Antimony, wrote in the sixth chapter of his *Labyrinth*, that experience proceeds from the many experiments made by science, and that where there is science, there is experience while on the other hand, where there is experience there is science: however, he says that science ought to precede experiment.[40]

Grévin continued by asking whether enough observations had been made on the internal use of antimony to reason from them and to reach a general rule. Here Paracelsus (referred to earlier as an authority) was subjected to criticism for his belief that antimony purifies the human body in the same way that it refines gold.[41]

> Gold and silver are bodies that do not live, they are terrestrial, cold and dry and immobile; the human body is living, it is full of heat and fecund humidity, it moves by itself and is nearly as far removed from the metals as is the earth.[42]

Grévin's work focused the attention of the Parisian Faculty of Medicine on this problem. On 3 August 1566 this august body decreed that antimony was a poison and dangerous to health. Grévin himself reported the text of this document in both French and Latin:

> In the Assembly of the entire College of the Faculty of Medicine called to give judgment on Antimony, it is advised by the authority of all those who have excelled in the art of medicine, confirmed by reason, and stated

---

[38] Ibid., fol. 12ᵛ.
. . . ie la voulu experiṁēter en moymesme, comme estant vne chose aussi facile à prēdre qv'vn grain de bled mis en poudre. I'en meslay doncques seulement trois grains auec vn peu de conserue de roses, dōt il me suruint en moins d'vne heure vn si estrange vomissement qu'encores que de ma nature ie sois facile à vomir, si est-ce qu'a chasque fois qu'il me prenoit, i'en estois au mourir. Or me print il par huict fois, & autant de fois me trauailla il par bas, dōt ie demouray quasi hors de moymesme, & me laissa vne grande foiblesse, laquelle me continua bien huict iours. Tout ce qu'il purgea ne fut qu'vne matiere aquueeuse: ce que i'ay de mesme obserué en quelques autres qui en ont pris: & ny a point de double que s'il fait ne soit semblable aux sains, aux intemperez & aux malades, si ce n'est qu'elle soit diuersifiee par le meslange de quelque humeur, lequel parauēture se sera ietté parmi. La vertu doncques cachee en l'Antimoine est de tirer force humiditez du corps, tant par haut que par bas. Ces choses ainsi deduites, il me sera plus facile de prouuer mon second poinct, qu'est le principal, & mōstrer que l'Antimoine est vn poison & non vn medicament.
[39] Ibid., fol. 27ᵛ.   [40] Ibid., fol. 28ᵛ.
[41] Ibid., fol. 24ᵛ (from the *De longa vita*).   [42] Ibid., fol. 29ᵛ.

many times in the past and now once again in the presence of the Advocate of the King: that Antimony is a poison which should be placed in the rank of simples which have a venomous quality, which cannot be corrected and which cannot be taken internally without great danger.[43]

De Launay did not hesitate to prepare a *Responce . . . touchant la faculté de l'Antimoine* (1566), in which he restated the importance of antimony and wrote of the value of alchemical procedures in medicine.[44] Grévin felt compelled to reply with *Le Second Discovrs . . . sur les vertus & facultez de l'Antimoine, Avqvel Il est sommairement traicté de la nature des Mineraux, venins, pestes, & de plusieurs autres questiõs naturelles & medicinales, pour la confirmation de l'aduis des Medecins de Paris . . .* (1567). By this time the Paracelsian theme of the debate was far more apparent. It was at this time that Grévin translated Jean Wier's *Cinq livres de l'impostvre et tromperie des diables: des enchantements & sorcelleries* (1567), which included a damning appraisal of Paracelsus and his followers. However, other French authors were beginning to present translations and commentaries on the Paracelsian system of medicine.

The first translation of a work by Paracelsus into French was *La grande, vraye et parfaicte chirurgie* (Anvers 1567, reprinted 1568) by Pierre Hassard, a physician and surgeon of Armentières, who had published earlier works on astrology, earthquakes, and the cure of venereal disease. In his preface (dated Brussels, 10 July 1566) Hassard pictured Paracelsus as a tireless scholar who had written hundreds of volumes on philosophy, medicine, astrology, theology, political justice, natural magic, and other subjects. His goal had been "to experiment on all things and by all things in order to find the true foundations of all arts and sciences, but principally Medicine and Surgery."[45] Even though Paracelsus's was the true natural magic and "la pure fontaine cabaline," Hassard placed no particular emphasis on chemistry.

Very different from the medical translation of Pierre Hassard was the *Compendium* of Paracelsian philosophy and medicine written by Jacques Gohory (1520–1576) under the pseudonym Leo Suavius in 1567 (re-

43 Jacques Grévin (1567), fol. 101r. The Latin text is given on sig. viir.
En l'assemblée de tout le College da la Faculté de medecine appellée pour donner iugement de l'Antimoine, il a esté aduisé par l'authorité de tous ceux qui ont esté excellens en l'art de medecine, confirmee par raisons, deduictes souuentesfois, derechef encores depuis peu de temps en la presence de l'Aduocat du Roy: que l'Antimoine est vn poison, lequel doit estre mis au rang des Simples qui ont qualité venimeuse, & lequel ne peut estre tellemēt corrigé par aucune correction, que sans danger tresgrand on le puisse prendre dedans le corps.
44 Loys de l'Aunay (1566). See especially p. 46, where he wrote of "vne alchimie freschement descendue du ciel . . . ."
45 Paracelsus (1568), sig. A5v. I used a microfilm of this work from the Bibliothèque St. Geneviéve, Paris. The first edition of 1567 was also published at Anvers by Guillaume Silvius. On Hassard, see R. Halleux (1983), 33–63 (45–7). Halleux also discusses other early Flemish Paracelsians in this paper.

printed 1568).[46] A diplomat and an advocate at the Parlement of Paris, Gohory was at the same time a literary figure with a special interest in the occult arts. He wrote on music and also has acquired a special place in the history of French literature for his translations of Machiavelli and *Amadis de Gaule.* His translation of the tenth book of the latter appeared in 1555.[47] The work contained descriptions of charms and enchantments and discussions of the quest for the Holy Grail and the magic of Merlin. How could anyone doubt that a work with so much occult material contained deep mystical significance? Those persons who were well-read in cabala and occult physics would easily note his enigmas and hieroglyphics. Gohory's interest was foreshadowed by an earlier text in which he sought to decipher the Sibylline mysteries by the use of numerological and cabalistic techniques.[48] No less open to mystical interpretation was his translation of Francesco Colonna's (1433–1527) *Hypnotomachie, ov Discours du Songe Poliphile* (1561) with its allegorical illustrations and its dream setting – a form familiar to anyone who knew the alchemical and Hermetic literature.[49]

One need not be surprised then to find that Gohory's account of the work of Paracelsus should be centered less on practical medicine than on the occult interpretation of the Paracelsian description of the cosmos. Indeed, he took the opportunity to attack the French translation of Paracelsus by Hassard whenever possible. In addition to Hassard, he cited the work of Thomas Erastus and attacked the Paracelsian texts published by Gerhard Dorn, whose reply, oddly, was appended to the second edition of Gohory's *Compendium.*[50]

Gohory had surely read the recently published Paracelsian *Philosophia ad Athenienses* (1564) because in the *Compendium* he discussed in detail the generation of the four elements from the *mysterium magnum* and then described the Paracelsian account of the spirits of the universe associated with the elements: the Nymphs, Tritons, Lorinds, Durdales, and Melo-

[46] A good survey of the literature is found in Owen Hannaway's biography of Gohory in the *Dictionary of Scientific Biography*, vol. 5, pp. 447–8. The basic study is E. T. Hamy (1899), pp. 1–26. Jacques Gohory's relationship to Paracelsism, neo-Platonism, and Hermeticism is discussed in D. P. Walker (1958), pp. 96–106 and in Walter Pagel (1962), pp. 128–9. Gohory's place in the history of sixteenth-century chemistry is discussed by J. R. Partington (1961), vol. 2, pp. 162–3.

[47] I.G.P. [Jacques Gohory, Parisien] (1555); see the "Epistre dv Tradvctevr," sig. à iiiʳ, in which the mystical significance of the work is discussed.

[48] Jacques Gohory (1550).

[49] Jacques Gohory, tr. (1561); see sig. a iᵛ in which Gohory points to the obscure meanings and hieroglyphic characters of the text. This work, completed in 1467 but not published until 1499, is discussed in its Renaissance context by Ioan P. Couliano (1987), pp. 40–2.

[50] In 1571 Gohory also founded a small philosophical society, the Lycium Philosophal San Marcellin, at his home in the Faubourg Saint-Marcel, where the members prepared Paracelsian medicines and carried out alchemical experiments; Gohory discussed Paracelsian medicine with Jean Fernel, Ambroise Paré, Jean Chastellan, and Leonardo Botal.

synes.[51] Interested at all times in the work of Johannes Trithemius, Gohory suggested that Paracelsus had learned of these spirits from his mentor and that he had taken the three principles from the works of earlier alchemists, suggesting that Ioannes Valentianus might be a likely source.[52] The *Compendium*, a short work of only fifty pages, presents a poor account at best of the Paracelsian system. Gohory wrote with approval of the macrocosm–microcosm analogy[53] and rejected the Galenic humors.[54] Potable gold and antimony were praised as medicines, and as one might expect, great stress was placed on the importance of magic, cabala, charms, amulets, and talismans.[55] Unfortunately, he presented very little in defense of any of this.

Included in the volume was the text of Paracelsus' *De vita longa*, which appeared with Gohory's commentary. Like so many of his contemporaries, Gohory was impressed with the accounts of the wonderful cures of Paracelsus. But because he was neither a physician nor a chemist, we find here little practical information. Rather, Gohory discussed Paracelsus as a Renaissance magus, and he found in the *De vita longa* a text that he could compare with earlier discussions of the prolongation of life by Roger Bacon and Marsilio Ficino.[56] To this extent the work of Gohory does not fall into the mainstream of Paracelsian thought. Walker has perhaps correctly categorized this author as one of the "Demonic magicians" in the Hermetic tradition rather than a chemist or chemical philosopher.[57]

In addition to the praise of Paracelsus by Gohory and Hassard, the year 1567 witnessed the publication of Jacques Grévin's second discourse on antimony, which was in reply to de Launay, and his translation of Jean Wier's *Cinq livres de l'impostvre et tromperie des diables: des enchantements & sorcelleries*. In the *Cinq livres* the chemists were pictured as the followers of Paracelsus, and "they are true imitators of their master in their arrogance, vainglory and presumption. They cry out and speak loudly their promises and use great words to impress others."[58] These chemists rely on the book by Paracelsus called the *Paragranum*, use

[51] Leo Suavius [Jacques Gohory] (1568), pp. 22–4.
[52] Partingon (1961), vol. 2, p. 162.
[53] Suavius (1568), p. 32.   [54] Ibid., p. 33.
[55] Ibid., pp. 275ff. See the chapter titled "De vera magia carminibus & characteribus adversus Wieri aliorumque calumnias."
[56] Roger Bacon, a major source, is referred to throughout Gohory's work. The comparison of Paracelsus with Ficino is found in ibid., pp. 199ff.
[57] D. P. Walker (1958), pp. 96–106.
[58] Jean Wier, *Cinq Livres de l'impostvre et tromperie des diables: des enchantments & sorcelleries* . . . , trans. Jacques Grévin (Paris: Iacques du Puys, 1567), fol. 105ᵛ. Wier's view of Paracelsus is most accessible in *Histoires Disputes et Discours des Illusions et Impostures des Diables, des Magiciens infames, sorcieres et Empoisonneurs: des Ensorcelez et Demoniaques* (2 vols., Paris: Aux bureaux du Progrès Médical and A. Delahaye et Lecrosnier, 1885), pp. 260–2. This is a reprint of the 1579 ed. and includes two dialogues on sorcerers and their punishment by Thomas Erastus.

quotes from it to attack the ancient and sacrosanct art of medicine, and then proceed to present new principles and words that cannot be defended by reason.[59] The claims of the Paracelsians that the true medicine was known to Adam and to some of the prophets of old are to be rejected. For Wier, although some chemical medicines were of value, at best "chemistry . . . is only a small part of medicine."[60]

Wier's appraisal was much to Grévin's liking, and he quoted it at length in his Second Discourse against de Launay.[61] By this time he was also able to cite the translation of Paracelsus's *Grossen Wundartznei* by Pierre Hassard[62] as well as the new edition of the *De longa vita*. On the basis of these texts he accused de Launay of not understanding Paracelsus, even though his adversary gave credit for his text primarily to Mattioli. Surely de Launay's preparation of antimony was very different from that described by Paracelsus.[63] Not only was de Launay ignorant of the work of Paracelsus, he apparently knew little of alchemy, logic, or medical practice.[64] He was an empiric who experimented on his patients, no better than an assassin.

But Grévin was not ready to damn the medical use of alchemy altogether.

> I confess that by the means of alchemy one can accomplish many beautiful cures. I approve, praise and exalt highly the extraction of quintessential oils since in them the virtues and faculties of things are purer and thus less impeded by corporal excrements.[65]

Chemicals have a more prompt action than the mixtures of the apothecaries, and even antimony had some virtues useful for exterior use. Thus, Grévin returned to his attack on de Launay four years later in his *De venenis libri duo* (1571); it is clear that by this time Grévin had read widely in the chemical and Paracelsian literature.[66] His views, however, had not altered: Chemistry is useful to the physician, but it is far from being the basis of a new science and medicine that the Paracelsists would wish.

The exchange between Grévin and de Launay had centered on the internal use of antimony in medicine, but it also served to introduce Paracelsus to the French medical community. The four tracts by Grévin and de Launay had appeared at the same time as Pierre Hassard's Paracelsian translation and Jacques Gohory's Paracelsian *Compendium*. Taken as a whole, these works presented the positions for and against chemistry as a medical and cosmological system, the use of chemicals inter-

---

59 Ibid., fol. 106^r.   60 Ibid., fol. 106^v.
61 Grévin (1567), fols. 101^v–102^v.
62 Ibid., fols. 91^v–93^r. Here Grévin refers to the Hassard translation regarding the purifying action of antimony on gold.
63 Ibid., fols. 90–3.
64 Ibid., chaps. 1 and 2, fols. 27ff.   65 Ibid., fol. 94^r.
66 Jacques Grévin (1571), pp. 260–70.

nally in the body, and the work of Paracelsus himself in translation into French and Latin. Above all, the Paracelsian medical faculty had entered the debate by banning the internal use of antimony by physicians.

Chemical practice

The authors of contemporary tracts on the plague turned again to Paracelsus as an authority. Pierre Hassard praised Paracelsus as "the incomparable doctor and prince of Philosophy, Medicine and Surgery" in his translation of Paracelsus's *De la Peste* (1570).[67] But Hassard also took the opportunity as translator to reply to Gohory's criticism of his translation of *La grande, vraye et parfaicte chirurgie*. Rather than being a true compendium of Paracelsian philosophy, he said, Gohory's little book seemed to be more of a "derision ou deprauation." The great German disciples of Paracelsus, Adam of Bodenstein and Gerhard Dorn, had already replied to Gohory, and Hassard felt it necessary to point out that his critic did not understand what Paracelsus had meant.[68]

The text of Paracelsus's *De la Peste* discussed the place of man in the cosmos and made the point that magic is for the benefit of man. It is not evil or a form of enchantment. "The Magician governs the heavens and the stars."[69] The Creator God "is the parent or generator of the Microcosm" and "this is the anatomy that the physician must know – that of comparing the Macrocosm and nature together."[70] For those who aspire to be true physicians or surgeons, advice is given that they must master both astronomy and the spagyric art (chemistry).[71]

Nicholas Hovel's *Traité de la Peste* (1573) was an original work, but it was no less Paracelsian in spirit. Hovel compared the ability of antimony to purify metals with its medical use in ridding the human body of all superfluities and excrements – as the learned Paracelsus had written.[72]

In 1575 Alexandre de la Tourette prepared a work on potable gold that appeared at both Paris and Lyon in separate editions. Here he wrote of *aurum potabile* as a cure for all diseases. (This subject would become a focus of debate that divided chemists and Galenists for the next century.) La Tourette took this opportunity to praise both alchemy and Paracelsus. At the start he wrote of the wonderful three principles.[73] Above all the physician should have a knowledge of mercury and sulfur and their properties of purging and coagulating,[74] which give these two

[67] T. Paracelsus (1570), p. 4 ("Epistre Dedicatoire").
[68] Ibid., p. 11.   [69] Ibid., p. 31.
[70] Ibid., p. 116.   [71] Ibid., p. 134.
[72] Nicholas Hovel (or Hoüel) (1573), p. 44.
[73] Alexandre de la Tourette (1575), fol. 8v.
[74] Ibid., fol. 9r.

chemicals the ability to "conserve the body in incorruptibility: for which reason they are called by physicians the true balm of nature."[75]

Because gold is the source of the principles in their purest form and best balance, it is essential for the physician as the most powerful medicine for all manner of disease. Many people have written on this subject, he said, but none more effectively in our age than

> the great Philosopher, Theophrastus Paracelsus, a Swiss, who merits being in the first rank, as being the true monarch of all philosophy and medicine, both in true theory and in good practice and in certain experience, having cured in his time all illnesses which academic physicians consider even today to be incurable.[76]

Although la Tourette did not present a way to make *aurum potabile*, he offered the reader an apology for alchemy, which for him was not a means for making gold or silver but was a fundamental science,

> which teaches us how to separate the elements of every mixture produced by nature: and to collect each of them in its proper vessel. In addition, alchemy is an art which shows the means of separating the subtle from the gross, the pure from the impure; and of taking from each natural mixture its pure and distinct essence, in which lies all the virtue of the mixed substance. Or one might define it in this way: Alchemy is a science, by which we learn to know the first matter of all the bodies of the world, be they animal, vegetable or mineral . . .[77]

La Tourette was answered the same year by L. S. S. (or S. L. S. as given in the catalog of the British Library) in a tract criticizing the chemists who claimed to have the secret of making *aurum potabile*. L. S. S. defended the philosophy and medicine of the ancients against the Paracelsians. He praised chemistry but was strongly opposed to the "new inventions" of Paracelsus and his followers who used "strange and fantastic words" such as *spagyry* for chemistry and spoke of sulfur, mercury, and salt as the true elements of all bodies. Here they strayed too far from the true and ancient philosophy. Although it would be appropriate to make corrections in the traditional works, it was wrong to try to overturn them.[78]

L. S. S. was aware of Gohory's edition of the *De vita longa* and attacked the Paracelsian internal use of antimony.[79] As for la Tourette's potable gold, he caustically questioned whether la Tourette had presented the king with an actual gold solution, or whether he had only given him an apology for it on paper.[80]

Similar to the criticism of L. S. S. was that of Bernard Palissy (ca. 1510– ca. 1590) who has been most frequently discussed as a master potter

[75] Ibid.
[76] Ibid., fol. 14^v.   [77] Ibid., fol. 27^r.
[78] L. S. S. (S. L. S. in the British Library catalog) (1575), fol. 5^r–5^v.
[79] Ibid., fol. 6^v.   [80] Ibid., fol. 27^r–27^v.

who specialized in enameled ware.[81] His books show him to have been
dissatisfied both with the educational establishment and with the views
of the chemists. His comments on agriculture emphasize the importance
of fertilizers due to their vital salt content, a concept to be found in the
work of Paracelsus.[82] In the *Discours Admirables* (1580) will be found
Palissy's "Traité des Metavx et Alchimie," in which he displayed his
extensive knowledge of current chemical theory but firmly rejected
transmutation. Also in the *Discours Admirables* is the "Traité de l'Or
Potable," in which he rejected the medicinal value of gold in any form.
To those who suggested that Paracelsus had used potable gold to cure
lepers, Palissy answered that "perhaps Paracelsus pretended that his
medicine was drinkable gold, and that he never had any."[83] Nor is
antimony of any use for the physician because "its action is poisonous,
and by its poisonous nature it affects all parts of the stomach, the belly
and the whole body . . ."[84]

The significance of chemistry as a practical art was becoming ever
more evident. Jacques Besson, best known for his *Theatrum instrumen-
torum et machinarum* (1578), published his *Art et Moyen de Tirer Hvyles et
Eaux, de tovs Medicaments simples & Oleogeneux*, which described distillation equipment and gave directions for the preparation of various oils
and waters.[85] And Ambroise Paré (ca. 1517–1590) added a twenty-
eighth book, on distillation, to his surgical works (1575):

> . . . it now seemes requisite that we speake somewhat of Chymistry and
> such medicines as are extracted by fire. These are such as consist of a
> certaine fift essence separated from their earthy impurity by Distillation, in
> which there is a singular, and almost divine efficacy in the cure of diseases.
> So that of so great an aboundance of the medicines there is scarse any
> which at this day Chymists doe not distill, or otherwise make them more
> strong and effectuall than they were before.[86]

If distillation promised great benefits for the pharmacist and surgeon,
it seemed no less promising for agriculture to Bernard Palissy (1499 or
1510–1589).[87] In his *Discours admirables* (1580) he included essays on salts
and marl, stressing the life-giving properties of salt and pointing out
that it increased crop yields when spread on fields. Indeed, he claimed
that the reason manuring is beneficial is that salt is released from the

---

81 Discussions of the work of Palissy are still colored by the study of Henry Morley (1852)
    even though there are a number of more recent studies. A helpful introduction to the
    literature prior to 1957 will be found in Palissy (1957), pp. 257–64. Of special value for
    the historian of chemistry is Partington (1961), pp. 69–77.
82 See Debus (1968), 67–88.
83 Palissy (1961), pp. 228–9; Palissy (1957), p. 115.
84 Palissy (1961), p. 230; Palissy (1957), p. 116.
85 Jacques Besson (1573).
86 Ambroise Parey (Paré) (1634), p. 1093.
87 I discussed the Paracelsian background of Palissy's agricultural writings in my "Palissy,
    Plat and English Agricultural Chemistry in the 16th and 17th Centuries" (1968).

substance through rain and the normal weathering process. These views had been expressed earlier by Paracelsus.

Joseph Duchesne (or Quercetanus) (ca. 1544–1609),[88] one of the most influential of the early French chemists, published his first work in 1575 as a reply to Jacques Aubertus who had earlier that year published a short tract on the origin of metals and on chemical medicines.[89] Aubertus was openly anti-Paracelsian in tone and was shortly taken to task by Duchesne.

Like many other French chemists, Duchesne was a Calvinist who had lived away from his homeland for many years in this period of religious warfare. He took his medical degree at Basle and then moved first to Cassel and then to Geneva, where he was granted citizenship in 1584 and where he served as a diplomat to the Council of the Two Hundred. He did not return to France until Henry of Navarre took Paris in 1593. At that time he was appointed physician in ordinary to the king.

Duchesne's response to Aubert was a short work in which he argued against the Aristotelian position of his opponent. Chemistry should be accepted by all as the true key to nature, for it

> . . . openeth unto us so many works of the almighty God, it laieth open so many secretes of nature, and preparations of herbes, beastes and minerals hetherto unknowen, and sheweth the uses almost of all things, which were hidden and laid up on the bosome of Nature, that they shew themselves unkinde toward man, that would have this art buried.[90]

However, at no time was Duchesne to be a blind follower of Paracelsus, though he clearly admired the work of the man.

> As touching *Paracelsus*, I have not taken upon mee the defence of his divinitie, neither did I ever thinke to agree with him in all points, as though I were sworne to his doctrine: but . . . he teacheth many things almost divinely, in Phisicke, which the thankfull posteritie can neither commend and praise sufficientlie . . .[91]

Although he favored the use of the Paracelsian chemical remedies, Duchesne argued that there was much to be learned from the work of Hippocrates and Galen. The Galenists should not charge the chemists with confining themselves to the prescription of metals and minerals because the chemists, no less than the high doctors of Paris, appreciated the values of traditional *materia medica*. His reply to the charge that the chemicals of this new sect were too violent and sharp was that if properly prepared they are "sweet and familiar to our nature."[92]

[88] On Duchesne, see Allen G. Debus's short biography in the *Dictionary of Scientific Biography* (1971). Duchesne's considerable influence on English chemistry and medicine is discussed in Debus (1966), pp. 87–101.

[89] Iacobus Aubertus Vindonis (1575).

[90] Joseph Duchesne (1575), pp. 2–3. Here I cite the English translation (1591), fol. 1.

[91] Ibid.

[92] Duchesne, English, fols. 6ʳ–6ᵛ; Latin, pp. 20, 22.

Aubert had argued against alchemy, stating that it was customarily accepted that metals were engendered by the stars through astral influences, a force that the alchemist could not duplicate. Duchesne countered that the true efficient cause of the generation of metals "is heate, by force whereof mettales congealed in the bowels of the earth are disposed, digested and made perfect."[93] This was a natural process that might be duplicated in the laboratory, and which seemed to negate Aubert's argument.[94]

Duchesne's reply was published with his *De mineralium, animalium, et vegetabilium medicamentorum spagyrica praeparatione & usu*, a practical guide to chemical preparations that included compounds of antimony for internal as well as external use in medicine.

The following year Duchesne published his *Sclopetarius*, which centered on the problem of poisoning from gunshot wounds, a practical concern to the many Renaissance surgeons attached to armies. Here Duchesne asked why these wounds so often infected the body with deadly poisons. The ingredients of gunpowder were often used separately as medicines, so they could not be the cause.[95] German soldiers, when wounded, mixed no small portion of gunpowder in a cup of wine "and as a holsome medicine drinke it up."[96] But if gunpowder is not the cause, one should ask if it is the leaden shot. But this could not be because "lead doth greatly agree with our nature, and is verie holsome thereunto: for it greatly auaileth to the consolidation and drying of sores . . . and in the use thereof, there appeareth no one signe of venome." Indeed, some soldiers carried bullets in their bodies for years with no signs of illness. Therefore, wrote Duchesne, "I plainly confesse that lead being plainly and simplie in his owne nature considered, cannot bring any venome to the wound, except it be outwardly poisoned, which thing is not heard to be done . . ."[97]

At this point the chemist in Duchesne asserts himself. Lead is composed of an impure and combustible sulfur and "a great store of grosse, unclean and dross mercury." It is therefore "most easily imbibed with any liquor." The reason then for the poisoning of gunshot wounds is the imperfect nature of the metal which takes on its deadly nature in the manufacturing process,[98] thus,

> . . . we conclude that the shot may be poisoned . . . by often dipping and quenching them in mercuriall waters and deadly iuices, through $\tilde{y}$ which their substance may be altered, & spoiled, and so they doo venime and infect the wound with their euill disposition . . .[99]

[93] Duchesne, English, fol. 14ᵛ; Latin, pp. 53–4.
[94] Duchesne, English, fol. 15ʳ; Latin, p. 57.
[95] Joseph Duchesne (1590), p. 6.
[96] Ibid., p. 7. [97] Ibid.
[98] Ibid., pp. 7–10.
[99] Ibid., p. 10.

As for those Galenists who would confine themselves to medicinal preparations of the ancients and wished to reject the new chemicals, Duchesne replied,

> . . . to what purpose is it that they object unto us ẙ sulphurie metaline & venemous stinckes (as they call them) by whose smell and drawne breath (for these are their contumelius words) they be almost strangled that come into the dennes of those *Cyclops*? But is it unknowne unto those slaunderers and sicophantes, that the olde Phisitions made verie many medicines of most filthie thinges, as of the filth of eares, sweate of the body, of womens menstrewes (and that which is horrible to be spoken) of the doong of man, and other beastes, spittle, urine, flyes, mise, the ashes of an Owles head, the hoves of Goates and Asses, ẙ wormes of a rotten tree, and the scurfe of Mules, as may be gathered out of the writings of *Galen*, *Aetii*, *Aegineta*, *Diosc. Plinius*, *Serap*: to passe the metalines which it is evident they did also use.[100]

Duchesne advocated a careful diet and the evacuation of humoral excess through the proper application of medicines, which for the most part were chemically prepared. He warned against the use of hot oil for amputations, advocating the constant use of running water instead. Here again chemical remedies were prescribed to help "stay the blood."[101]

Duchesne's attack on Aubert was criticized by John Antony Fenot in 1575, and Aubert, himself, replied the following year.[102] In 1579 the Parisian physician Germain Courtin published an attack on Paracelsus, the three principles, potable gold, transmutation, and the whole of pyrotechny.[103] Another attack on Paracelsian medicine was made by Toussaint Ducret, a physician of St. Marcel who published a treatise on gout in 1575 that was specifically directed against the Paracelsians. An ardent Galenist, Ducret dedicated his book to Thomas Erastus whose four part attack on Paracelsus was already considered the most scholarly defense of traditional medicine. Although Ducret was concerned about the views of Paracelsus on tartar as the cause of diseases that affected the joints, he launched into a far reaching attack on the Paracelsian system as a whole. Paracelsus had denied the existence of both the four Aristotelian elements and their attendant humors;[104] instead he had postulated three other elements, stating that all things that burn are sulfur, anything that crosses over to smoke or fumes is mercury, and ashes are in fact salt. In a lengthy discussion, Ducret denied the truth of these three as elements. He also rejected the belief of Paracelsus that metals are generated from the action of the heavens (as the father) on the earth mother and that the growth process is similar to the development of a fetus. As for the belief that a chemist can duplicate and hasten this

---

[100] Ibid., p. 74.   [101] Ibid., pp. 19, 31.
[102] Joannes Antonins Fenotus (1575); Iacobus Aubertus Vindonis (1576).
[103] Toussaint Ducret (1575), p. 90.   [104] Ibid., pp. 104–5.

process in his laboratory, it was simply not true. Ducret flatly denied the possibility of transmutation.[105] In short, he felt that the views of Paracelsus were inept and absurd regarding basic medical and scientific doctrines, the cause of disease, and the preparation of medicines.[106]

During these years some of the work of Gerhard Dorn, a German Paracelsist who had earlier replied to Jacques Gohory, was published in France. His mystical *La Monarchie du Ternaire en Union, Contre la Monomachie de Binaire en Confusion* appeared in 1577,[107] and his edition of Paracelsus's *De Restituta utriusque Medicinae vera Praxi* appeared at Lyon the following year with his commentary on the text and a vignette portrait of Paracelsus on the title page, the first portrait of him published in France.[108]

The works of one of the most vocal French Paracelsists, Bernard George Penotus, began to appear in the final decades of the sixteenth century. Born at Port-Sainte-Marie in Guienne sometime between 1520 and 1530, Penotus studied at Basel and lived to about the age of ninety. Late in life he became disillusioned with both alchemy and Paracelsus.[109] Penotus published a number of works in Latin and German, some of which were translated into other languages. His subjects were alchemy and chemical medicine. Among his works is one ascribed to Paracelsus (probably incorrectly) titled the *Centumquindecim curationes experimentaque* and published first at Lyon in 1582. This work was translated into English by John Hester and published in 1596 after Hester's death (ca. 1593), along with translations of the *Secrets* of Isaac Hollandus and the *Spagericke Antidotarie* of Joseph Duchesne.

In his extensive "Apologeticall Preface" to his *Curationes*, Penotus complained bitterly of the dishonesty of the Galenists:

> For when as reports are spread of the straunge cures of sundrie grieuous diseases, which are wrought by the benefite of tinctures and vegetall and minerall spirites, by the cunning and labour of those whom the common sort at this day cal Chymists or Alchimists: by and by on the contrarie part they crie out that those colliar phisitians can do no good but kil al men that put themselues into their hands with their venemous medecines, so that they ought to bee driuen out of the commonwealth, and that they are deceiuers, and that their extractions and preparations, their subtile, and thinne spirit wil profit nothing, and that the spirit of Vitriol is poison, the essence of Antimonie and Mercurie is nothing, the extraction of Sulphur is nothing worth, neither the liquor of gold: and to be briefe, that al things are contrarie to the nature of man, and more to be auoided then the eies of a basiliske. And yet they in the meane time like cunning and craftie theeues priuily, and with fair promises picke out from the poore Chymists

[105] Ibid., p. 137.   [106] Germain Courtin (1579).

[107] Recently reprinted with a preface by J. P. Brach (Paris: Gutenberg Reprints). I have not seen this edition which is described in a Gutenberg catalog ca. 1985.

[108] Paracelsus (1578).

[109] On Penotus, see J. R. Partington (1962), vol. 2, pp. 161, 269–70.

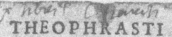

THEOPHRASTI
GERMANI,
PARACELSI, MEDICO-
RVM ET PHILOSOPHO-
rum omnium, in vniuerfum
facilè Principis.

*De reſtituta vtriuſque Medicinæ vera
Praxi.*

LIBER PRIMVS.

*Gerardo Dorn Doctore Phyſico, ac interprete Ger-
manico, in hunc ordinem recolligente.*

Ad Illuſtriſſ. ac Potentiſſ. Princip. D. FRANCISC.
VALESIVM, Andegauorum, Biturigum,
Alençonium, Turonenſium, &c Ducem.

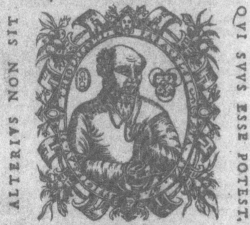

ALTERIVS NON SIT QVI SVVS ESSE POTEST.

LVGDVNI,
PRO IACOBO DV PVYS.

M. D. LXXVIII.

Cum priuileg. Cæſareæ ac Regiæ maieſt. ad decennium.

The first portrait of Paracelsus to be published in France. From the title page of
Paracelsus, *De restituta utriusque medicinae vera prax, liber primus, Gerardo Dorn
interprete* (1578). Courtesy of the Wellcome Institute Library, London.

the secrets of Phisicke, and secretly learn those things that they forbid the common people as poisonous afterwardes challenging them for their owne practises.[110]

Addressing the Galenists, he pointed to the experimental nature of the work of the chemists:

> I say euery Paracelsian which doth but onely carry coales vnto the worke, can shewe you by eie three principles of *Theophrastus* physicke. Haue you tasted the most sharp salt? or the most sweet oile? or the balme that most delicate liquor? All those being hidden in euerie thing that is created, you haue not once perceiued. . . . Is it not a great follie to write against a thing, and not to vnderstand it wel before? Such as are addicted to *Paracelsus* doctrine, when they perceiue you haue no stronger weapons then those you haue hitherto gathered, they will conclude that you rather confirme and establish Paracelsus physicke, then confute it.[111]

Penotus claimed that most dangerous diseases had been cured by properly prepared chemical medicines and that the chemists could not be praised sufficiently.

> We haue brought into physicke, essences, oiles, balmes, and salts, all which the Alchymists schooles haue founde out. And how great light is come vnto physicke onely by true distillation, it is knowen vnto all men, and daily experience teacheth, how great commodity hath redounded thereby vnto the sicke.[112]

He warned against the "counterfeit Paracelsian" who offered dangerous remedies never prescribed by the true Paracelsian. Here he may have been referring to the case of Roch le Baillif which had resulted in a new confrontation between the Medical Faculty at Paris and the French Paracelsians.

Le Baillif and the Parisian Galenists

Known also as the sieur de la Rivière, Roch le Baillif was a native of Normandy. In 1578 he published a short summary of Paracelsian medicine, *Le demosterion*, in which he praised the still living Adam of Bodenstein, Gerhard Dorn, and Pierre Hassard and listed a series of certain cures discovered by the chemists, including leprosy, dropsy, paralysis, and gout.[113] He was aware of his alchemical heritage and listed famous masters of the art down through history to Jacques Gohory.[114]

---

[110] Paracelsus (1596), sig. A3ᵛ.   [111] Ibid., sig. A4ʳ.

[112] Ibid., sig. B1ʳ.

[113] Roch le Baillif (1578), from the "Au lecteur." The present account of le Baillif's career is based primarily on Hugh Trevor-Roper (1972), vol. 2, pp. 227–50. See also Dietlinde Goltz (1972), 337–52.

[114] Le Baillif (1578), sigs. e iiᵛ–e ivᵛ.

Those who seek certainty, he said, should turn not to Galen but to Paracelsus, because his is the true medicine and "Science is the creation of God, and is therefore certain and true."[115] Here "medicine" is printed in the margin to indicate to the reader that "Science" is the true medicine. Galen had been badly informed, but Paracelsus had founded his new medicine on the four columns of philosophy, astronomy, alchemy, and virtue.[116] We need not be surprised to see the four humors rejected here and the Paracelsian principles extolled. Are not all things of a ternary Creation?[117] The Creation had occurred in terms of number, weight, and measure and consisted of matter, form, and privation. We should then expect to see that matter is composed of three, not four, components: sulfur, salt, and liquor (mercury).[118] Most of *Le demosterion* is composed of three hundred aphorisms, which offer a short compendium of Paracelsian dogma, and the remainder of the book is devoted to tracts on chiromancy, conjuration, the baths of Brittany, and a lexicon of Paracelsian terms.

The same year that he published *Le demosterion*, le Baillif left Brittany for Paris where he was appointed médecin ordinaire to Henry III. Here he began work on two other tracts, one on the plague and the other on man and his essential anatomy, both published in 1580. The first tract began with a defense of the three principles as the components of matter,[119] and the second had little to offer on traditional anatomy. Rather, le Baillif wrote of man as a Godly creation and then proceeded to discuss the relationship of the macrocosm to the microcosm.[120] He was willing to accept the elements as the great world but remained adamant that the principles were all that were necessary to understand the components of our world.[121] He went on to discuss the importance of the archeus in the digestive process and digressed to point out the significance of physiognomy and chiromancy in reading the bodily interior.[122]

Le Baillif's stay in Paris was short and disastrous. First he was accused of coining false money, and then his medical views became the object of concern to the members of the Parisian Medical Faculty, who had the right to limit practitioners in the City to graduates of the Paris school. Ordered to halt both his practice and his lecturing (1578), he refused and was summoned to appear before the parlement. In an emotional three-day trial le Baillif and his counsel, a distinguished attorney, Étienne Pasquier, defended Paracelsian medicine.[123] The Galenists hoped to use his case to put an end to this medical heresy. And indeed, the trial dealt

---

[115] Ibid., p. 4. [116] Ibid., p. 2.
[117] Ibid., p. 14. [118] Ibid.
[119] Roch le Baillif (1580), fol. 4v–5r.
[120] Roch le Baillif (1580), fols. 9r–11r.
[121] Ibid., fols. 13r–14v. [122] Ibid., fols. 18r, 22v.
[123] On Pasquier and the trial, in addition to Trevor-Roper see D. Thickett (1979), pp. 64, 71, 217.

with Paracelsism far more directly than had the antimony edict of 1566. They had no trouble convicting le Baillif because "to every question proposed to him, he always sang one of his songs . . . [one needed] to know of his three principles, Salt, Sulphur and Mercury; or the separation of the pure from the impure; or of the microcosm."[124]

The trial was a victory for the medical establishment, and on 2 June 1579, le Baillif was ordered to leave Paris. Before doing so he prepared his *Sommaire Defence*, dated 15 July 1579,[125] in which he appealed to the Paris Faculty of Medicine on behalf of the many physicians who placed confidence "in the very learned Paracelsus."[126] Forbidden to practice medicine in Paris, he wrote this work to show publicly that gout, dropsy, epilepsy, paralysis, pthisis (tuberculosis), gravelle (urinary calculus), and quartan fever are curable.[127] The rest of the work is a defense of Paracelsus and his view that medicine cannot be understood or practiced without a knowledge of alchemy, a fact known not only to Dioscorides, Rhazes, Avicenna, and Arnald of Villanova but also to men of his own time such as Fernel, Wecker, Adam of Bodenstein, and "The learned Andernach, the premier [physician] of our time who extracts his excellent remedies in this way."[128] Le Baillif then returned to Brittany where he established a medical practice at Rennes. Although he continued to write, he no longer played a significant role in the developing debate.

The Galenist victory was anything but decisive. In fact, the interest in Paracelsus and chemical medicine continued to grow if we judge by the increasing numbers of tracts issuing from the shops of the printers. For example, Antoine de Fregeville (1588) prepared a *Palinodie chimique* in which he pointed out the errors of the chemists and the alchemists,[129] and Jean Suau argued against the presumption and intolerable imposture of the spagyrists, who claimed to have prepared both a new medicine and a new philosophy, in his tract on the plague (1586).[130]

An important proponent of Paracelsian medicine was Claude Dariot (1530 or 1533–1594) who studied medicine at Montpellier, but who, as a protestant, fled France after the St. Bartholomew's Day Massacre. He was admitted to citizenship at Geneva in 1573 and served as the town physician of Beaune. Interested in astrology, Dariot had published a brief guide to that subject in 1557 in Latin, which was to go through a number of editions in French and English by the end of the century.[131]

---

124 Trevor-Roper (1972), p. 236.
125 Roch le Baillif (1579), sig. ã iiii[r]. The British Museum copy of this rare tract is incomplete, ending at sig. c i.
126 Ibid., sig. ã iii[r].
127 Ibid., sig. ã iii[v]–a iiii[r].
128 Ibid., sig. b iiii[r]–b iiii[v].
129 Antoine de Fregeville Du Gault (1588).
130 Jean Suau (1586), p. 1.
131 Information on pharmaceutical practice in Renaissance Montpellier is to be found in Louis Dulieu (1973).

As a physician Dariot was a Paracelsian. In 1582 he published his *De praeparatione medicamentorum*, a collection of three tracts, the first of which discussed the principles of Paracelsian thought and argued that in reality they differ little from those of Galen and Hippocrates. He paid tribute to Severinus and Guinter, who had been trained in traditional medicine but who had learned to appreciate the chemical medicine of the Paracelsians. Unfortunately, he noted, many of the chemical directions presented by Paracelsian authors, including Paracelsus himself, were difficult to follow. Even Guinter was at fault here.[132]

Turning to his own search for truth, Dariot referred to his extensive reading of the alchemical literature. He had read Hermes, Geber, Arnald of Villanova, and Raymond Lull and had found that they all wrote "in hidden words" of medical secrets.

> Since that time our Paracelsus, a great physician and an accomplished philosopher, has written fully and in many places, but very obscurely, this being the cause of the vexation for many enemies of science who have held this against him. . . . How much better it would have been if the physicians of his time, rather than persecuting him and driving him from their company, would have received him and exhorted him to write his secrets more clearly.[133]

Although chemistry remained an unknown science to many, Dariot noted that it was becoming more widespread among the learned. Referring to his own training at Montpellier, Dariot recalled that:

> In my time, I have seen at Montpellier (living Messieurs Rondelet, Saporte and Schirron, learned physicians) medical doctors and scholars, who worked to separate the oily and more subtle substances from fragrant simples, from aromatics and diverse fruits, and these were replaced in use by the said Sieur Rondelet (the first of his time) and Saporte.[134]

It was necessary then to write clearly and more openly for the many who are becoming interested in the subject.

> I will try to write the truth without any mixture or disguise, the method of preparation of each [substance I describe] according to the way I made it myself and experimented with it.[135]

Dariot refused to agree with those who argued that the cure by similitude advocated by Paracelsus conflicted with the views of the ancient physicians. In this case Paracelsus had referred to neither the primary nor the secondary qualities of the Aristotelians but to substances and virtues. Dariot interpreted Paracelsus as having presented three classes of disease, which corresponded to the principles: salt, sulfur, and mer-

---

[132] I have used the French translation of the Dariot's *De praeparatione medicamentorum* (1608), separate pagination, pp. 4, 13.

[133] Ibid., p. 12.   [134] Ibid.

[135] Ibid., p. 13.

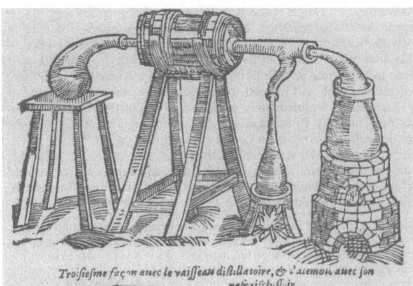

Troifiefme façon auec le vaiffeau diftillatoire, & l'alemou auec fon rafraifchiffoir.

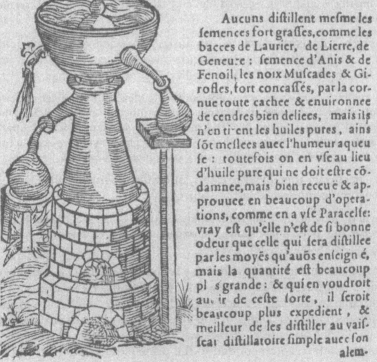

Aucuns diftillent mefme les femences fort graffes, comme les bacces de Laurier, de Lierre, de Geneure : femence d'Anis & de Fenoil, les noix Mufcades & Girofles, fort concaffés, par la cornue toute cachee & enuironnee de cendres bien deliees, mais ils n'en tirent les huiles pures, ains fôt meflees auec l'humeur aqueufe : toutefois on en vfe au lieu d'huile pure qui ne doit eftre côdamnee, mais bien receuë & approuuee en beaucoup d'operations, comme en a vfé Paracelfe: vray eft qu'elle n'eft de fi bonne odeur que celle qui fera diftillee par les moyês qu'auôs enfeigné, mais la quantité eft beaucoup pl s grande : & qui en voudroit auoir de cefte forte, il feroit beaucoup plus expedient, & meilleur de les diftiller au vaiffeau diftillatoire fimple auec fon alem-

Distillation equipment from Claude Dariot, *Traittez de la preparation des medicamens* in *La Grande Chirvrgie de Philippe Aoreole Theophraste Paracelse grand Medecin & Philosophe . . .* (3rd ed., 1608). From the collection of the author.

cury. Therefore, when Paracelsus wrote that like cures like, he understood that a diseased substance is cured by a similar substance: Salt is cured by its like, sulfur by its like, and mercury by the same.[136] It seemed clear to Dariot that chemical concepts were an integral part of medical theory.

Dariot was also concerned with the question of the elements and the principles. Again he denied any conflict between the ancients and the chemists. Paracelsus himself had taught how to separate earth, water, air, and fire from bodies; and the Aristotelian matter, form, and privation could be compared with the Paracelsian principles. For Dariot the example of a burning twig could be used to establish the two systems at the same time,[137] not just one system or the other.

Much of Dariot's *Treatise on the Preparation of Medicines* was devoted to a description of practical chemical techniques and to the actual chemical procedures for the new medicines. Of special interest is Dariot's description of antimony. He began by noting that, among the ancients of the time of Galen, antimony was used only as an external medicine and never taken orally.[138] However, this had changed with the alchemists, who likened the human body to gold, each being perfect in its own realm. Because antimony was used to purge gold of its impurities, they thought that antimony might purge the body of man of its illnesses and bring it back to perfect health.[139] Paracelsus himself had sought the proper preparation of this substance.

In addition to its original Latin edition, Dariot's work on medicinal preparations appeared several times in French translation and was usually published together with his tract on gout and his translation of Paracelsus' *Grossen Wundartznei*. The *Discours de la Govtte* appeared first in 1588. In it he wrote of the importance of the ancients in showing us the road to truth which had since been traveled by many others. Personally he had "read and reread" Paracelsus. But medicine did not appear in perfected form at one moment, there remained a need for constant work and for honest doctors to publish what they discovered.[140]

Also in 1588 Dariot completed his translation of Paracelsus's *Greater Surgery*, the *Grossen Wundartznei*, from the Latin translation of Josquin d'Alhem (1573), not from the original German.[141] Once again he refers to the difficult nature of the alchemical texts, which he ascribes to their original hieroglyphic form. Over the years a few alchemists had maintained an understanding of these characters – knowledge they had passed on only to their disciples – and it was the glory of Paracelsus to have found and to have collected these secrets.[142] Here we encounter

---

[136] Ibid., p. 16. [137] Ibid., pp. 21–2.
[138] Ibid., p. 135. [139] Ibid.
[140] Dariot, . . . *de la goutte* in *La Grand Chirvrgie* (1608), p. 7 (separate pagination).
[141] No reference is made to the earlier French translation by Pierre Hassard.
[142] *La Grand Chirvrgie*, trans. Dariot (1589; ed. used Montbeliart, 1608), sig. ‡5r.

the basic Paracelsian belief that chemistry and medicine could not be separated:

> It would seem to be impossible to separate the preparation of remedies from this science . . . that is to say, separate medicine from alchemy. Alchemy teaches how to prepare remedies and if one tried to separate the one from the other he would do nothing but obscure medicine which would be a great folly since the very foundations of medicine would be overturned.[143]

This emphasis is strengthened by his lengthy annotations, which are clearly indicated to the reader: comments on the results of his own medical practice and on theoretical problems concerning the Paracelsian principles and the relationship of the two worlds.[144]

Conclusion

Only twenty-two years separated the completion of Dariot's translation of the *Grossen Wundartznei* (1588) from the decree of the Parlement of Paris against the internal use of antimony (1566). Yet, in this short period, the medical world of Europe was rent with dissension. In France, in particular, Paracelsus became a widely known philosopher-physician. The debate between de Launay and Grévin raised questions about the safety of the internal use of metallic derivatives and led to a debate on the internal use of the new medicines and to the charge that Paracelsus had been a sorcerer. Some of those writers who were influenced by the Paracelsian corpus – such as Pierre Hassard, G. B. Porta, Joseph Duchesne, and Bernard Palissy – sought practical information in fields as varied as medicine and agriculture. Surgeons were particularly interested in new chemically prepared salves and balms. Other practitioners such as Jacques Gohory found in the Paracelsian texts a continuation of the traditional mystical world view of the Hermeticists and the alchemists.

The attack on Roch le Baillif by the Medical Faculty of Paris in 1579 led to a new confrontation, this time an attack on Paracelsian medicine as a whole rather than on the internal use of antimony. But although the Medical Faculty of Paris was successful in its suit, forcing a royal physician to return to the provinces, the Paracelsian medical heresy was becoming more widespread. New translations were made, and chemical medicines were being applied in ever more fields: as a remedy for fevers, gout, plague, and gunshot wounds. Those physicians who hoped to discover a universal medicine for all diseases saw hope in the alchemical and Paracelsian promise of an *aurum potabile*.

---

[143] Ibid., p. 22.
[144] Excellent examples are Dariot's annotations on pp. 245–52.

In all these areas the medical profession in France, as in other European countries, was fractured. The work of an author practically unknown before 1566 had rapidly become the center of a medical storm. As early as 1580 André du Breil referred to the dangers of the Paracelsists, who sought to overturn the foundation of traditional medicine.[145] For him they were fellow travelers of the alchemists who were properly classed among the empirics. In fact, they were neither true empirics nor philosophers; rather, they were like those who call themselves Christian but who in reality carry out the work of the devil.[146] Perhaps even more interesting was the fact that news of the medicine was known beyond the medical profession. In his *Apologie de Raimond Sebond* (1580) Michel Eyquem Montaigne asked "Combien y a il que la medecine est au monde?" He then noted:

> They say that some newcomer called Paracelsus is changing or reversing the entire order of the old rules, maintaining that, up to the present, medicine has merely served to kill people. He will be able to prove that easily enough I believe, but it would not be very wise for me, I think to test his new empiricism at the risk of my life.[147]

Roch le Baillif had been appointed médecin ordinaire to Henry III, and the followers of Paracelsus throughout Europe were to be found at the courts of protestant princes. It was not too surprising then that when Henry IV took Paris in 1593, he had with him physicians who favored the new chemical medicine. This would accelerate a debate that was already well underway.

[145] André du Breil (1586), sigs. a vi[v]–a viii[r]. On du Breil, see Alison Klairmont Lingo (1985–6).
[146] Du Breil (1586), pp. 33–7.
[147] Michel de Montaigne (1987), pp. 150–1. For the original text, see Michel Eyquem de Montaigne (1976), vol. 2, pp. 286–347 (actually 348–9).

3

Paris and Montpellier: the great chemical debate

Il faut les bruler & enfumer ainsi que renards en leur
tasnier; ou comme fraislons en leurs trous & fourneaux;
ou les boüiller auec leurs huilles distillees & alambi-
quees, comme on faict les choux en Dauphiné, qui est la
plus seure voye que l'on puisse tenir, & le meilleur eui-
dent que l'on puisse choisir pour deliuer d'vne tant pernicieuse & detestable secte de Chimistes, & pseudo-em-
pyriques, & distillateurs Paracelsistes, . . .[1]

Thomas Sonnet, Sieur de Courval (1610)

Alchemy, chemistry, and Paracelsian medicine were attracting increasing interest in the late sixteenth and early seventeenth centuries. Neither the 1566 decree prohibiting the internal use of antimony nor the
legal defeat of le Baillif in 1579 had reduced the flow of books on chemical medicine from the printers' shops.

Traditional alchemical texts on transmutation remained popular, and
living authors turned to this subject as interest in all things chemical
spread. Gaston Duclo (born ca. 1530) published a number of alchemical
works and prepared a lengthy refutation of Thomas Erastus' attack on
transmutation (1590), which was later included in Zetzner's *Theatrum
Chemicum* (1602). The Sieur de Nuisement, receiver-general for the
County of Ligny and Barrois, prepared a treatise on the *Traittez du vray
sel secret des Philosophes, et de l'Esprit general du Monde* (1621) that described a vitalistic philosophy in a world containing spirit, soul, and
body.[2] This work was to become a favorite of seventeenth-century alchemists. Jean Collesson wrote *L'Idee Parfaicte de la Philosophe Hermetiqve*
(1630), which described the theory and practice of the philosophers'
stone, a work that was to be reprinted in the eighteenth century.[3] Similarly, René De La Chastre, a gentlemen of Berroyen, offered the reader a
*Prototype ov Tres Parfait et Analogiqve Exemplaire de l'Art Chimicq; a la Phys-
iqve ov Philosophie de la science Naturelle. Contenant les Cavses principes &*

[1] Thomas Sonnet (1610), pp. 239–40.
[2] Sieur de Nuisement (1621); see particularly chaps. 1–3.
[3] M. I. Collesson (2nd ed. 1631; 1st ed. 1630).

demonstrations scientifiq . . . (1620).[4] The words in the title might make the modern reader think that this work is indeed an experimental chemical treatise leading to an overall philosophy of natural science, but this is not the case. La Chastre's text is a traditional alchemical description of nature's perfection of gold and how the operator might duplicate its process in his laboratory.

A work that went through numerous editions in Latin, French, German, and English well into the eighteenth century was Jean D'Espagnet's *Enchiridion Physicae Restitutae*, published first at Paris in 1608. President of the Parlement of Bordeaux, D'Espagnet sought to re-establish ancient philosophy in its purity, which meant for him a turn toward Hermes and the pre-Socratic philosophers as well as a careful study of the alchemical tradition. D'Espagnet devoted much space to the divine harmony of the world, the Creation, and both the Aristotelian elements and the Paracelsian principles. It was a natural philosophy that borrowed from contemporary chemistry as a means of explanation, as we can see in the following example:

> The lower Region of the Air is like unto the neck or higher part of an *Alembick*, for through it the Vapours climbing up, and being brought to the top, receive their condensation from Cold, and being resolved into water, fall down by reason of their own weight. So Nature through continued distillations by sublimation of the water, by cohobation, or by drawing off the liquor being often poured on, the body doth rectify and abound it.[5]

D'Espagnet accepted the sun as the source of the vital spirit "which flows as a rivulet from that General, and doth work all things in this Microcosm or little World MAN, according to an Analogie with the Sun in the Macrocosm or greater world."[6] The earth is the "womb of the World, the vessel of Generation, the mother of a multiplied, and almost numberless issue . . ."[7] Overall, the work was a typical theoretical and alchemical approach to nature. Although it might well have been presented as an alternative to the work of the ancients, D'Espagnet preferred to offer it as a purification of ancient philosophy.

Blaise de Vigenère (1523–1596), like Gohory, belongs as much to the world of literary history as to the history of science. He was born of a noble family and served the nobility in the foreign service and as a private teacher. As a scholar he prepared translations of and commentaries on ancient texts and histories. However, Vigenère also had an interest in the occult side of the sciences. His *Traicte dv Feu et dv Sel* was

---

4 René De La Chastre (1620).
5 Jean D'Espagnet, (1651), p. 52; *La Philosophie Natvrelle Restablie* . . . (1651), pp. 75–6. The dedication to this French translation is by Jean Bachou. Thomas Willard is currently preparing an annotated edition of the English translation of D'Espagnet's work.
6 D'Espagnet (English), p. 81; (French), p. 119.
7 D'Espagnet (English), p. 87; (French), p. 129.

published posthumously in 1608; and though this text was later appro-
priated for Zetzner's six-volume alchemical collection, the work itself
emphasized traditional alchemical thought. He began with the Creation
and turned to the elements. True understanding was to be had only
with the aid of the cabala and natural magic, which is "nothing else
properly (as *Orpheus* saith) but a forme of marriage of the starry heaven
with the earth, whither hee darts his influences, by which shee im-
pregnes comming from the Intelligences who assist therein . . ."[8]

Blaise de Vigenère fully accepted the analogy of the macrocosm and
the microcosm:

> For, as God hath made the Sunne, Moone, and Stars, thereby to declare to
> the great World, not only the day, night, and seasons, but the change of
> times, and many signes that must appeare in the earth. So hath he man-
> ifested in the little world Man, certaine draughts and lineaments, holding
> place of lights and starres, whereby men may attaine to the knowledge of
> very great secrets, not common, nor known of all.[9]

Again we read of a living cosmos for the "Intelligences of the superiour
world do distill and breath as it were, by some channels their influences,
whereby the effects come to struggle and accomplish their effects here
below . . ."[10] Of great importance in the air was saltpeter, which was
said to have a disposition midway between seawater and fire in the form
of sulfur, being therefore both inflammable and salty, and for this reason
accounting for the thunder and lightning in the skies and for the explosion of gunpowder here on earth.[11]

Traditional alchemy did indeed flourish during these years (and we
shall have occasion to refer to it often), but though the words *alchemy*
and *chemistry* were used interchangeably, the medical chemistry of the
Paracelsian physician was far removed from the work of the goldmaker
by the closing decades of the sixteenth century. It was the medical debate relating to chemistry in France that would raise new questions that
went beyond the points at issue with Grévin, de Launay, and le Baillif.

The Parisian debate

In 1593 Henry of Navarre ended a long period of civil war by taking
Paris, a military and political event that had unexpected medical and
chemical results. The French physicians who were interested in the
work of Paracelsus and the application of chemistry to medicine were
almost all Huguenots. These protestants, many of whom had been in
exile for more than twenty years since the St. Bartholomew's Day mas-

---

[8] Blaise de Vigenère (1642). I have examined this edition, but here I cite the English
    translation (1649), p. 34.
[9] Ibid., p. 8.   [10] Ibid.
[11] Ibid., p. 41.

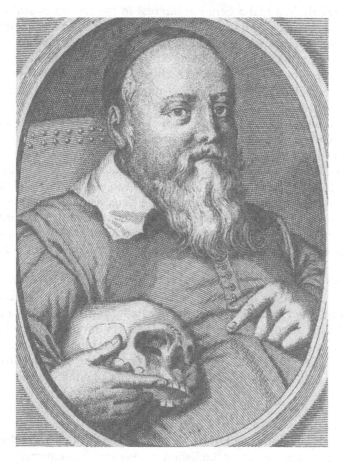

Sir Theodore Turquet de Mayerne (1573–1655). From the collection of the author.

sacre felt that they could return to France now, even to Paris itself. If they were aware of the hostility of the Parisian Medical Faculty to chemistry and the Paracelsians (and they surely must have been), they must also have known that the new king, Henry IV, favored the new medicine. Even the ill-fated Roch le Baillif had been appointed médecin ordinaire to Henry III, and chemical physicians were being welcomed to the service of the rulers of the principalities of Europe at a time when they remained anathema to many of the medical schools on the Continent.

In 1594 Jean Ribit, sieur de la Rivière (ca. 1571–1605), a Huguenot, was appointed first physician to the king.[12] Critical of the many unlearned Paracelsists he had met on his travels throughout Europe, Ribit de la

[12] Hugh Trevor-Roper differentiated between Jean Ribit, sieur de la Rivière and Roch le Baillif, sieur de la Rivière in his "The Sieur de la Rivière, Paracelsian Physician of Henry IV" (1972), vol. 2, pp. 227–50.

Rivière nevertheless had a genuine interest in the new chemically prepared drugs, which seemed to offer much for the future of medicine.
Ribit's appointment was symptomatic of change in the new reign, so it is
not surprising to find him appointing chemists as royal physicians. The
two most prominent were Joseph Duchesne and Theodore Turquet de
Mayerne (1573–1655). We have already noted the long stay of Duchesne
in the Swiss cantons, and the case of Mayerne is similar.[13] Mayerne also
was of Huguenot stock; his parents had fled to Geneva after the St.
Bartholomew's Day massacre, and it was there that he was born. He
attended Heidelberg and then Montpellier, which was becoming a center for Paracelsian and chemical medicine. There he took his medical
degree in 1597 before moving to Paris where Ribit de la Riviere obtained
a post for him as médicine ordinaire to the king, as he had earlier done
for Duchesne. Mayerne proceeded to organize a series of lectures on
chemical medicine for surgeons and apothecaries (1599) and quickly
became widely known as one of the foremost proponents of the new
medicine.

It should be noted that the chemical physicians associated with the
court were developing into a formidable medical group. As Rio Howard
pointed out, the Parisian Medical Faculty had declined from seventy or
eighty physicians in the mid-sixteenth century to about forty in the
1590s.[14] It was not until forty years later that their numbers increased to
roughly one hundred, the size usually given for the seventeenth century. During this period of decline the number of court physicians increased.

Before the reign of Henry IV there were on average some fifteen to
twenty-five physicians for the king and another five to ten for the members of the royal family. With the accession of Henry of Navarre the post
of médecin ordinaire was established to assist the premier médecin.
These two physicians then arranged for the appointment of eight regular physicians, who served by quarter, plus fifteen consulting physicians for the king alone. This total of twenty-five for the king and ten or
more for the royal family is comparable to the number of physicians in
the Parisian Medical Faculty. If one takes into account the fact that the
premiers médecins of Henry IV and Louis XIII were interested in chemical medicine and sought to expand their own medical establishment,
we can see the basis for a serious clash, relating to both authority and
method.

The controversy was exacerbated by the changing tone of the chemists. With the exception of Gohory most of the chemical works published
in France prior to 1600 dealt primarily with the internal use of chemical

---

13 On Mayerne, see Thomas Gibson (1933). For his relationship to Ribit de la Rivière, see
    Trevor-Roper (1972). His connection with Hermetic philosophers is borne out in a
    paper by John H. Appleby (1979).
14 Rio Howard (1981).

preparations, and the anger of the Galenists was directed primarily at the compounds of metals and minerals.

Significantly, it was Joseph Duchesne who added a new dimension to the debate. His earlier works had for the most part dealt with the chemical aspects of medical practice though he had not hesitated to debate the origins of metals with Jacques Aubertus in 1575. But his interests were far-ranging and in 1587 he published his *Le Grand Miroir dv Monde*, a five-book poetical account of the universe that began with God and the Creation and proceeded to describe the three worlds: intellectual, celestial, and elementary. In this ambitious project he discussed the heavens, the stars, the angels, and the oceans, as well as the theory of sympathetic action. In the six-book second edition (1593), he promised in the preface another four books, the last of which would describe man, the microcosm in which "we see the various paths of the celestial stars in the movement of the breast and the vital parts" whereas "in the lower abdomen are the nutritional parts which belong to the elementary and corruptible world . . ."[15] Each book in verse was accompanied by an even longer prose commentary relating to the difficult passages for those not learned in "philosophie diuine & humaine."[16]

In the fifth book Duchesne discussed the elements, from which he eliminated fire at the start:

> Chasque corps a sa forme, & propre & naturelle:
> Mais le feu n'est doué d'une nature telle,
> Doncques il n'est pas corps: tout corps de soy reçoit
> Toute espece, qu'en luy estre engrauee on void
>
> . . . .
>
> Ainsi doncques le feu ne subsistant de soy,
> Perd nom de corps, par la categorique loy.[17]

In Genesis, Moses spoke only of two productive elements, water and earth. Duchesne agreed that air should not be given the name of element or principle.[18] Air, in fact, is nothing but "a sublimation of water."[19]

In addition to these two elements, there are in all things the three principles:

> De toute chose ainsi separer tu verras,
> Deschainant les liens qui nouënt la nature,
> Ceste actiue liqueur, qu'on appelle Mercure,
> Qui flamme ne conçoit: ce bel huile coulant,
> Qui de soulphre a le nom, d'autant qu'il est bruslant:
> Est ce sec agissant terre pure & luisante,
> Qu'on dit sel, côme vn sel fondât dans l'eau bouillante.[20]

15 Joseph Duchesne (1593), sig. ¶ viii^r.
16 Ibid., title page.
17 Ibid., p. 428. 18 Ibid., p. 429.
19 Ibid., p. 434. 20 Ibid., p. 433.

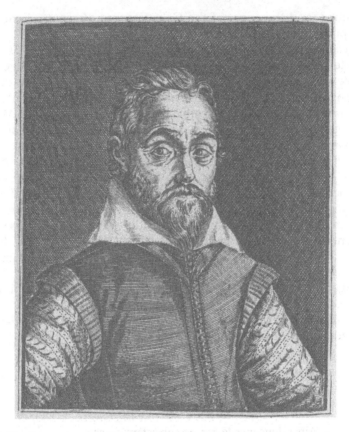

Joseph Duchesne (ca. 1544–1609). From his *Recueil des plus curieux et rares secrets* (1641). Courtesy of the Wellcome Institute Library, London.

In his notes on the elements Duchesne described chemistry as the true natural philosophy, a viewpoint that he ascribed to Theodore Zwinger: "I call chemists those who by virtue of the fire know how to separate heterogeneous or dissimilar bodies, and to join the homogeneous or similar ones."[21] Chemists are the men who could properly present the secrets of natural philosophy to the eyes of others. There are both natural and supernatural chemistries. The common chemists know neither the principles nor the causes of things . . . "they amuse themselves by making various fires, by amassing pots and bottles, by wasting their coals, and by making poor use of their time."[22] Those who merit the name "operateurs & artisans" extract oils and other substances from simples, and if they mix medicines, they are called empirics.

> Those who study how to reduce things to their causes and natural principles by the strength of their spirit and who discourse on the properties of

21 Ibid., p. 529.   22 Ibid., p. 532.

Nature are properly Physicians or Natural Philosophers: but because they use their hands, one may also properly call them mechanics and artisans.[23]

Duchesne's poetical account of the universe may not have been widely read among physicians, but in 1603 he published a new work, this time on theoretical medicine, the *De priscorum philosophorum verae medicinae materia*. Here was a strong plea for the superiority of chemical medicine from one of the royal physicians. It appeared at a time when both chemistry and the medical establishment surrounding the king seemed to threaten the Parisian Medical Faculty. Although Wightman ignored the political factors, he was quite right in his analysis, stating that "the point at issue was no longer metallic or any 'new' remedies, but whether or not the rising science of chemistry should be allowed to play any part in the ancient discipline of Medicine."[24] Although there had been almost continuous debate between the Parisian Medical Faculty and the chemists for forty years, Duchesne's work of 1603 sparked a new debate that was to continue into the third quarter of the seventeenth century and was to have an undercurrent of medical politics in addition to the question of theoretical orthodoxy.

The opinions of Duchesne that were so offensive to the members of the Parisian Medical Faculty were primarily expressed in the *Liber De priscorum philosophorum verae medicinae materia* of 1603 and the *Ad Veritatem Hermeticae medicinae ex Hippocratis veterumque decretis* of the following year.[25] Here was to be found a defense of chemistry, the new remedies, and a chemical interpretation of nature and medicine. As in his earliest works, Duchesne did not reject the ancients, only their modern disciples.

> If *Hypocrates* or *Galen* himselfe, were now againe aliue, they would exceedingly reioyce to see art so inlarged & augmented by so great and noble addition, and would patronize and upholde with their owne hands, that which was hidden from the old fathers in former ages: and reiecting many of those things, which before pleased them, yeelding to reason and experience, would gladly imbrace the new.[26]

Duchesne called the Galenists of his day dogmatists and contrasted them with the spagyrists. The dogmatists, he said, turn to Galen "and

---

[23] Ibid.

[24] W. P. D. Wightman (1962), vol. 1, p. 258.

[25] In addition to the original editions, the Latin editions of Duchesne (1613) and (1605) have been used. A French edition of the first title is Duchesne (1626). The English translation is by Thomas Tymme (or Timme) and should be used with the Latin since though it is substantial, it is incomplete.

General accounts of the Parisian debate can be found in A. G. Chevalier (1940); Lynn Thorndike (1959), vol. 6, pp. 238–53; Wightman (1962), vol. 1, pp. 257–63; and Pascal Pilpoul (1928), pp. 35–9.

[26] Duchesne (English, 1605), sig. B2v.

as if by a royal edict where the sentence is firm and without doubt, pronounce that contraries cure."[27] But the spagyric chemists place their faith in reason and experience rather than books. They seek the internal essence of bodies. "C'est icy le noeud de la matiere, l'occasion de la diuersité, & le fondement de toute spagyrie."[28]

Although Duchesne was no more a blind follower of Paracelsus in 1603 than he had been a quarter century earlier, it is clear that he approved of many concepts that were generally accepted by the Paracelsians. Like them he based his cosmology on the Creation story in Genesis in which God played the part of a divine alchemist.

> We holde by *Moses* doctrine that GOD in the beginning made of nothing a *Chaos*, or *Deepe*, or *Waters*, if wee please so to call it. From the which Chaos, Deepe, or waters, animated with the Spirits of God, God as the great workemaister and Creator, separated first of all *Light* from *Darknesse*, and this *Aetheriall Heauen*, which wee beholde, as a fifth Essence, or most pure Spirite, or most simple spirituall body. Then hee diuided Waters, from Waters; that is to say, the more subtill, Aiery, and Mercuriall liquor, from the more Thicke, Clammy, and Oyely, or Sulphurous liquor. After that, he extracted and brought forth the *Sulphur*, that is to say, the more grosse Waters, from the drye parte, which out of the separation standeth like salte, and as yet standeth by it selfe apart. . . . This was the worke of God, that hee might separate the Pure from the Impure: that is to say, that he might reduce the more pure and Ethereal Mercury, the more pure and inextinguible Sulphur, the more pure, and more fixed salte, into shyning and inextinguible Starres and Lights, into a Christalline and Dyamantine substance, or most simple Bodie, which is called *Heauen*, the highest, and fourth formall Element. . .[29]

Salt, sulfur, and mercury were for Duchesne the active elements. The traditional elements "haue only passiue qualities."[30] Fire is denied once again the status of element because "*Moses* in the first Chapt. of his *Genesis* . . . maketh no mention of Fier. . . And therefore we acknowledge no other Fier than Heauen, & the fiery Region which is so called of burning."[31] Here Duchesne was repeating what he had said in *Le Grand Miroir dv Monde* (1587) though both Paracelsus and Jerome Cardan had, still earlier, rejected fire as a true element.[32] As for air, Duchesne now accepted it as a third element even though it "cannot be separated by itselfe, but doth eyther vanish into ayre, or else remayneth mixed Sul-

---

[27] Duchesne (French, 1626), p. 4; (Latin, 1613), sig. A3r.

[28] Duchesne (French, 1626), p. 6; (Latin, 1613), sig. A3v. The following discussion of Duchesne is based largely on Debus (1965), pp. 90–6.

[29] Duchesne (English, 1605), sig. H1r; (Latin, 1605), p. 144.

[30] Duchesne (English, 1605), sig. G2v.

[31] Duchesne (English, 1605), sig. G3r; (Latin, 1605), p. 137.

[32] Jerome Cardan (1934), p. 15. See also Cardan (1580), pp. 45–6, and (1557), p. 21, chap. 2. John Woodall referred to the *Meteorem*, cap. 1, as evidence of Paracelsus's support of three rather than four elements (1617), pp. 309–10.

phur and Mercury. . ."[33] It would seem that air was required to make a ternary system: ". . . aier and earth, two extreames are fitlie ioyned together, by a thyrd, which is water, a meane between them both."[34]

As Duchesne spelled out in the *De priscorum philosophorum*, there are three active and three passive elements; but the three principles of the chemists are the true elements that must be understood by all natural philosophers. "There are three principall things mixed in euery Naturall bodie: to wit, *Salte, Sulphur,* and *Mercurie*. These are the beginnings of all Naturall things."[35] As in alchemical tradition, these three principles were not our modern laboratory reagents but were sophic substances "which neuerthelesse hath some conscience and agreement with comon Salt, Sulphur, and Mercurie."[36]

Constantly seeking triads, Duchesne compared the *tria prima* with body, soul, and spirit "for the body is attributed to salt: the spirit to Mercurie: and the soule to sulphur: eueryone to their apt and conuenient attribute."[37] These principles also had more recognizable attributes. Mercury "is a sharpe liquor, passable, and penetrable, and a most pure & *Aetheriall* substantiall body"; sulfur "is that moyst, sweet, oyly, clammy, original"; salt "is that dry body, saltish, meerly earththy, representing the nature of *Salt*."[38]

All three principles must be present in all things, and because he had used the Platonic argument of the mean to show the need for three of the Aristotelian elements, he turned to it again:

> For as a man can neuer make a good closing morter, of water and sand onely, without the mixture of lime, which bindeth the other two together like oile and glue: so Sulphur as the oily substance, is the mediator of Salt and Mercurie, and coupleth them both together: neither doth it onely couple them to death, but it also represse and contemperate the acrimonie of Salt, and the sharpnesse of Mercurie, which is found to bee very much therein.[39]

These three could be seen in the air: The winds give evidence of spiritous mercury and sulfur is the basis for comets and lightning, and salt is seen in the thunderbolt as the "stone of lightning." In the vegetable kingdom, mercury could be seen in leaves and fruits; sulfur in flowers, seeds, and kernels; and salt in wood, bark, and roots.[40] A similar breakdown could be found in the animal kingdom.[41] For those who sought

33 Duchesne (English, 1605), sig. G2^r.
34 Duchesne (English, 1605), sig. G3^r.
35 Duchesne (English, 1605), sig. B3^r.
36 Duchesne (English, 1605), sig. H3^v; (Latin, 1605), p. 150.
37 Duchesne (English, 1605), sig. P4^v; (Latin, 1613), p. 28.
38 Duchesne (English, 1605), sig. D1^v; (Latin, 1605), p. 131.
39 Duchesne (English, 1605), sig. T4^v; (Latin, 1613), p. 108.
40 Duchesne (English, 1605), sig. I3^v; (Latin, 1605), p. 166.
41 Duchesne (English, 1605), sig. K2^v; (Latin, 1605), pp. 172–3.

other guides, Duchesne noted that tastes are due to salt, "odours in Sulphur: colours out of both, most chiefely out of Mercurie: because Mercurie hath the volatile Salt of al things, ioyned unto it."[42]

Thomas Erastus had argued against the Paracelsian principles in his *Disputationes de medicina nova Paracelsi* (1572–4) from the standpoint of fire analysis, which he insisted (correctly) did not separate bodies into their elementary components as the chemists alleged. Duchesne, however, followed chemical tradition in insisting that chemists could correctly "anatomize" bodies with fire into salt, sulfur, and mercury. "And yet those naturall substances, are not said to be begotten, by such separations, as if they were not before: neyther yet as being before, are they corrupted by the arte of separation, but they were in compounde, and after separation, they ceased not to bee, and to subsist."[43]

As there were thought to be three principles upon which to base natural philosophy, so medicine must be based on three rather than four humors: chyle, blood (venous), and

> The third of the humours, is that which after sundry reterations of the circulations, made by the much vital heate of the heart, doth very farre exceede in perfection of concoction: the other two, which may be called the elimentary or nourishing humour of life, and radical Sulphur: the which is dispearced by the arteries throughout the whole body, and is turned into the whole substance thereof . . . .[44]

Duchesne suggested that because there was a continual circulation of the elements in the macrocosm,[45] there must also be circulation of the blood in man. However, his concept of a circulation of the blood was not the same as the circulation Harvey postulated a quarter century later. Duchesne, thinking as a chemist, had in mind the circulating currents evident in a heated liquid. In this case his overall view of blood flow remained essentially Galenic.[46]

Duchesne's medicine was dominated by his acceptance of the macrocosm–microcosm analogy and his search for chemical analogies. The distillations and condensations that he recognized in the atmosphere as the causes of rain were the same as those that caused catarrh in man. By analogy he reasoned that in the macrocosm the true source of wind,

---

42 Duchesne (English, 1605), sig. T3ᵛ and T4ʳ; (Latin, 1613), p. 106 (incorrectly numbered 116).
43 Duchesne (English, 1605), sig. G3ʳ.
44 Duchesne (English, 1605), sigs. Liʳ–Liᵛ; (Latin, 1605), p. 179.
45 Duchesne (English, 1605), sig. C4ʳ; (Latin, 1605), p. 128.
46 The concept of the circulation of the blood as a chemical distillation has been discussed in some detail in regard to the work of Cesalpino by Walter Pagel (1951) and (1967), pp. 169–209. For further details on this problem and the relation of Duchesne and Fludd, see Allen G. Debus (1961). In brief, with the exception of a reference that suggests that all of the blood circulates in the body as in a chemical pelican, Duchesne discusses in detail only the venous system. He states that the blood that is carried to the heart by

sleet, and snow is the condensation of mercurial vapors, which in man cause ringing in the ears, paralepsy, apoplexy, and similar illnesses.[47] In short, what we learn of one world must be applicable to the other.

Duchesne insisted that all those who accepted the Galenic dictum that contraries cure would "neuer easily finde out a remedie for sicknesse," and that, indeed that was not the true meaning of Hippocrates' words. Rather, like cures like and the best medicines are those prepared by chemical means.[48] The preparation of medicines was the main use of chemistry, not the transmutation of base metals to gold. Yet, even metallic perfection could be achieved by the operator; and he gave the directions presented by Paracelsus for the transmutation of lead to antimony.[49]

Duchesne insisted that he was not a Paracelsian. For him, chemical medicine was the true medicine of Galen and Hippocrates.[50] He affirmed that the principal object of his *De priscorum philosophorum* concerned the Galenic *materia medica*, and he sought primarily to embellish Galenic remedies with some chemical ornaments "plus beau, plus riche & plus vtile."[51] He wrote that Paracelsus should not be given full credit for this chemical philosophy because he was only one of many who had taught it over the centuries, going back to the greatest antiquity.[52] At the same time Duchesne was convinced that there were new diseases in the seventeenth century that had been unknown by the ancients, and new remedies were required for them. Because these new diseases were often localized, it was imperative that all true physicians be well traveled. In no other way could they learn of these current medical problems.[53]

If Duchesne did not consider himself a Paracelsian, others did, and the reaction of the Parisian Medical Faculty to his works was swift. The elder Jean Riolan (1539–1606), censor of the faculty, produced in 1603 an *Apologia pro Hippocratis et Galeni Medicina*. The ensuing debate is very

the vena cava is there circulated and distilled over in a purer form to the brain where it is redistilled or circulated a second time. In the Tymme translation (sig. K4v; Latin, 1605 pp. 177–78) Duchesne states that "the same blood being carried into the heart by the veyne called *Vena Caua*, which is as it were the Pellican of nature, or the vessel circulatory, is yet more subtilly concocted, and obtaineth the forces as it were of quintessence, or of a Sulphurus burning Aquavita, which is the original, which is the original of natural & unnatural heat. The same Aquauita being carried from hence by the arteries into the *Balneum Maris* of the Braine, is there exalted againe, in a wonderful maner by circulations: and is there changed into a spirit truly ethereal and heauenly, from whence the animal spirit procedeth, the chiefe instrument of the soule . . ."

47 Duchesne (French, 1626), pp. 183–4.
48 Duchesne (Latin, 1613), pp. 14–15; see also (English, 1605), sig. N4r.
49 Duchesne (English, 1605), sigs. I1v–I2r; (Latin, 1605), pp. 157–8.
50 Duchesne (French, 1626), pp. 104–5; (Latin, 1605), pp. 69–70.
51 Duchesne (French, 1626), pp. 8–9; (Latin, 1613), sig. A4v.
52 Duchesne (French, 1626), pp. 26–7; (Latin, 1613), pp. 4–8.
53 Joseph Duchesne (1618), pp. 151–4.

complex, and its chronology has best been described by Pascal Pilpoul, Lynn Thorndike, and W. P. D. Wightman.[54]

Duchesne was defended in print by his protégé and friend, Theodore Turquet de Mayerne, in an *Apologia. In qua videre est inviolatis Hippocratis & Galeni legibus, remedia Chymici preparata, tuto usurpare posse* (La Rochelle, 1603) in which he insisted that the use of chemically prepared remedies should not be considered an attack on the ancients. However, Mayerne had been spreading his views on chemistry in a series of lectures to young surgeons and apothecaries, and his defense of Duchesne was considered highly offensive by the members of the faculty. Jean Riolan's son, Jean Riolan the younger (1577–1657), answered in an *Ad Famosam Turqueti Apologiam Responsio* (Paris, 1603). In a decree against Mayerne, the Parisian Medical Faculty declared that he was

> unworthy of practising medicine because of his rashness, his impudence, and his ignorance of the true principles of medicine. [The Medical Faculty] urges all physicians who practise medicine wherever they may be to distance themselves from Turquet and to reject similar opinions.
>
> It exhorts them to remain faithful to the doctrine of Hippocrates and Galen. . . .

Those who did not adhere to this decree would be deprived of their university degrees and the privileges of the academy and would be expelled from the Order of the Doctors Regent.[55] Martin Akakia III, who had also studied at Montpellier, replied to the pamphlet by Riolan, as did Joseph Duchesne in his *Ad veritatem Medicinae hermeticae ex Hippocratis veterumque decretis stabiliendam* (1604).

Turquet left for England in 1606 and was incorporated M.D. at Oxford. He was to become physician to both King James and Queen Henrietta Maria as well as president of the Royal College of Physicians. There he became interested in the long-delayed pharmacopoeia of the college. He pressed for its publication (1618) and was largely responsible for the inclusion of chemical preparations in the volume. As I have shown elsewhere, the acceptance of chemical remedies was accomplished with far less debate in England than in France.[56]

To return to the French scene, Duchesne turned to others for support. Israel Harvet published a *Defensio Chymiae* against the *Apologia* of Riolan the elder, to which were added notes by Guillaume Baucinet (Paris, 1604). In this he asked why it should be that the school at Paris was the only one in the world that still neglected and condemned the art of chemistry? By doing so they condemned many of the most prominent physicians of their age: Sylvius, Fernel, Andernach, Crato, Schegkius,

[54] Pilpoul (1928), passim; Thorndike (1941), vol. 6, pp. 238–53; Wightman (1962), vol. 1, pp. 256–63.

[55] Pilpoul (1928), p. 36.

[56] Here see Debus (1965).

Mattioli, Gesner, and Zwinger.[57] Even though Erastus had attacked Paracelsus, he had not rejected all aspects of the use of chemistry in medicine.[58] Harvet went on to defend the use of chemical salts, citing passages from Hippocrates and Galen in favor of cure by similitude.[59] Riolan the younger replied to Harvet as "Joannes Antarvetus" in an *Apologia, pro iudicio Scholae Parisiensis de Alchimia. Ad Harveti & Baucyneti recoctam crambem* (Paris, 1604), in which he made the point that the school at Paris did not repudiate all chemical preparations,[60] only those of chemists who claim to separate pure essences from noxious poisons but discard the valuable medicinal substances and prescribe the poisons.[61]

A persistent problem for the medical faculty was Petrus Palmarius (Pierre Paulmier) (1568–1610), a Parisian physician and a member of the faculty who wrote in support of the faculty while advocating the use of chemical medicines. As early as 1591 he had been censured for proposing to give a course on spagyric chemistry to apothecaries,[62] and in August 1603 an arrêt was issued against him. Six years later he published his *Lapis philosophicus Dogmaticorum*, in which he wrote of the superiority of the ancient medical authors and their modern supporters and at the same time defended the use of chemically prepared drugs, insisting even that antimony could be used internally for very difficult cases. Predictably Paulmier was condemned by the faculty. He was banned from the faculty and ordered not to be reinstated for at least two years, and then only after asking pardon for his offenses.[63] He defended himself in a short reply.

This controversy continued until the death of Duchesne in 1609. Jean Riolan the elder died in 1606, but his son and other members of the faculty answered every tract printed in favor of chemical medicine.

In 1605 Jean Riolan the younger published three works supporting the position of the faculty, and the debate soon spread beyond French borders. Editions of the chief tracts appeared in Germany, and an English translation of key sections of Duchesne's *De priscorum philosophorum* and *Ad vertitatem hermeticae medicinae* was made by Thomas Tymme in 1605. Perhaps any debate so important to one of the most famous medical schools of Europe was bound to attract widespread attention. In any case, when Andreas Libavius revised his well-known *Alchymia* (1597) for

---

[57] Israel Harvet (1604), p. 1.
[58] Ibid., p. 4.
[59] Ibid., pp. 38–45.
[60] Ioannis Antarveti (1604), p. 6.
[61] Ibid., p. 22.
[62] Pilpoul (1928), p. 35.
[63] Ibid., p. 38. L. W. B. Brockliss [(1978), 242] notes that his censure was not as severe as it might have been because he renounced the theories of the chemists and argued only that some distilled remedies were superior to the traditional ones.

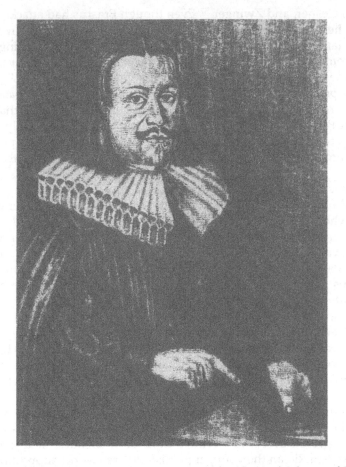

Andreas Libavius (1540–1616) by Fennitzer in the National Library of Vienna. From a photograph. Copyright: National Library of Vienna.

publication in 1606, he also wrote a *Defensio alchemiae et refutatio objectionum ex censura Scholae Parisiensis.* Both here and in his lengthy *Alchymia triumphans,* published the following year, Libavius discussed the history of the Parisian debate in great detail.

By this time Libavius was established as an authority on chemistry and medicine.[64] Born at Halle in 1540, he had taken his medical degree at Jena where he was appointed professor of history and poetry (1586–91). Later he served as the town physician in Rothemburg, involving himself in numerous debates. In many ways he was a defender of tradi-

[64] On Libavius I follow my earlier account: Debus (1977), vol. 1, pp. 168–73. In addition see Wightman (1962), vol. 1, pp. 259–63; Partington (1962), vol. 2, pp. 244–67; Thorndike (1923–58), vol. 6, pp. 238–53; and Owen Hannaway (1975), pp. 75–151. See also Allen G. Debus (1971), 185–99, and (1972), vol. 1, pp. 151–65.

tion, and in the conflict over logic he defended the Aristotelians against the Ramists. His position in respect to chemistry was more complex. He objected strongly to the introduction of mysticism and occultism into the sciences and medicine. In his later years he was one of the most vocal opponents of the Rosicrucian tracts; but as early as 1594, in his *Neoparacelsica,* he wrote against the Paracelsian system of nature. Still, Libavius was a strong advocate of chemistry, not only for the preparation of chemical medicine but also for the transmutation of base metals to gold. Both goals seemed to him to be legitimate for the practical chemist.

For Libavius, alchemy (or chemistry) was a divine art, but was known imperfectly because of authors who purposely misled their readers.[65] He defined alchemy as the perfection of magisteries and the extraction of pure essences from mixed substances by separation.[66]

Libavius had a special interest in the application of transmutation to medicine. In reviewing the Parisian debate he took the side of Duchesne. Like him, he discussed the various medical sects, which for him were the Galenists, the chemiatri, and the Paracelsians.[67] The Paracelsians were to be rejected. Their works were founded on paradoxes, absurdities, and madness; and they themselves were infected by the magic they found in their master's *Philosophia sagax,* which was filled with necromancy and the search for power by summoning of evil spirits.[68] If this was not bad enough, information gathered in this fashion had become the basis for a system of terrestrial and celestial phenomena. But their work could be easily dismissed as worthless because of their insistence on the truth of the macrocosm–microcosm analogy. It was not true that all the things of the great world were also found in man; indeed, there could be no mixture of the great and small worlds.[69] To be sure, he added, Paracelsus had described the three principles that were essential for any chemist, but he had taken these from Aristotle.[70]

As for the Galenists, they were not as bad as they had often been described by the chemists.[71] Their works remained the basis of medicine, and many of them judged the works of Galen open-mindedly rather than insisting that Galen's pronouncements be followed to the letter in every case.

Libavius divided the iatrochemists, who were of more interest to him, into two groups. The first group was comprised of those authors who

---

65 Andreas Libavius (1606), sig. A2ʳ.
66 Ibid., sig. B5ʳ. "Alchemia est ars perficiendi magisteria, & essentias puras è mistis separato corpore, extrahendi."
67 Libavius, *Commentariorum Alchymiae,* signs. Aa2ᵛ–Aa5ᵛ.
68 Ibid., sigs. Aa2ᵛ–Aa3ʳ.
69 Ibid., sig. Aa3ᵛ.
70 Libavius (1606), p. 109.
71 Libavius, *Commentariorum alchymiae,* sig. Aa2ᵛ.

argued for the traditional theoretical medicine of the ancients with the addition of whatever was to be found of use in the armory of chemically prepared medicines. Among these authors he recommended Avicenna, Mesue, Rhazes, Albertus Magnus, Arnald of Villanova, Raymond Lull, and Philip Ulstadius. These men confined themselves to directions for the preparation of medicines and had not meddled with chemical cosmology or mystical descriptions of the macrocosm and the microcosm. His second group, the Hermetic physicians, were those authors who searched for catholic principles and wrote at length of an all-encompassing universe based on the macrocosm and the microcosm. They claimed to be the only true chemical physicians whereas in reality, Libavius said, they are but sophists who pay lip service to Hippocrates as they distort everything with their chemical explanations. No matter what they might say, these authors are among the greatest enemies of the Galenists.[72]

Considering himself one of the rational iatrochemists, Libavius said that the Parisian Medical Faculty had rightly condemned the Paracelsians and the Hermetic physicians but that they had gone beyond reason in their attack on Joseph Duchesne and Turquet de Mayerne. Indeed, he felt the faculty had wrongly attacked the use of chemistry in medicine.[73] The benefits of this subject for the physician were too well known to be denied. There is no doubt that Libavius wanted to enlist the benefits of chemistry in the support of medical knowledge while maintaining the firm basis of ancient medical theory.

In his final antichemical blast, the elder Riolan penned an *Ad Libavi Maniam* (1606) accusing Libavius of inconsistency in accepting both chemical medicine and the ancients. He suggested that alchemy might be diabolic in origin[74] and added that because it was an art with much that was bad and little good, it might well be rejected.[75]

In 1610 Thomas Sonnet, sieur de Courval and doctor of medicine, upheld the view of the Parisian Medical Faculty in a work against medical charlatans, specifically referring to chemists and Paracelsists in his title. Although he did not believe that antimony was useless in all cases, Sonnet agreed with Grévin that it was a very dangerous poison.[76]

The empirics, Sonnet felt, were a dangerous lot. Among them were the alchemists and the distillers,[77] but the principal empiric authors were the Paracelsists. Paracelsus had denied the existence of God and

[72] Ibid.
[73] Ibid., sig. Aa4r.
[74] Jean Riolan (1606), p. 24. The possible relationship of alchemy to witchcraft and black magic was frequently discussed in the early modern period. As an example see Martin Antoine Del Rio (1599) and Reginald Scot (1584).
[75] Riolan (1606), p. 26.
[76] Thomas Sonnet (1610), pp. 138–9. This work has recently been discussed by Alison Klairmont Lingo (1985/86).
[77] Sonnet (1610), p. 178.

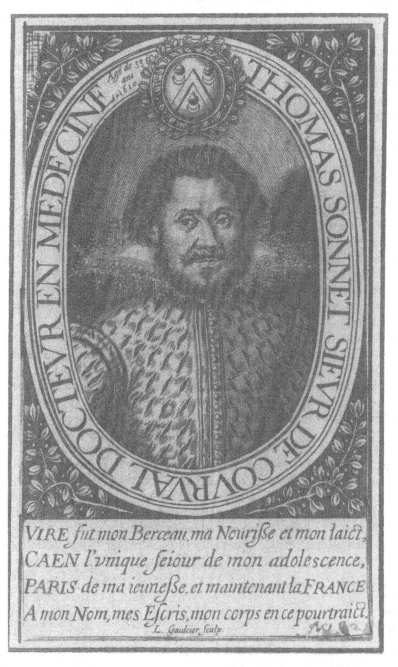

Thomas Sonnet, sieur de Courval (1577–1627). Courtesy of the National Library of Medicine, Bethesda.

had introduced many errors, blasphemies, and absurdities into theology, medicine, and philosophy,[78] such as horrendous suggestions that
a man could be made in a glass cucurbit from human sperm, a "passage
more impious, villainous, and detestable has never been written nor
pronounced by an author."[79] And could it really be believed that Solomon and St. John in the *Apocalypse* had metaphorically described and
set forth all the secrets of alchemy, that God was the first alchemist, or
that Tubal Cain was an alchemist because he fashioned iron and brass?[80]
Men who believe such ideas should be destroyed; they should be
smoked out of their dens like foxes or "boiled with their distilled oils and
alembics, as one prepares cabbages in Dauphiné . . ."[81]

Regardless of the distaste of Sonnet and the opposition of the Parisian
Medical Faculty, chemists continued to promote all aspects of their art.
Gabriel de Castaigne, almoner to the king, wrote a work on chemical
medicines (1611, 1615) that included an alchemical text by Jean Saunier
from the early fifteenth century, letters from Alexandre de la Tourette
dated 1579,[82] and a defense of potable gold. In 1613 Godfrey Roussel
wrote on the secrets of pharmacy and distillation, "vulgairement nommé
Alchemie ou Spargerie." This work again promoted potable gold as a
universal cure.[83]

Perhaps more practical was Jacques Pascal, master apothecary of
Beziers, who compared chemical pharmacy with that of the Galenists
(1616). He discussed his examination of the substances he had found in
other pharmacists' shops. These had been filthy and impure.[84] Accordingly, he denounced his competitors and praised chemistry as the proper method of preparation because, he said, chemical medicines are separated from their terrestrial and excrementitious parts by a very exact
method of preparation, which render them spiritous in nature.[85] Chemical methods permit the use of small quantities of medicines, which
cause no trouble to the patient.[86] Pascal noted that the use of heat in
distillation separated bodies into their principles "or pure substances
which are sulphur, salt and mercury: that is to say, to oil, salt and
water."[87] Pascal's work was approved by de Ranchine, professor of medicine and chancellor of the University of Montpellier,[88] but Pascal was

[78] Ibid., pp. 184–5.
[79] Ibid., p. 185.
[80] Ibid., pp. 231–2.
[81] Ibid., p. 239.
[82] Gabriel de Castaigne (1661), pp. 83–5.
[83] Discussed in Lynn Thorndike (1958), vol. 7, p. 166.
[84] Jacques Pascal (1616), sigs. ã 2 – ã 3.
[85] Ibid., p. 7.
[86] Ibid.
[87] Ibid., p. 124.
[88] Ibid., sig. ē 1ᵛ.

well aware that the acceptance of chemistry by Galenic pharmacists would be a slow and difficult process. He wrote that many physicians feared that if the chemical art were introduced as he felt was necessary, it would prove prejudicial to the traditional practice of medicine because it would be a blow to the common pharmacy from which they took their remedies.[89]

Although Pascal was protected by the chancellor of the University of Montpellier, other practitioners were not. Pierre Reneaulme, a physician of Blois, was attacked by the Parisian Medical Faculty for having used chemical drugs, even antimony, and then forced to recant and to promise in the future to use only those traditional drugs approved by the faculty (1609).[90] Six years later the Gardes Apothecaries de Provins requested that action be taken against those pharmacists who persisted in selling antimony and other chemical drugs. A new decree was forthcoming (18 October 1615) forbidding the sale of chemical medicines.[91]

The chemical philosophy and the new philosophy

Although the Paracelsian chemical philosophy was well known to present a chemical interpretation of the universe that was opposed to Galenic medicine and to Aristotelian philosophy, the debate in France until about 1625 centered on medical and pharmaceutical problems, particularly the medicines derived by chemical means from metals and minerals. The broader cosmological problems became a matter of greater concern in ensuing years.

Joseph Duchesne's philosophical work, *De priscorum philosophorum verae medicinae materia*, was translated into French as the *Traictè de la matiere, preparation et excellente vertu de la medecine balsamique des anciens philosophes* in 1626. This work went far beyond medicine in its assumption that chemistry was the basis of all natural philosophy. Only two years before, the *Basilica Chymica* of Oswald Crollius (1560–1609) had been translated as *La royale chymie* by I. Marcel of Boulene. This translation was reprinted in 1627, 1633, and 1634. Here was to be found Croll's lengthy Admonitory Preface, ostensibly an introduction to the *Basilica* itself (which was a chemical formulary) but was in fact a discussion of the Paracelsian chemical interpretation of the macrocosm and the micro-

---

[89] Ibid., p. 122.
[90] Pilpoul (1928), p. 37.
[91] Ibid., pp. 38–9. The text of the document is presented here (39):
Censuit unanimi omnium consensu, ista medicamenta chymica damnanda, Pharmacopoeis et aliis omnibus interdicenda. Itaque idem collegium omnes judices precatur, ut in conseruere animadvertant qui ejusmodi medicamenta proescribent, administrabunt et voenalici exhibebunt.

cosm. The Admonitory Preface remains today perhaps the best introduction to the chemical philosophy of nature penned in that period.

The Rosicrucian texts added further interest to a chemically oriented
medicine. Published first in 1614 and 1615, the *Fama fraternitatis* and the
Confessio called for a new Christian learning to replace the works of the
ancients.[92] The unknown author took it for granted that everyone
agreed that the basis of natural philosophy was medicine, a godly art.
The Rosicrucian Order had been supposedly founded by Christian Rosenkreutz, who was said to have lived in the fifteenth century. He had
learned great truths in the Near East in the course of an interrupted
pilgrimage to Jerusalem. He had described these secrets in his great
book *M*, which was available to the Rosicrucian brotherhood, who made
it – along with Holy Scripture and nature – the basis of their studies.
The brotherhood acknowledged that Europe had many learned authors,
but they mentioned only Paracelsus, whose works were in their hidden
vaults alongside the Bible and the work of their founder.[93]

How wonderful it would be, the author of the *Fama* added, if the true
scholars of Europe united for the benefit of mankind. This could be done
if all those who wanted to join in this reformation of learning would
publish their intent to join the Rosicrucian brotherhood.[94] No true scholar would be ignored because both the *Fama* and the *Confessio* were to be
published in five languages. Those who were approved for membership
would be contacted.

In fact, nine editions of these works were published in four languages
between 1614 and 1617, and an English translation appeared in 1652. In
less than ten years several hundred books and tracts debated the merits
of the Rosicrucian "Manifesto."[95] It is difficult today to understand why
this appeal should have attracted such attention, but it did. In his own
utopian work, the *Christianopolis* (1619), Johann Valentin Andreae (1587–
1654) commented:

> What a confusion among men followed the report of this thing, what a
> conflict among the learned, what an unrest and commotion of impostors
> and swindlers, it is needless to say. There is just one thing which we
> would like to add, that there were some who in this blind terror wished to
> have their old, and out-of-date, and falsified affairs entirely retained and
> defended with force. Some hastened to surrender the strength of their
> opinions, and after they had made accusation against the severest yoke of
> their servitude, hastened to reach out after freedom.[96]

Of special interest is the fact that in 1623 Paris was visited by men who
announced themselves to be members of the Rosicrucian brotherhood

[92] [Rosicrucians] (1652), pp. 1–2.
[93] Ibid. pp. 36, 5, 10.
[94] Ibid., p. 31.
[95] A listing of the early Rosicrucian texts is to be found in F. Leigh Gardner (1923).
[96] Johann Valentin Andreae (1916), pp. 127–38.

and who promised to show all of their secrets to those who wanted to be initiated. Placards were posted at the Louvre and elsewhere:

> We being deputies of the principal College of the Brothers of the Rose Cross, are making a visible and invisible stay in this city through the Grace of the Most High, towards whom turn the hearts of the Just. We show and teach without books or marks how to speak all languages of the countries where we wish to be, and to draw men from error and death.[97]

Incensed by this act, young Gabriel Naudé (1600–1653), a medical student, wrote in fifteen days his *Instrvction a la France svr la Verité de l'Histoire des Freres de la Rose-Croix* (1623), in which he castigated the French for their willingness to embrace new and often ridiculous opinions. From his point of view the Rosicrucian texts were more absurd than any he had seen – and indeed, they seemed to him to have grown out of the pernicious heresies of Paracelsus.[98] Yet, no matter how heretical and arrogant Paracelsus might have been, Naudé was anxious to rescue him and others from the charge of necromancy. True, Paracelsus had claimed the power

> to ripen fruits in an instant; to make one horse travell further in a day, then another shall in a month . . . in a word, to do whatever seems, and ever hath been thought impossible. But I extreamly wonder since he pretended to the absolute knowledge of all those kinds of Magick, why he never did anything by the assistance of them. . . . Though therefore he might justly be condemn'd as an Archheretick for the depravednesse of his opinion in point of Religion, yet do I not think he should be charg'd with Magick. For this consists not in the *Speculations* and *Theory:* which every one may explicate according to this fantasie, but in the practice of the *Circle* and *Invocations* . . .[99]

It is interesting to note that René Descartes (1596–1650) returned to Paris in 1623 after years of travel and service in the mercenary armies of Europe. He, too, was aware of the Rosicrucian tracts, and his friends thought that he had become a member of the secret order.[100] This charge was made frequently until the end of the century.

Although we are accustomed to think of Descartes primarily in terms of the mechanical philosophy, his work also reflects important aspects of other Renaissance philosophies. Like the Paracelsians, Descartes was thoroughly disappointed by the traditional learning of the schools. He had studied literature, languages, rhetoric, mathematics, theology, phi-

---

[97] Gabriel Naudé (1623), p. 27. I have used here the translation of Frances A. Yates (1972), p. 10.
[98] Naudé (1623), p. 42.
[99] Gabriel Naudé (1657), pp. 187–8, and (1659), pp. 268–88. It is interesting to note that Naudé was trained as a physician and that he was a friend of the arch-Galenist, Gui Patin. In 1628 Naudé wrote a defense of the medical school in Paris [De antiquitate & dignitate Scholae medicae Parisiensis]. See Jack A. Clarke (1970), pp. 10–12.
[100] Here I follow William R. Shea (1979), 29–47 (32–3).

losophy, and all the other sciences, but he had found no certainty in any
of them. After his years of study and meditation he had come to the
conclusion that "as far as all the opinions I had accepted were concerned, I could do no better than undertake once and for all to be rid of
them in order to replace them afterwards either by better ones, or even
by the same, once I had adjusted them by the plumb-line of reason."[101]
His doubts vanished when he realized that he could begin to reestablish
certainty by accepting only a belief in himself and in God. Impressed by
mathematical proofs he sought a system that would be as sure in the
world as mathematics was within its own realm. His hope was to de-
duce the true system of the universe much as a geometrician developed
his propositions and theorems. This is the Descartes we usually think of,
a philosopher seeking a mathematical and mechanical interpretation of
natural phenomena.

But there is evidence that Descartes knew the mystical texts of his age
as well. In his *Discourse on Method* (1637) he wrote that as a student he
"had gone through all the books I could lay my hands on dealing with
the occult and rare sciences."[102] He felt that he knew their true worth so
that he would not be "misled either by the promises of an alchemist or
the predictions of an astrologer, the impostures of a magician, or the
tricks or boasts of any of those who profess to know more than they
do."[103]

But Descartes' dissociation from the occult may not have been as
sharply defined as he would have had his readers believe. William Shea
has recently reexamined the seventeenth-century evidence relating to
the vision that Descartes had had of a new science. While stationed as a
soldier in Germany in 1619, Descartes wrote in his notebooks of universal harmonies in a fashion more attuned to Hermetic thought than to
mechanical philosophy. These notebooks also attest to his interest in the
prolongation of life, in sympathetic action, and in the importance of
medicine.

Additional evidence of Descartes's discovery of his new method while
in winter quarters in Germany was found in manuscripts seen by Leibniz in 1675.[104] Descartes described a revelation that occurred on the
night of November 10–11, 1619 "which he imagined could only have
come from on high." In a first dream he was frightened by ghosts and a
high wind, which prevented him from going where he wanted to go. He
awoke in fear, confessed to God, and then fell asleep again. A second
dream ended with a piercing noise, and he awoke again only to see a
large number of fiery sparks all around him in the room. In a third

101 René Descartes (1968), p. 37.
102 Ibid., p. 29.
103 Ibid., p. 32–3.
104 Shea (1979), p. 43–4.

dream he saw two books before him: a dictionary, which he interpreted as the sciences gathered together, and a collection of poems, which he judged to be the "union of philosophy and wisdom." A poem was handed to him, and he saw that it was the "Est et Non" of Pythagoras, meaning truth and error in human knowledge and the profane sciences. He took the clap of thunder that he heard to be "the signal of the Spirit of Truth descending on him to take possession of him." A dream sequence of this sort is far removed from the more sober attitude we might wish for in a philosopher like Descartes; rather, it is similar to the alchemical dreams that were common from late antiquity to the seventeenth century.

In his article Shea notes that the young Descartes can be contrasted with the mature scholar who authored the *Discourse on Method*. But this is true only in part. If we go beyond the famous "Cogito, ergo sum" and turn to the less commonly read fifth and sixth books of the *Discourse*, we find material that is not often discussed by philosophers. Descartes's interest in the creation of the universe by God working on the initial chaos[105] is reminiscent of Paracelsus. The sixth book contains evidence that for Descartes his method would go far beyond theory; here we find that the goal of science is to present a practical philosophy not far removed from the similar goals of Francis Bacon, and the natural magicians.[106]

Most surprising is the fact that the ultimate goal of Cartesian practical philosophy was not to elucidate physical problems at all; rather, the aim of science is

> . . . principally for the preservation of health, which is undoubtedly the first good, and the foundation of all the other goods of this life; . . . if it is possible to find some other means of rendering men as a whole wiser and more dexterous than they have been hitherto, I believe it must be sought in medicine.[107]

But Descartes viewed the medicine of his day as a defective science even though it was a noble one. To improve medicine then, no less than for the Paracelsians, was to be his goal in life.

> . . . I will say simply that I have resolved to devote the time I have left to me to live to no other occupation than that of trying to acquire some knowledge of Nature, which may be such as to enable us to deduce from it rules in medicine which are more assured than those we have had up to now; . . .[108]

[105] Descartes (1968), pp. 62–4.
[106] Ibid., p. 78.
[107] Ibid.
[108] Ibid., p. 91.

It is interesting to see that in 1651 the French translator of D'Espagnet's alchemical *Enchiridion Physicae Restitutae* (1608) discussed recent
mystical contributions to a revised natural philosophy. Referring first to
Francis Bacon, Robert Fludd, and the German authors Gorleus and Tau-
rellus, he wrote that France had produced Peter Ramus, Jean D'Espagnet, and – René Descartes. He thought that one could rightly place a
high value on Descartes' philosophy, which is "both inventive, subtile,
and filled with truth." Yet, recognizing the value of his work, he continued, "we do not detract from the work of D'Espagnet who was the
first in France to attempt to restore the true philosophy of the ancients."[109] This mid-century evaluation of the contributions of D'Espagnet and Descartes as comparable in value may seem odd today, but
again it points to the different standards of that period.

Numerous alchemical classics were translated into French in the early
decades of the seventeenth century. In 1624 the *Twelve Keys of Philosophy*
by Basil Valentine appeared in French, and other titles by this author
were published in succeeding years. On 23 August 1624, fourteen alchemical theses were posted in Paris.[110] Among them were rejections of
both the four elements and the three principles, in place of which was
postulated a five-element–principle system: earth, water, salt, sulfur,
and oil (or mercury or acid spirit). The sublunary world was affirmed to
be composed only of earth and water because, it was said, air does not
differ from water and fire cannot be distinguished from the empyrean
heaven. Transmutation among the elements and principles was denied,
and Aristotle was faulted on many points, among them his rejection of
atoms. Understandably, Aristotelian philosophy was attacked but so
were the Paracelsian chemical philosophers.

The defense of the theses was scheduled for the following day, at the
house of François de Soucy, formerly the hôtel of Queen Marguerite. A
thousand people assembled for the event.[111] Jean Bitault was named the
defender; Anthoine Villon, known as the soldier-philosopher, was
named as judge and moderator; and the chemical physician Etienne de
Clave was to serve as president. However, the meeting did not proceed
because all three participants were arrested before it began. Their case
was heard by a Court of Request on August 28 and by September 6 the
doctors of the Sorbonne had officially condemned the theses. Not long
after this Jean-Baptiste Morin published his *Refvtation des Theses* in which

109 D'Espagnet (French, 1651), isg. ē ii ʳ.
110 This episode is discussed at length by the editor in Mersenne, *Correspondence*, vol. 1
     (1945), pp. 167–8. These theses are described by Mersenne in *La verite de sciences.
     Contre les septiques ou Pyrrhoniens* (1625), reprinted (1969), pp. 79–80. The theses are
     also found in Jean Baptiste Morin (1624), pp. 11–17. Useful for an account of the
     meeting and the proceedings against Bitault, Villon, and de Claves is the account in
     Mercure Française (1625), pp. 503–12.
111 Ibid., p. 504.

he condemned Villon and de la Claves as atheists who had forged a "new Philosophy."[112] Their rashness had been stopped only by an arrêt of parlement.

The main figures of this Hermetic conference were no more silenced by this action of the parlement than the earlier chemists had been. François de Soucy was shortly to write a *Sommaire de la Medecine Chymique* (1632) in which he promised to present clearly those subjects of which others had written obscurely. Although he devoted some space to the theoretical basis of the three principles, the bulk of his book was devoted to practical chemical recipes.[113]

De Clave prepared one of the more popular chemical textbooks, the *Cours de chimie* (1646), but he also wrote a *Novvelle Lvmiere Philosophique des Vrais Principles et Elemens de Nature* (1641), in which he rejected the element theories of both Aristotle and Paracelsus.[114] De Clave thought there was little point in refuting Aristotle unless something better could be offered. To be sure, the four elements were unsatisfactory because neither air nor fire was a true element.[115] Moreover, the Aristotelians had ignored the true chemical anatomy and resolution of the chemists, which was essential for determining the true elements. In fact, he said, element theory was chaotic: The Aristotelians spoke of four elements, the Paracelsians of three principles, and others of an almost infinite number. Some chemists accepted the three principles plus the elements water and earth, but water and earth were excremental, not pure, simple, and harmonious, and therefore could not be included.[116] Although de Clave spoke of the need for chemical analysis, he remained closely restricted to logical arguments and to the commentaries on Aristotle prepared at the University of Coimbra in Portugal.[117] In the end he defined an element as "a simple body which enters into the mixture of composite bodies and to which they can finally be resolved."[118]

The condemnation of alchemy by the Parlement of Paris showed clearly that chemistry was seen as a threat to natural philosophy as a whole, not just to the medical establishment.

Concerned by what appeared to be an increasing interest in Rosicrucian and alchemical mysticism, Marin Mersenne (1588–1648) examined both subjects in his *Quaestiones celeberrimae Genesim* (1623) and his *La verite des sciences* (1625). He had followed closely the increasing tide of French publications on alchemy as well as the Du Soucy conference and

---

[112] Morin (1624), p. 4.
[113] François Du Soucy (1632).
[114] Estienne de Clave (1641), sig. Aii^v.
[115] Ibid., pp. 143–4.
[116] Ibid., pp. 144–7.
[117] References to the Coimbra commentaries are frequent and run throughout de Clave's volume.
[118] Ibid., p. 260.

the resultant condemnation of the alchemical theses. During these years Mersenne also became aware of the folio volumes of Robert Fludd (1574–1637)[119] who sought to replace the Aristotelian world view with his own alchemical vision of a macrocosm–microcosm universe.

We would expect the work of Mersenne – who was a friend and correspondent of Descartes, Gassendi, and most of the savants of his day whom we could classify among the early mechanists – to emphasize mathematics as a key to understanding natural phenomena. Indeed, most of *La verite des sciences* is a description of this subject. He asked how one could understand Holy Scripture or even Plato or Aristotle without it? Without mathematics one could not properly interpret any branch of knowledge; indeed, it was as essential to the investigation of medicine as it was for astronomy.[120] Even Paracelsus (in the *De ente astrorum*) accepted this, continued Mersenne, and surely chemists required a mathematical understanding of the proportion of saltpeter in excrement, of sal ammoniac in bone, and of salt, sulfur, and mercury in all things that exist.[121] For Mersenne these subjects were all basically mathematical.

In this lengthy work of over a thousand pages Mersenne began with a two-hundred page attack on the alchemists in which he discussed his views in dialogue form among an alchemist, a skeptic, and a Christian philosopher. At the outset the alchemist argued that

> We can take pride in the fact that there is no science as certain as ours because it teaches by experience which is the mother, the source and the universal cause of all knowledge: and it is for the lack of this that Aristotle and the other philosophers have wondrously failed in their philosophy. . .[122]

The skeptic found nothing certain in the sciences,[123] and for him this was no less true in mathematics and astronomy than it was in chemistry and Paracelsism. The alchemist replied that the chemical operations in the laboratory and the equipment needed for the art made this subject the basis of knowledge: "there is nothing but truth in all the operations of chemistry: because you see all that which enters there is true, palpable and real."[124] For the Christian philosopher the words of the alchemist were unconvincing[125]; even the chemists' principles could not

---

[119] On Fludd, see Allen G. Debus (1977), vol. 1, pp. 205–93.
[120] Mersenne (1969), 233–5, 242–3, 525. The standard study of the scientific work of Mersenne, and surely one of the most important works on seventeenth-century French science, is still Robert Lenoble's *Mersenne ou la naissance de mecanisme* (1971).
[121] Mersenne (1969), p. 566.
[122] Ibid., pp. 1–2.
[123] Ibid., pp. 29ff.
[124] Ibid., p. 41.
[125] Ibid., p. 56.

be confirmed, and salt, sulfur, and mercury were not the first principles because they could be resolved into two bodies: water and earth.

Mersenne's rejection of the views of the alchemist was mild but firm. For the Christian philosopher the recent condemnation by the Sorbonne was a just one because these doctors had rightly questioned the theological implications of the alchemical theses.[126] The Christian philosopher was especially alarmed by the alchemical revival of atomism.[127] The alchemists' vaunted "observationally" based system of elements and principles ran the risk of being ruled out of consideration should salt, sulfur, or mercury be decomposed into other substances.[128] Then they could not possibly be considered elemental.

Mersenne's Christian philosopher was willing to admit that alchemy offered much of value, but the secret tradition must be abandoned. There should be an academy for alchemy in every kingdom, or even in every province, to improve the health of man through the development of medicines as well as to police the field by seeking out and punishing charlatans. Alchemical language should be reformed to eliminate strange and enigmatic terms such as "Christian-cabalistique," "Divino magique," and "Physico-chymique" and replace them with words "that signify clearly the operations of Alchemy in the way that the terms in Philosophy signify those things that we have in the spirit."[129]

Mersenne's reformed alchemy would steer clear of religious, philosophical, and theological questions, which were of absolutely no concern to it.[130] He noted that there were some people for whom the subject served as a counter-church and who argued that the most ancient theology, magic, and pagan fables were best explained by the science. Many, indeed, held to the chemical interpretation of the Creation. These dreams and speculations must be rejected if alchemy was to gain the approval of the Catholic Church. Mersenne's alchemist was at last won over:

> I promise to follow your advice because I know that true Spagyry has no need of being explained by Sacred Scripture or by fables: and that which we do is to give luster to our science, and to put a stop to the scorn of the ignorant . . .[131]

Mersenne's views of a reformed alchemy stripped of religious overtones and mystical analogies was anathema to Hermetic philosophers such as Robert Fludd, whose work on the macrocosm and the microcosm initiated a long exchange of philosophical tracts and volumes be-

[126] Ibid., pp. 82–3.
[127] Ibid., p. 81.
[128] Ibid., p. 56.
[129] Ibid., p. 107.
[130] Ibid., p. 107.
[131] Ibid., p. 119.

tween Fludd and Johannes Kepler, then with Mersenne, and finally with Mersenne's friend Pierre Gassendi.[132] Kepler, Mersenne, and Gassendi all emphasized the importance of mathematics as a key to the understanding of nature – but not in terms of the universal harmonies described by Fludd. Mersenne's *La verite des sciences* forms part of this debate in that he felt that the claims of the alchemists must be overturned prior to the establishment of a truly new science founded on mathematics.

Medical chemistry and Paracelsism in the 1630s

Although direct translations from the work of Paracelsus remained uncommon, C. de Sarcilly published a group of Paracelsian treatises in 1631, in which he noted that interest in Paracelsus began about 1558 when Mattioli and Gesner wrote of chemical medicines.[133] No one, Sarcilly added, had done more to spread interest in this medical system than Peter Severinus; it was after his time that the Galenists began to band together in opposition.

> We see how they use cabal and artifice to maintain and conserve themselves in their absolute empire; It is by these means, each one in his own place, with Princes and Magistrates where they have entry, favor and credit, and even with private persons, they detract with scorn Chemistry, its remedies and its Sectators.[134]

The Galenists demanded that the chemists, with their antimony, mercury, and poisons, should be sent to the hangman as murderers and that this should be the fate of all those who dared to give metallic things to the human body. They were quick to falsely cite cases of those who died by such remedies. In this way they incited terror and panic, which certainly resulted in horror and suspicion of chemical medicine.[135]

Even though chemical physicians had cured the pope, the emperor, and all of the electors of the empire by the true *aurum potabile*, this was nothing to the Galenist.[136] For Sarcilly, one should not try to combine Galenist and chemical medicine because they are opposed.

> From this results the erroneous belief that one can bring into agreement the two professions of medicine. But because these two have totally different principles and foundations it is necessary to repeat one's work every day. And such physicians are like hermaphrodites who have both sexes, but who are never able to reproduce.[137]

[132] I have discussed these debates in *The Chemical Philosophy*. See note 113. See also Wolfgang Pauli (1955), pp. 137–240; Lisa Cafiero (1965).
[133] Paracelsus (1631), p. 20.
[134] Ibid., pp. 25–6.
[135] Ibid.
[136] Ibid., p. 27.
[137] Ibid., p. 28.

Pierre-Jean Fabre (1588–1658) presents us with a particularly interesting blend of alchemist and practical physician, who is only now beginning to be understood, through the research of Bernard Joly.[138] Born in the South of France at Castelnaudary, Fabre spent most of his life there as a local physician. He took his medical degree at Montpellier and ministered to Louis XIII during one of his trips to the South.

To many of the physicians of his time he was known as an authority on the plague, for which he recommended chemical medicines. His treatise on the plague (1653) was reprinted as late as 1720.[139] Yet, the great bulk of Fabre's writings show him to have been strongly attracted to the mystical and religious aspects of chemistry. His *Hercules piochymicus* (1634) interpreted the labors of Hercules as an alchemical process, and in his *Alchymista Christianus* (1632) he pointed out the similarities of Christianity and alchemy.[140] He saw valid correspondences between the sacraments and chemical operations: Calcination symbolized penitence, fire and water corresponded to baptism, and the philosophers' stone could be compared to nothing less than the eucharist. Assuming this, Fabre thought that true alchemists were like priests, the spirit of mercury was like the angels, the earth was like the Virgin Mary, and the life-giving properties of salt gave it a valid connection with Christ. These correspondences could be visualized because they were sculpted on the great churches of France whose artist-architects had presented their esoteric knowledge to the viewer.[141]

Unlike most other Paracelsians, Fabre most frequently wrote in Latin. An exception was his *L'abregé des Secrets Chymiques* (1636), in which he pointed to the uniqueness of chemistry whose subject matter encompassed all nature.[142] We could use it not only as a key to the animal and vegetable kingdoms but also as a guide to understanding heaven, which we could comprehend only by the intellectual operation of our souls. This could not be excluded from the domain of alchemy.[143] Because of correspondence, Fabre continued, alchemy was understood properly as the most important and basic of the sciences.

> . . . Alchemy is not only an art or science for teaching metallic transmutation, but it is also a true and solid science which teaches us the central core of all things and this in divine language one calls the Spirit of life. God infuses this Spirit among all the elements for the production, nourishment

---

[138] Bernard Joly (1988). Joly refers to two earlier important studies on Fabre: Auguste Fourés (1891), pp. 140–58, and René Nelli (1958), pp. 36–50. I have seen neither of these.

[139] Pierre-Jean Fabre, *Traité de la Peste selon la doctrine des médecins spagyriques* (Toulouse, 1653). This was reprinted as *Remèdes curatifs et préservatifs de la peste* in 1720 at Toulouse.

[140] Pierre-Jean Fabre (1632).

[141] Joly (1988), vol. 1, p. 31.

[142] Pierre Jean Fabre (1636), p. 8.

[143] Ibid., p. 9.

and maintenance of natural things. It is to be found at the center of all things, making a body incorruptible, permanent and fixed, able to resist all sorts of changes which it will have to endure for the benefit of the diverse generations which will be hatched from its center.

Alchemy then teaches us about this divine and spiritual substance in all things; and it demonstrates by its chemical operations how to extract and separate it from the elementary entanglement and corruption, in order to free its powers and virtues which are nearly infinite and God given. [Alchemy then] merits truly the name of unique natural philosophy since it shows the basis, the foundation and the root of all created things and it teaches the purification and exaltation of the same; from whence comes the metallic transmutation of metals, the fertility of vegetables and the prolongation of life . . .[144]

No less interested in the universal spirit of life was Henri De Rochas, a physician and royal councillor, whose *La Vraye Anatomie Spagyrique* (1637) described the chemists' universal life spirit as having been created by God and pervading all parts of the three worlds: supercelestial, celestial, and elementary.[145] It was subtle and penetrating, and united easily with the soul, germ, or seed of corporal things. Because it was communicated through heavenly influences, it reached all bodies able to receive it and became materialized. For this reason the universe as a whole and all things in it are alive.

It follows then that the entire universal world is endowed with life, since each part of it is accompanied by a vital action; and one after another each individual and each species has its proper life, but these are only participating lives in the universal life of the world in which are hidden and contained all the invisible seeds.[146]

The following year Rochas published *La physique Reformee* (1638), in which he turned to chemistry again as the key to natural philosophy. The work itself was based primarily on Holy Scripture and chemistry. In it he defended astrology, opposed the Galenists by accepting the Paracelsian dictum that like cures like, and discussed the powder of sympathy.[147] He wrote that with distillation it was possible to obtain the first principle of all things [water in vegetables; phlegm in animals; and mercury in metals].[148] He went on to discuss sulfur and mercury and then to categorize four fundamental diseases: those associated with the three principles, and a fourth, poison.[149]

Another popular author was Jean d'Aubry, abbé of Notre Dame de l'Assomption, conseiller and medecine ordinaire to the king, whose

[144] Ibid., p. 10.
[145] Henry De Rochas (1637), pp. 242–3.
[146] Ibid., p. 248.
[147] *La physique Reformee* is discussed at length in Thorndike (1923–58), vol. 8, pp. 274–7.
[148] Henry de Rochas (1638), p. 151.
[149] Ibid., p. 516.

works on medicine were published in a number of editions over a thirty-year period. D'Aubry defined a number of types of medicine, among them theurgic, mathematical, harmonic, fantastic, magical, empirical, dietary, surgical, philtric, Galenic, and chemical.[150] He was careful to point out that when he spoke of chemistry, he did not mean the art that tinges metals and stones or coagulates mercury to make false money.[151] He was still less interested in chrysopoeia, which teaches true metallic transmutation. Rather, he was interested in the practical aspect of Galenic medicine. This is an art, he wrote, that had many followers at Montpellier but was quite different from "Medecine Paraseltique" which "finds in the microcosm all the rarities of the heavens, the marvels of the earth, and the mysteries of nature."[152] He thought it unfortunate that few understood the writings of Paracelsus. "I have seen at Montpellier (the town of my birth) many Doctors so fearful that they condemn Paracelsus, and then when I ask them in what consists the theory of Paracelsus, they frankly admit that they understand nothing."[153] D'Aubry discussed the work of Paracelsus at length and emphasized the importance of the Archeus "which gives life, birth and the characteristic qualities to all created things."[154] In addition to giving his own views on theoretical medicine, D'Aubry referred to his cures in a book of consultations.

Quite different in his approach was Fabius Violet, sieur de Coqueray, whom Pagel has singled out for his discussion of gastric digestion. Pointing to Violet's discussion of acetum esurinum as a digestive factor in the stomach, Pagel believed Violet to be more decisive than Paracelsus though not as definite as van Helmont who had identified the acid as hydrochloric.[155] Violet was a close follower of Paracelsus in rejecting humoral medicine and in attributing disease to a coagulation of sulfur and mercury brought about by salt. He had a special interest in the Paracelsian "tartaric" diseases and discussed illnesses caused by obstruction.

Medicine, Violet contended, was founded on four columns: philosophy, astrology, alchemy, virtue and duty. The first column must be proven by demonstration.[156] It must be based on man and the matter he consists of, as well as the four contraries and the relationship of the elements. The physician, he said, knows that sulfur, salt, and mercury are the principal constituents of all things, also that man has within him arsenic, vitriol, acid, tartar, and sulfur, and that man is properly called

150 Jean d'Aubry [ca 1660], pp. 1–36.
151 L'Abbe Jean d'Aubry (1638 [?]), p. 12.
152 Ibid., p. 14.
153 D'Aubry [ca. 1660], p. 14.
154 Ibid., p. 1.
155 Walter Pagel (1958), pp. 161–4.
156 Fabius Violet (1635), pp. 17–53, based on Paracelsus' *Paragranum*.

the microcosm of the great world.[157] He thought that the connection between the two worlds required the true physician to understand astrology; but alchemy was required also, in part to prepare the necessary medicines for his art but also to understand how food and drink are converted into blood and flesh through internal purifications and separations. Violet asked the reader to think of the pear or the prune, both astringent and disagreeable to the taste when green, but after the internal alchemists have cooked them to perfection they demonstrate their goodness.[158] Violet attacked the Galenists, who refused to stain their hands with coals, cinders, or the materials required for luting. In the end the alchemist has far greater satisfaction in knowing that his was the true medicine created by God.[159]

An author who deserves greater attention than he has received is David de Planis Campy (1589–ca. 1644), who produced some ten works on medical chemistry and traditional alchemy. He was a councillor and Chirurgien ordinaire to Louis XIII, and his works were collected and published in a folio volume in 1646. Planis Campy wrote in open admiration of Paracelsus. He accepted the relationship of the macrocosm and the microcosm and the doctrine of signatures.[160] He argued that God had provided mankind with remedies for all illnesses and that the Paracelsian cure by similitude was not opposed to the Hippocratic or Galenic theory of cure because it did not refer to either first or second qualities but to substances and virtues.[161] Nor were the three principles contrary to Hippocratic principles. The four elements were the "peres producteurs" of the entire "body Physic," but all bodies could be reduced to the three principles, which were the basis of the three fundamental classes of disease.[162] "It is invariably accepted among chemists that all bodies are composed of the three principles, and that all illnesses come from their corruption, not only in regard to animals, but also vegetables and minerals."[163]

In his *Bouquet Chymique* (1629) Planis Campy referred to *Ecclesiasticus* 38 in his assertion that "I say then that the Hermetic Medicine is true because it is the creation of God."[164] He wrote that chemistry has an ancient history going back to the time of Tubal Cain and Hermes,[165] and alchemy is a science that teaches the means of separating the elements of each mixed body produced by nature and of separating the pure from the impure. By its means physicians could learn of the first matter of all

157 Ibid., p. 22.
158 Ibid., pp. 36–7.
159 Ibid., p. 43.
160 Robert Multhauf (1954).
161 David de Planis Campy (1646), p. 67.
162 Ibid., p. 68.
163 de Planis Campy (1646), *Le Bouquet Chymique in Les Oevvres*, pp. 409–10.
164 Ibid., p. 392.
165 Ibid., p. 394.

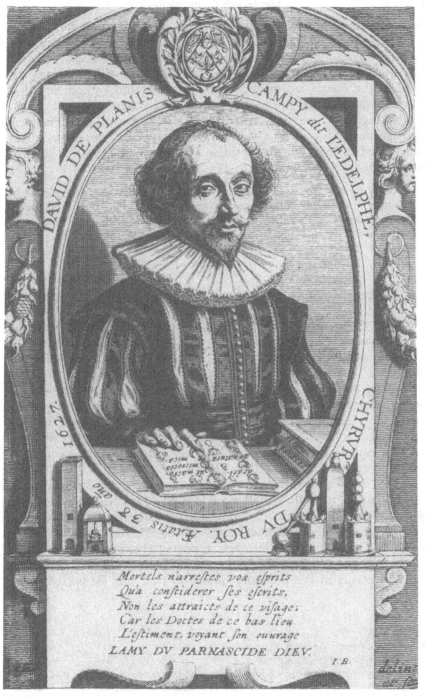

David de Planis Campy (1589–ca. 1644). Portrait from *L'hydre morbifique exterminee par l'Hercule chymique. . .* (1628). From the collection of the author.

the bodies of the world, be they animal, vegetable, or mineral. But the goal of chemistry was "to prepare medicines in such strength that they are more agreeable to the taste, more healthful to the body, and less dangerous in their operation."[166] Much of the *Bouquet Chymique* is devoted to the discussion of chemical operations and equipment, after which the author turns to recipes for distilled waters, oils, salts, pills, tablets, unguents, liniments, and plasters. The success of these chemical remedies in treating seven diseases thought not long before to be incurable argued strongly for the adoption of chemical medicine in place of the ancients.

> O happy innovation! since it has disentangled us from the chaos of error and ignorance in which the common opinion had confined us. O happy chemical remedies! by your introduction we have seen all illnesses held for incurable by the common treatment now totally exterminated by your usage.[167]

Guy de la Brosse and the Jardin des Plantes

Although the medical student who was interested in chemistry would have had no trouble pursuing his interests at Montpellier, the situation was quite different in Paris. Not only had the Parisian Medical Faculty relentlessly pursued chemical physicians and purveyors of chemical medicines, they had also opposed all attempts to teach chemistry to medical students or to anyone else associated with the medical profession. Pierre Paulmier had been censured for suggesting that apothecaries take a course in spagyric chemistry (1591), and Turquet de Mayerne had suffered the same fate for his desire to give such a course to young surgeons and apothecaries (1603).

Early in the seventeenth century Jean Beguin arrived in Paris, possibly from Sedan. Here, with the influence of Ribit de la Rivière and Turquet de la Mayerne, he was granted permission to establish a laboratory and give lectures on pharmaceutical preparations.[168] His *Tyrocinium chymicum* (1610), based on these lectures, appears to have been derived ultimately from the *Alchymia* of Libavius,[169] but there is a direct connection with Paracelsus in the prefatory quotation from the *De tinctura physicorum:*

---

[166] de Planis Campy (1646), p. 75.
[167] de Planis Campy (1628), sig. vii[r,v].
[168] The classic account of the work of Beguin and the various editions is that of T. S. Patterson (1937). See also the discussion in Partington (1962), vol. 3, pp. 2–4, and Helène Metzger (1923), pp. 35–44. A discussion of the literature as a whole is in P. M. Rattansi's biography in the *Dictionary of Scientific Biography*, vol. I (1970), pp. 571–2.
[169] A. Kent and O. Hannaway (1960).

First, you must learn Digestions, Distillations, Sublimations, Reverbera-
tions, Extractions, Solutions, Coagulations, Fermentations, and Fixations;
and you must also know what Instruments are required for use in this
Work; as Glasses, Cucurbits, Circulatory Vessels, Vessels of *Hermes*,
Earthen Vessels, Balneums, Wind Fornaces, Fornaces of Reverberation,
and other such like: as also a Marble, Mortars, Coals, &c. So may you at
length proceed in the Work of Alchimy, and Medicine.

But as long as you shall by Phantasie and Opinion adhere to feigned
Books, you will be apt for, and Predestined to none of these.[170]

For Beguin "Chemistry is the Art of dissolving natural mixed bodies,
and of coagulating the same when dissolved, and of reducing them into
salubrious, safe and grateful Medicaments."[171] Indeed, there was no
doubt that "The intention of this Artist, is to prepare most sweet, most
wholsome, and most safe Medicaments."[172] But, he said, the Galenic
apothecaries argue that the chemists' drugs "are venomous and plainly
repugnant to humane Nature, as being Metallick and taken from Minerals; and generally are more sharp, more corrosive, and more hot than is
convenient, and also very strongly smell of the fire."[173] Although the
chemist readily admitted the use of metals and their derivatives, rather
than using them crudely as had the ancients and some of the moderns,
he prepared them in a form freed from "all venomous malignity."

The profitable must be separated from the unprofitable; the venom from
the salutary Mummy; and the Kernel and Marrow uncased from Rindes,
Shells, Husks, and Feces. So at length from thence may Remedies be taken
apt for the Cure of the most deplorable diseases, quickly, safely, and
pleasantly, if they be adhibited by learned, expert, and circumspect Physicians, and according to the prescribed Rules of *Therapeia*.[174]

Galenists complained that the use of fire made medicines more caustic
and dangerous,[175] but even Galen wrote that fire meliorates many
things.[176] If this condemnation of fire were to hold true "then can neither our Meats, or Drinks, or vulgar Medicaments be safe and
wholsome; since, in preparing them, oftentimes a greater degree of fire
is required than for Spagerick Remedies . . ."[177] In fact, he said, the use
of fire makes medicines more valuable than the common ones because it
separates the pure from the impure.

---

[170] John Beguinus (1669), sig. b2r&v. This quotation had been dropped from the French
and Latin editions by 1615, but Russell's translation was based on the earliest editions
of the text, which included practical admonitions to the reader.
[171] Ibid., p. 1.
[172] Ibid., p. 3.
[173] Ibid., p. 4.
[174] Ibid., p. 5.
[175] Ibid., p. 8.
[176] Ibid., p. 9.
[177] Ibid., p. 10.

Having defended the use of chemistry in the preparation of medicines, Beguin went on to discuss the various operations of the chemist: solution, calcination, extraction, coagulation, lutation, distillation, and others. Through all of this his allegiance to the three principles was evident. The remainder of the book was devoted to specific preparations.

Primarily a practical work, Beguin's *Tyrocinium* must have been one of the most successful publications of the century; Patterson traced forty-one editions in the period 1610–90. Later editions were expanded, updated and used as textbooks by teachers of chemistry throughout Europe. Beguin was thus a notable figure for having developed the first successful course of chemistry in France and for having written a textbook that became the model for the many similar works that were to follow.

Beguin had been able to give his course because of the support of the physicians at the court, who favored chemical medicine. Rio Howard has shown that the Parisian Medical Faculty numerically had reached a nadir in the early decades of the century, at a time when the number of court physicians was increasing.[178] The first physicians to the king under Henry IV and Louis XIII sought to increase their influence in the medical community. Ribit de la Rivière attempted to establish licensing boards for physicians in provincial towns, and these were to be staffed by intendants named by him. Needless to say, the medical faculty resisted this plan, which was nonetheless approved by Henry IV.[179]

Under Louis XIII the number of physicians at court increased to eighty or a hundred, more than were on the faculty itself. The physicians of Henry IV had included the three most prominent chemical physicians in France: Joseph Duchesne, Theodore Turquet de Mayerne, and the premier médecin, Ribit de la Rivière. It would clearly be incorrect to characterize the court physicians as a group solidly committed to Paracelsian and Hermetic mysticism. Some were, but others were interested only in practical processes for a limited number of medicines, and still others were members of the medical faculty. Nevertheless, the court physicians were a group apart from the medical faculty; they were led by a few men who were anxious to establish an independent power of their own and included a number of influential chemists.

Both the father and the grandfather of Guy de la Brosse (ca. 1586–1641),[180] who was to become the founder of the Jardin des Plantes in

178 Howard (1981), see note 14.
179 Ibid.
180 On Guy de La Brosse, see Howard, ibid., as well as her "Guy de La Brosse and the Jardin des Plantes in Paris" (1981b), *La Bibliotheque et le Laboratorie de Guy de La Brosse au Jardin des Plantes à Paris* (1983), and "Guy de La Brosse: Botanique et chimie au debut de la revolution scientifique" (1978). Here I have worked from a photocopy of the galley proofs kindly sent to me by the author. See also Henry Guerlac (1972), vol. 1, pp. 177–99. See also E. T. Hamy (1900) and (1897).

Paris, had been among the court physicians. Guy de la Brosse's father, Isaïe de Vireneau, Sieur de la Brosse (d. ca. 1610), had an interest in medicinal plants as well as chemistry, for which he too had been condemned by the medical faculty (1607).[181] Very little is known of Guy's life, but a contemporary listed him along with the doctors of Montpellier, even though there is no record of his ever having attended that famous medical school. What we do know of him relates primarily to his plan to establish a royal garden of medicinal plants.[182]

La Brosse's project was first drafted in 1616. He sought a teaching and research institution in which lectures would be given twice a week from May to September. There was to be a resident *droguier* from whom students would learn both the preparation of herbal remedies and the technique of distillation. The consummation of his plan was long delayed even though he had the support of Jean Héroard (1551–1628), who served as premier médecin of Louis XIII after 1616.[183] Héroard was another graduate of Montpellier (1575) who was reputedly sympathetic to the use of chemical remedies.

The views of la Brosse can be found in his *De la natur, Vertu et Vtilité des Plantes* (1628), which devotes one substantial book out of five to a general discussion of chemistry.[184] Here he wrote that chemistry was much in vogue among the Germans and that those who subscribed to that medical sect were called Paracelsists, chemists, or Hermeticists:

> but on the other hand it is greatly despised and lamented by the Sanguinary [blood letting or Galenist] sect, not only because these delicate persons fear that they will soil their hands with coals, but also because they fear the labor and the cost: idleness and avarice have so corrupted their mercenary souls, that they would rather abandon their profession than lose a denier . . .[185]

La Brosse thought highly of Paracelsus and Severinus but felt that most of the other followers of Paracelsus – Croll, Duchesne, Penotus, Dorn, Libavius, and others – had simply copied his words without turning to laboratory experiments.

La Brosse had a special interest in the three principles, but he discussed the elements as well, rejecting fire as one of the true chemical principles and explaining why chemists do not include air among their elements.[186] In effect, he continued the five-element–principle system of Duchesne: that is, salt, sulfur, and mercury with the traditional water and earth. Because of his special interest in botany, La Brosse faulted many chemists who seemed to turn exclusively to remedies derived

---

181 Here I follow Guerlac's account (1972), p. 180.
182 Ibid., p. 181.
183 On Héroard, see E. W. Marvick (1974).
184 This work has been examined in most detail by Rio Howard (1978).
185 Guy de la Brosse (1628), p. 293.
186 Ibid., p. 319.

from metallic substances. He argued that medicinal substances must be found elsewhere as well – clearly meaning plants.

The Parisian Medical Faculty perceived La Brosse's plan to be a rival to their own, and in 1618 Jean Riolan proposed a botanical garden in Paris that would be the equal of the already famous garden at Montpellier.[187] This project led nowhere, so in 1626 Louis XIII gave his assent to the La Brosse plan. There was to be an intendant (La Brosse was named to this post in 1633), an assistant to the intendant, and three pharmacist demonstrators to show the uses and chemical properties of plants.[188] A superintendant chosen from the physicians of the royal household was to supervise the staff of the Jardin. The first person named to this post in 1626 was Jean Héroard. Progress was slow, and the official establishment of the Jardin did not occur until 1635. It was another five years before the opening ceremony took place. At this time La Brosse had but one more year to live. Another eight years passed before the first professor of chemistry was appointed, the Scot, William Davidson (Davisson). He was followed by Nicolas Lefèvre, then Christofle Glaser, and Moyse Charas, all of whom prepared chemical texts that were widely read and influential. In the second half of the seventeenth century, through the work of these teachers and authors Paris became a center for the teaching of chemistry, even though the subject remained anathema to the members of the medical faculty.

Théophraste Renaudot and the Bureau d'Adresse

With the appointment of Davisson as professor of chemistry at the Jardin des Plantes in 1648, the teaching of chemistry was well established in Paris, though not at the university. However, this did not lessen the opposition of the medical faculty, whose members continued to thunder against the chemists and their chemicals, especially against the many antimonial preparations, which were gaining popularity.

In the fourth decade of the century a new champion of chemicals arose in the person of Théophraste Renaudot (1584–1653).[189] A protestant, he had taken his degree at Montpellier where he had matriculated in 1605. It would have been impossible for him to have attended Paris, where proof of one's Roman Catholicism was required.[190] Unlike many others, after receiving the licentiate, which permitted him to practice, he had gone on to take the doctorate (12 July 1606). After a period of travel he returned to his home, Loudon, where he married and set up his practice.

---

[187] Guerlac, (1972), p. 181.
[188] Ibid., p. 189.
[189] On the various activities of Renaudot, see especially Howard M. Solomon (1972).
[190] Ibid., p. 5.

At Loudon Renaudot became aware of the problems of the poor, and at this time (1611) he met Armand-Jean du Plessis de Richelieu, later to be named cardinal. The following year (1612) Richelieu called a meeting in Paris to discuss the problems of the poor. Renaudot was invited and while there he was given the title of royal physician in reward for offering his ideas on poor relief to the Crown.[191] In 1618 he was given the additional title of commissaire des pauures du royaume. These were honors that did not require his attendance at court, and Renaudot remained for most of the year at Loudon. Nevertheless, it seemed wise to convert to Catholicism, which he did sometime before 1626, when he finally moved to Paris. As a royal physician he was able to set up practice even though the Parisian Medical Faculty tried to enforce its right to limit physicians in Paris to its own graduates. He became an active supporter of Richelieu, who saw to it that Renaudot's titles were reconfirmed in 1617, 1618, 1621, 1628, 1629, and 1630.

In Paris, Renaudot was in a position to establish his Bureau d'Adresse (1630 or perhaps a year or two earlier), which he hoped would go far to solve the problems of the poor.[192] In part this was a clearing house for the unemployed, who could register and hope to find a suitable employer. Unfortunately, it seemed a threat to the traditional journeyman system of the guilds. In addition to this practical function, the Bureau d'Adresse provided medical assistance. Free medical consultations were being provided to the poor as early as 1632.[193] At first this service was confined to medical consultations on Tuesday afternoons, when the physicians would examine patients, prescribe treatment, and refer them to a physician who would treat them gratuitously. In addition Renaudot inaugurated a system of low-interest loans to aid the poor; a printing shop that published the *Gazette* (1631), one of the first French newspapers; and a long-running series of conferences which are of interest in reference to the development of European scientific academies.

Frances Yates has shown that French literary academies had a long history,[194] with roots in the fifteenth-century Florentine Academy of Marsilio Ficino and Pico della Mirandola. We have already noted the group surrounding Jacques Gohory in France in the late sixteenth century, which dabbled in Paracelsian medicine.

The conference established by Renaudot met regularly between 22 August 1633 and 1 September 1642 on Monday afternoons.[195] Any subject was open for discussion other than those concerned with religion and matters of state. Any and all persons were admitted and allowed to

[191] Ibid., p. 39.
[192] Ibid., p. 40.
[193] Ibid., p. 46.
[194] Frances A. Yates (1947).
[195] See the collection of 287 conferences: E. Renaudot, ed. (1666). These conferences were partially translated into English (1664) and (1665).

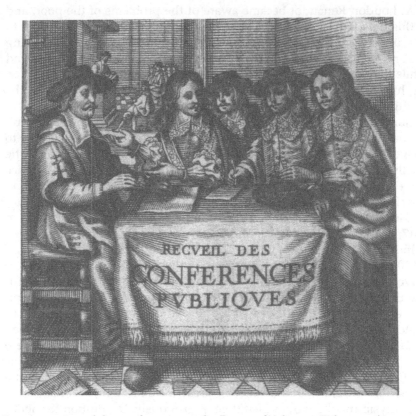

Representation of the conferences at the Bureau d'Adresse. Title page from vol. 1, [Eusèbe Renaudot, ed.], *Recveil General des Qvestions traitées és Conferences du Bureau d'Adresse* (1666). Courtesy of the British Library.

speak. Also, weekly reports of the conferences were available in printed form. Interesting though these accounts are, the views expressed cannot be associated with any specific individuals. Although we know that Jean-Baptiste Morin, Tommaso Campanella, and Ètienne de Clave were present on occasion, we know nothing of any other participants.

The sciences and medicine were particularly well represented among the subjects discussed. The Aristotelian elements, motion, the vacuum, the descent of bodies in free fall, and even the motion of the earth were discussed, as well as specific diseases, diet, bloodletting, the Bezoar-stone, and purging. Of more concern to us were the discussions related to Paracelsism, chemical remedies, and cure by similitude.

In the conferences no effort was made to reach a consensus. The reader of the weekly report was simply presented with the different views that were offered. Thus, in regard to cure by similitude, one speaker suggested that since the chemical principles had been over-thrown, "all the remedies founded thereupon ought to be suspec-ted."[196] A second speaker suggested that there was no real difference between the chemists and the Galenists on this point because "when the Chymists say, That *Similia curantur similibus*, they speak not of diseases, as the Galenists do . . . but of the part diseased . . ."[197] A third speaker contended that remedies prepared from metals and minerals have more venomous qualities than those prepared from plants and animals, and that because their preparation results from fire, they acquire even more dangerous qualities.[198] The fourth speaker commented that even if chemical remedies were to be separated from poisons, one could point to similar dangerous qualities in the traditional *materia medica*. The final participant rather eloquently stated that

> Chymistry, which opens the means thereunto by the solution of all Bodies, ought to be cherish'd, and not condemn'd, as it is by the ignorant or malicious, who must at least acknowledg it one of the members of Phys-ick, as belonging to Pharmacy, which consists in the choice and prepara-tion of Medicaments, and is part of the Therapeutical Division. But we say rather, That the three parts of Medicine, or its three ancient Sects, are the three parts of the World, *Europe, Asia*, and *Africa*; and Chymistry is that new World, lately discover'd, not less rare and admirable than the others, provided it be as carefully cultivated, and rescu'd out of the hands of Barbarians.[199]

Other topics discussed by the savants at various times included miner-al waters, atoms, natural magic, the powder of sympathy, cabala, sym-pathetic action, the philosophers' stone, and the quintessence. In a dis-cussion of the generation of metals, one participant remarked that the presence of sulfur represented the male sperm and mercury the mater-nal blood.[200] Relying on the belief that metals were gradually perfected in the earth, this speaker insisted that the imperfect metals differed from gold and silver only in accidental degrees. Therefore, "by power of heat in the bowels of the earth, Iron the most imperfect and lightest of all Metals is turned into Steel and Copper, afterwards into tin, and lastly, being more depurated into Gold and Silver."[201]

The Rosicrucians were debated in a general discussion, in which the second discussant claimed that some people maintained that Paracelsus learned all that he knew from the secret book *M* of the legendary found-

[196] Ibid., p. 38. For the French text, see E. Renaudot, ed. (1666), *Recveil General*, vol. 4, pp. 96–107.

[197] Renaudot (1665), p. 38.

[198] Ibid., p. 39.

[199] Ibid., p. 40.

[200] Ibid., p. 157.

[201] Ibid., p. 158.

er of the order, Christian Rosenkreutz.[202] This led to a follow-up conference titled "What Paracelsus meant by the Book *M*."[203] In reports of these sessions one finds little to encourage the would-be believer. One participant suggested that

> . . . if you look to the bottom of all, you will see their hands foul'd with coals or dung, their faces discolour'd by the Arsenical Exhalations of the Minerals they prepare in their furnaces, and yet the most pitiful wretch of them all will swear that he knows the great work.[204]

There is little doubt that Théophraste Renaudot had already become an important figure in the realm. He had been trained first as a physician and thought of himself as such. His degree was from Montpellier, and many of his assistants at the Bureau had similar academic ties. They all had an interest in chemistry and often prescribed antimony to their patients. Because of these factors, Renaudot and his medical activities were viewed with alarm by the members of the Parisian Medical Faculty.

The medical community at Paris – other than the court physicians – was for the most part quite as conservative as we have indicated. Lectures at the medical school were based on Hippocrates, Galen, and the "other princes of medicine."[205] The medical faculty itself extended far beyond the two professors (until 1634) of medicine to include all the medical doctors in the city; and as we have seen, these were usually limited to graduates of Paris.[206] In this way the members of the professional medical community were also members of the educational community.

The Parisian Medical Faculty claimed that only their graduates could practice throughout France; the practice of those who had been trained elsewhere was, or should be, limited only to the towns in which they were trained. With the exception of the royal physicians, the medical faculty strove to keep the medical community free from "foreign" influences,[207] which meant that even graduates of Montpellier were forbidden to practice in Paris even though that school had received from the popes at Avignon the right to allow its graduates to practice *"hic et ubique terrarum."*[208] Montpellier was suspect not only for its long interest in

202 Renaudot (1666), vol. 5, pp. 494–513; Renaudot (1665), p. 324.
203 Renaudot (1666), vol. 5, pp. 543–52; Renaudot (1665), pp. 326–8.
204 Ibid., p. 325.
205 Solomon (1972), p. 163.
206 Ibid., 164. In his studies of the teaching of medicine at Paris in the seventeenth and early eighteenth centuries, L. W. B. Brockliss (1978) used the extensive surviving medical theses of the period to show that traditional Galenism did not begin to decline until after the mid-seventeenth century and that it was only in the final decade of the century that iatrochemistry seemed to be predominant due to an interest in the then current acid–alkali theory. One notable exception is to be found in an earlier thesis by Pierre Yvelin (1633) who championed all metallic remedies (p. 243).
207 Solomon (1972), p. 165.
208 Ibid., p. 166. On the history of medicine at Montpellier, see Louis Dulieu, *La Medecine*

Cinamo mi, } ana drachmam vnam.
Seminis Fœniculi }
Fiat Electarium molle ad vfum.

Vinum Emeticum.

℞. Stibij optimi   libram vnam.
Nitri puriſſimi tantundem.

Puluerentur ſeorſim, dein commiſceantur & có-
iiciantur in mortarium æneum vel ferreum, mox in-
iecta pruna vel ferro candente materia incendatur,
quæ cum fragore & ſtrepitu exuretur, ſuperpoſita
trium digitorum interuallo patella ferrea, donec ſtri-
dor ceſſauerit.

Materia metallica inſtar vitri fuſi fuſce rubens ſe-
paretur ab impura craſſitie, & à nitro cruſtam albi-
cantem referente, & ter aqua tepida lauetur.

Cuius ſtibij vt iam dictum eſt præparati.

℞. Vnciam vnam.
Infunde in vini albi libris duabus, per duos treſ-
ve dies, vel plures.

Electarium è ſucco Roſarum.

℞. Succi Roſarum rubrarum recentium.
Sacchari optimi   ana libram vnam & Se-
miſſem.
Coquantur in Electarium Solidum igne lento.
Inſperge ſub finem trium Santalorum exquiſite
tritorum.   Ma-

Directions for the preparation of *Vinum Emeticum* as printed in the first edition of the *Codex medicamentarius* of the Parisian Medical Faculty (1638). This copy, originally owned by Jacques Mantel, refers in a marginal note to the condemnation of antimony by the Faculty. From the collection of the National Library of Medicine, Bethesda.

chemical medicine but also because it accepted protestant students. The Parisian Medical Faculty also attempted to maintain its authority over the surgeons and apothecaries of Paris, who understandably resented the interference.[209]

à Montpellier, 3 vols. [vol. I. Le Môyen Age, 1975; vol. II. La Renaissance, 1979; vol. III. L'Èpoch classique (Première Partie, 1983)].
209 Solomon (1972), pp. 168–9.

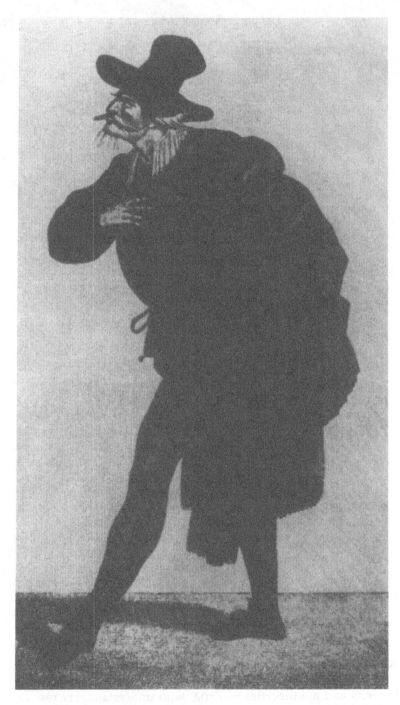

Hardouin de Saint-Jacques. From Francis R. Packard, *Guy Patin and the Medical Profession in Paris in the XVIIth Century* (1924). Courtesy of the Oxford University Press.

It was during the 1630s that Renaudot was giving free medical advice at the Bureau d'Adresse from ten to twelve o'clock every weekday morning. His medical staff was composed of physicians from non-Parisian schools, many of whom were protestants and advocates of chemical medicine. It seemed to the members of the Parisian Medical Faculty that their power was being directly challenged.[210]

A series of swift-moving events brought the matter to a head. For fifteen years the faculty had been at work on a pharmacopoeia, the *Codex pharmaceutique*. One of the approved purgatives contained antimony, *vin émétique*.[211] This had been accepted by a committee headed by Hardouin St. Jacques, dean of the Parisian Medical Faculty.[212] The question of whether this approval had been given properly was to plague the members of the faculty for decades and was a source of embarrassment to those members who opposed chemical remedies, especially antimony.

At this time the two sons of Renaudot, Isaac and Eusèbe, were medical students in Paris. Seeking to injure the father through his children, the faculty forced them to sign a disavowal of their father's activities in order to pass the first grade (1638).[213] This hardly affected Théophraste who had furnaces built at the bureau (September 1640), so that chemicals could be prepared there, and soon after obtained permission to build new facilities for the Bureau d'Adresse.[214] Renaudot was at the height of his power. He employed foreign-trained (non-Parisian) physicians whom he could license to practice throughout France through his power as commissaire general des pauvres; he attracted students of the Parisian medical school to his weekly conferences, students who would learn there of chemical medicines; he had obtained the right to set up his chemical laboratories; and he had a program of free medical consultations, which could serve as a teaching clinic. Furthermore, he had widespread support among the apothecaries and surgeons, whom he treated as equals.[215]

To extend his program of medical advice Renaudot prepared *La présence des absens*, a medical form that described symptoms and could be completed by anyone and set to the bureau. The bureau staff would then diagnose the patient in absentia and make recommendations for treatment by mail.[216] This made the bureau truly a medical center for the entire country, and of course, it was considered to be one more affront to the Parisian Medical Faculty. One of the faculty's most persistent defenders, Gui Patin (1601–1672; M.D. 1627) called for an all-out war against

---

210 Ibid., pp. 170–1.
211 Very popular in the seventeenth century, *vin emetic* was most frequently prepared by adding tartar emetic (tartar antimony) to sherry.
212 Ibid., p. 172; Pilpoul (1928), pp. 40–41.
213 Ibid., p. 44.
214 Ibid.; Solomon (1972), pp. 173–4.
215 Ibid., 174–5.
216 Ibid., p. 175; Pilpoul (1928), pp. 44–5.

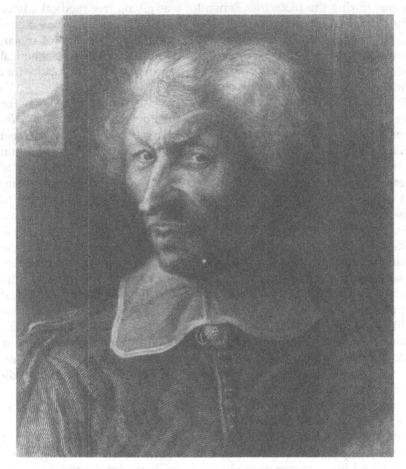

Gui Patin (1601–1672). Courtesy of the National Library of Medicine, Bethesda.

the "so-called physicians, promoters of insolent errors, empirics, cir-
culators [followers of William Harvey]: and especially against their chief,
Théophraste Renaudot."[217]

Patin was to have his way. An unyielding opponent of change and of
chemistry and chemical cures, he explained a decade later that chemistry was not necessary in medicine. Under the pretense of trying out
the virulent and pernicious metallic medicines on their patients, he
wrote, these chemists have killed more people than they have helped,
and antimony alone has killed more people in Germany than the king of
Sweden did with all of his armies (4 November 1650).[218] Patin kept track

---

[217] Ibid., p. 45. Many members of the faculty opposed the Harveyan concept of the
circulation as resolutely as they opposed the introduction of chemistry to medicine.
[218] Gui Patin (1846), vol. 2, p. 563. On Patin, see Francis R. Packard (1924).

of those killed by antimonial treatment in his *Le Martyrologue de l'Anti-moine ou le témoignage de la vertu émétique*, and he frequently referred with obvious pleasure to recent deaths caused by chemical physicians. Chemists, surgeons, and apothecaries, Patin hated them all; he was to oppose them until his death.

Three weeks after Renaudot had obtained permission to build furnaces at the bureau, he was officially informed by the medical faculty of the injunction against foreign physicians in Paris.[219] On 3 November 1640 Guillaume du Val became the new dean of the medical faculty, and one of his first acts was to set up a commission to investigate the activities of empirics in Paris, especially Renaudot. For the next three years Renaudot and his adversaries waged a pamphlet war, which Howard Solomon has followed in detail and which need not be repeated here.

Much of this debate concerned the history of the two chief medical schools, Paris and Montpellier, and the validity of their rights and privileges. Also of concern to both parties was the history of the use of chemical medicines both before and after the decree of 1566 against antimony. The Parisian Medical Faculty insisted on its right to grant permission to practice in Paris, and they remained firm in their opposition to chemical remedies, especially all forms of antimony. Thus, in an anonymous *Advertissement a Theophraste Renaudot Contenant Les Memoires pour jusitifier les Anciens droicts & privileges de la Faculté de Medecine de Paris*, the author [now generally considered to be Gui Patin though Jean Riolan is also a possibility (1640)] discussed at length the history of the actions taken by the faculty against the use of chemicals. The crime of which Montpellier was accused had been to try to avoid the censure of Paris by turning to chemistry and claiming that its medicines were better.[220] Renaudot had tried to introduce a medical schism into Paris, and the medical faculty had stood firm in its opposition to the teaching of alchemy and metals.[221]

In his *La Defence de la Faculté de Medecine de Paris . . .* (1641), René Moreau argued that though Renaudot had many impressive titles, not one of them gave him the right to practice medicine in Paris.[222] It was the faculty of medicine that decided who could practice. Moreover, Renaudot did not even confine himself to medicine but sold the *Gazette* and involved himself in a host of matters related to the bureau that are unworthy of a physician. Besides, he received his degree at the age of nineteen, too young for a medical doctor,[223] and was ignorant of medicine. As for the use of antimony, Moreau went to pains to show that graduates of Montpellier as well as those of Paris had condemned it.[224]

219 Solomon (1972), p. 177.
220 Anon. [Patin (?), Riolan Jr. (?)] (1641), p. 38.
221 Ibid., p. 56.
222 [Mr. Moreau, Doct. en Med.] (1641), p. 5.
223 Ibid., p. 19.
224 Ibid., p. 55.

These statements were made in a tract dedicated to Cardinal Richelieu, Renaudot's chief supporter. Indeed, it was already evident that were it not for Richelieu, Renaudot would not be able to carry out his plans.

The role of Richelieu reappeared when Isaac and Eusèbe were barred from their doctoral ceremonies on 26 January 1641 because of the "grave injuries of their father." At this point Richelieu summoned Du Val and asked him to call off the attack. Instead, the faculty in open session praised those who had written against Théophraste Renaudot[225]; and when Richelieu was out of Paris and Eusèbe attended him as a physician, the faculty refused to postpone Eusèbe's formal presentation until his return to the City. Finally, on 30 August 1642 the faculty offered to stop obstructing the brothers if they would once more renounce the Bureau d'Adresse. Richelieu was again called in to aid the brothers, who nevertheless were forced once more to renounce the work of their father.[226] When Richelieu died at the beginning of December, the Renaudots lost their patron. The medical faculty once again refused to admit the brothers to the doctorate.[227]

Early in 1643 a new dean of the medical school, Michel de la Vigne, sought and obtained the support of the University of Paris in their process against Théophraste Renaudot. At this point Louis XIII died (May 14), and the medical faculty called for injunctions against all of Renaudot's activities.[228] The court was now controlled by Anne of Austria, who was opposed to Richelieu and all his supporters. In August the suit against Renaudot was transferred from the Conseil du Roi to the prévôt of Paris. With this transfer Renaudot had essentially lost his case.[229]

In a final effort Renaudot appealed to the queen in *La requeste présentée à la Reyne*. This was answered by Patin in an *Examen de la requeste*. Renaudot replied to the *Examen*, but on December 9 he and his associates were ordered to cease their activities.[230]

A public session of parlement was held on 1 March 1644. Five lawyers represented Renaudot, his sons, the University of Montpellier, the Medical Faculty of Paris, and the University of Paris.[231] Chenvot, representing the faculty, attacked chemical medicine as no better than traditional medicine and as a system that ran the risk of killing some patients. He attacked Renaudot personally, noting that he had graduated too young by Parisian standards. Furthermore, he had created disorder in the medical profession. He was a protestant from Loudon, a town noted for devils. His given name was Théophraste, recalling not only the author

[225] Solomon (1972), pp. 179–80; Pilpoul (1928), p. 53.
[226] Solomon (1972), pp. 182–3.
[227] Ibid., p. 184.
[228] Ibid., p. 185.
[229] Ibid., p. 186.
[230] Ibid., pp. 186–7; Pilpoul (1928), p. 54.
[231] The trial is described by Solomon (1972), pp. 189–96.

of the ancient text of physiognomy but also Theophrastus Paracelsus, the originator of the chemical heresy in medicine. Beyond that, Renaudot was ugly and had a misshapen nose – unfortunate in a profession in which handsome practitioners were expected to inspire their patients. The legality of all his titles and offices were also questioned.

Renaudot's lawyer argued that scientific ideas were not proper for a legal case. More to the point was the argument that all of Renaudot's privileges had been accorded through the Conseil du Roi and that is where the case should be settled. But Renaudot no longer had significant support at court. Anne of Austria was hostile to him, and Richelieu's successor, Mazarin, was indifferent.

An arrêt of parlement demanded that Renaudot return his letters patent for the establishment of the Bureau d'Adresse. An inventory of its goods was to be made "in order to return and distribute them to whomever they belong."[232] He was allowed to keep his title as maître et intendant général des Bureau d'Adresse de France, but the title alone was meaningless. He was forbidden to practice medicine in Paris, but he was allowed to continue his publishing activities: The *Gazette* had been useful to the crown and it could remain so. On the other hand, the value of the public medical consultations he had established were recognized by an arrêt ordering the medical faculty to establish charitable consultations for the poor.

Needless to say, Patin was delighted. He composed two rondos *Sur le nez pourry de Theofraste Renaudot* and even commented on a quatrain of Nostradamus that seemed to prophesy this great victory of the faculty.[233] Happily he gloated that "Le pauvre diable est bien humilie."[234]

The triumph of antimony

With the father defeated and other successful actions taken against chemists, it finally seemed safe for the Parisian Medical Faculty to permit Isaac (1647) and Eusèbe (1648) to take their doctorates.[235] However, chemists and chemical physicians continued to publish, to the annoyance of Gui Patin and the traditional Galenists. A case of particular concern was that of Jean Chartier (1610–1662), a member of the faculty himself as well as professor of medicine at the Collège Royal, who wrote *La Science dv Plomb Sacre des Sages, ov l'Antimonie* (1651), in which he

232 Ibid., pp. 198–9.
233 [Gui Patin] [1644]. Here Patin referred to his adversary as an "Alchymiste, Charlatan, Empirique, vsvrier comme vn Iuif, perfide comme vn Turc, meschant comme vn Renegat, grand fourbe, grand Gazetier de France."
234 Pilpoul (1928), p. 55.
235 Solomon (1972), p. 217. Eusèbe (died 1679) was to become first physician to the Dauphin in 1672. His work on antimony (1653) is discussed later.

stated that although medicine was called the science of the gods by Hippocrates, chemistry was the part of medicine properly called the "Science Sacrée des Sages."[236] Antimony was known to the Hebrews, the Chaldeans, and the Arabs, and therefore should not be dismissed as a recent innovation in medicine. Nor was it a dangerous poison. Rather, it should be seen as the balm of life.[237] Even the medical faculty had recognized its value by including it in the *Codex*.[238]

For this breach of trust Chartier was attacked in a meeting of the full senate of the faculty by Dean Gui Patin and the Censors Jean Riolan, Jean Merlet, and René Moreau, all upholders of medical tradition. Chartier was saved from disgrace by François Vauthier (1589–1652), a physician of Montpellier and proponent of antimony, who was then the first physician to the king. However, with the death of Vauthier, Chartier was dismissed from his academic post and placed in prison.[239]

Chartier was attacked in print by Claude Germain, Doctor Regent en las Faculté de Medecine, in *Orthodoxe, ov de l'abus de l'Antimoine* (1652). Here Germain complained about the followers of Paracelsus, who had corrupted the purity of true medicine by their world view and their three principles. "To speak truly, I think it is foolish . . . to think that they would overturn the foundations of our philosophy and medicine in order to establish another one."[240] Yet, Germain was not as partisan as his colleague Patin because he believed that even Paracelsus was more judicious than his current followers.[241] As for chemistry, Germain considered it one of the most valuable parts of pharmacy because it had resulted in so many useful remedies. Those who sought to give it a divine origin had perhaps gone too far because they had taken too much of the credit from the Galenists. But those who rejected chemistry as an innovation did so unjustly because that would make it necessary to diminish the discovery of printing and the invention of paper, firearms, the compass, and the telescope; and in medicine one would have to condemn senna, rhubarb, and cassia because they had not been used by Hippocrates and Galen.[242]

Even the venerable Jean Riolan returned to the chemical battles in his *Cvrieuses Recherches svr les Escholes en Medecine, de Paris et de Montpelier* (1651), in which he again rehearsed the sins of the physicians of Montpellier. He noted with dismay that the alchemists had introduced their poisonous drugs into Paris in 1560.[243] These had come into com-

---

236 Jean Chartier (1651), pp. 2–3.
237 Ibid., p. 47.
238 Ibid., p. 51.
239 Pilpoul (1928), p. 64.
240 Claude Germain (1652), p. 224.
241 Ibid., p. 263.
242 Ibid., p. 392.
243 [Jean Riolan], (1651), p. 229.

mon use due partially to the recommendation of a Montpellier physician, de Launay. They had been rightly condemned at that time by the Parisian Medical Faculty, but Roch le Baillif, Pierre Paulmier, and others kept this medical heresy alive.[244] With each offense it had been necessary for the faculty to take action. Montpellier was defended by Isaac Cattier in 1653. He complained of Riolan's ignorance in not distinguishing between alchemy and chemistry. The latter's goal was the health of man. Cattier also made a distinction between the true and the false chemists, the latter being ignorant "puffers," greedy for gold, men who crowded the towns and filled their mansions with smoke, who ruined families and dishonored the art. The true chemist was a learned man, properly called a philosopher, who could be contrasted with the common sort of philosopher who did not have a real knowledge of nature.[245] Cattier also briefly related the history of the dispute over chemistry, emphasizing the inclusion of antimony in the *Codex*.[246]

The intensity of the debate increased when sixty-one members of the medical faculty signed a document attesting to the value of antimony (26 March 1652):

> We, the undersigned, Doctors of medicine of the Faculty of Paris, certify to all to whom it may concern, that the qualities of antimony are recognized by us to be very useful for the cure of a number of illnesses. We certify this on the basis of long usage and continual experience. Further we declare that this remedy which has for so long been charged with having a poisonous malignity has many rare virtues and that a physician can successfully employ it to combat a great number of diseases provided that he uses it with prudence and discretion.[247]

Among the signatories were Jean Chartier, Jean Thévart, and both Isaac and Eusèbe Renaudot.

François Blondel (ca. 1609–1682), who had taken his medical degree at Paris in 1632 and was no less opposed to the chemists than Patin, reacted against this declaration favoring antimony in a *Légende antimonial* (1653). Eusèbe Renaudot, on the other hand, used it defiantly to preface his extensive *L'Antimoine Ivstifié et L'Antimoine Triomphant . . .* (1653). Here Eusèbe distinguished the common chemists who sought only to isolate the three principles[248] from the "plus curieux artistes" who went on to prepare tinctures, waters, butters, oils, balms, and other necessary compounds for medicinal usage. These were the chemists who knew all the

244 Ibid., pp. 229–30.
245 Isaac Cattier (1653), pp. 194–5. Cattier received his medical degree at Montpellier in 1637 and practiced in Paris as médecin ordinaire to Louis XIV. He also wrote on the powder of sympathy (1651) and mineral waters (1663). Section CXXVIII (pp. 186–99) of his *Seconde Apologie* deals with "Charlatans, Chymiques."
246 Ibid., p. 195.
247 Eusèbe Renaudot [1653], sig. ē ii^r.
248 Ibid., p. 104.

possible antimonial preparations.[249] In a second section the author discussed the history of the debate, noting once again the decision to include "vin Emetique d'Antimoine" in the faculty's own *Codex*.[250]

L'Antimoine Ivstifié was attacked first by Jean Merlet in his *Remarques* (1654) and then by Jacques Perreau, Dr. Regent of the Medical Faculty, in his *Rabbat-Ioye de l'Antimoine Triomphant* (1654 and 1655).[251] Perreau noted that in the document supporting the use of antimony the signers did not include the dean, the censor, any of the previous deans, or the principal officers. Rather, they were a group of empirics, Paracelsists, and charlatans.[252] Antimony was a dangerous poison, the taking of which might well be compared with the taking of extreme unction.[253]

Gui Patin saw in this work of Eusèbe the treachery of his father, so he continued to speak out at any attempt to promote the use of chemistry in medical practice. Hearing that a new edition of Paracelsus was being prepared for publication at Geneva, he wrote (2 March 1655 to Falconel):

> What a shame that such a bad book is coming from the presses and the printers and that they cannot find something better: I would have preferred that they had printed the Koran which is not as dangerous and which at least would not deceive the whole world. *Chemistry is the false money of our trade.*[254]

An event in 1658 signaled the eventual closing of the debate. Louis XIV fell ill while he was with his army in Flanders.[255] He did not respond to the treatment prescribed by his physicians who proceeded to consult Du Sassoy, a local physician in Abbeville, who administered antimony to the king. The purge was a success, and Valot praised antimony as the cause of the cure. Gui Patin bitterly and angrily complained that in fact the king had had nine previous bloodlettings and that he was young and robust.[256]

In spite of repeated victories in the law courts, the old guard of the medical faculty was becoming less influential. On 18 December 1665 Jacques Thévart (1600–ca. 1674), who had earlier published on behalf of antimony and had been involved in a debate with François Blondel, requested that Parlement decree "the legal existence of antimony." The medical faculty met in full session to resolve the question; of the 102 physicians assembled, 92 voted in favor of placing *vin émétique* on the list of purgatives. On April 10 Parlement confirmed the decree.[257] Among

249 Ibid., p. 110.
250 Ibid., pp. 193–8.
251 Pilpoul (1928), pp. 74–7.
252 Jacques Perreau (1655).
253 Pilpoul (1928), p. 77.
254 Patin (1644), vol. 3, p. 47.
255 Pilpoul (1928), p. 82; Solomon (1972), p. 220.
256 Pilpoul (1928), p. 83.
257 Ibid., pp. 84–5; Solomon (1972), p. 220.

the dissenters, now reduced to a small minority, were Gui Patin and François Blondel. On 30 July 1666 Patin wrote that "these doctors say that a poison is not a poison in the hand of a good physician. They speak against their own experience because most of them have killed their wives, their children and their friends."[258] Like Patin, Blondel remained unrepentent and took legal action against Thévart and the new statutes and decrees of the medical faculty. An anonymous author attacked Thévart in a publication in 1655, and Thévart accused Blondel of writing the piece. This work identified the proponents of antimony as "heretics and disseminators of innovation and stated that antimony is a poison and that those who use it are ignorant empirics who do not know the good, true, and ancient dogmatic medicine."[259] Thévart replied once again that antimony had been known and used by the ancients.[260] Furthermore, the old decree of 1566 on which Blondel placed so much emphasis had proved injurious to chemistry in the new century.[261]

To be sure, occasional theses continued to be sustained both for and against antimony in the closing decades of the century, and Blondel was to reappear in opposition to antimony as late as 1681, but for practical purposes the antimony war had ended with the decree of the medical faculty of 29 March 1666.[262]

Conclusion

The century from 1566 to 1666 saw an almost continual debate between the chemists and the Galenists, the court physicians and the Medical Faculty of Paris, and between the medical schools of Paris and Montpellier. The Parisian Galenists repeatedly reaffirmed their claims through Parlement, and their members were quick to rise to any threat of medical heresy.

They forced Roch le Baillif to return to Brittany in 1579, and the statements favoring chemical medicine made by Joseph Duchesne and Theodore Turquet de Mayerne at the beginning of the seventeenth century were answered by the Jean Riolans, father and son. Members of the faculty who showed any tendency to favor chemical remedies, especially antimony, were censured or expelled, and the position of the faculty was unequivocally stated in the decree of 1615 forbidding the sale of chemically prepared drugs, in which antimony was singled out because of its special danger. For some people, the claims of the chemical philosophy seemed to go far beyond medicine. The Rosicrucian texts were viewed as

258 Pilpoul (1928), p. 87.
259 [Jacques Thévart] (ca. 1666), p. 8.
260 Ibid.
261 Ibid., p. 12.
262 For the debate in the period after 1666, see Pilpoul, pp. 87–93.

a threat to all persons interested in a new philosophy devoid of mysticism. These texts reflected an alchemical world view that Father Marin Mersenne was convinced had to be abandoned before a more mathematically oriented science could develop. Although he admitted the value of chemistry, he thought that this value was limited to the preparation of some medicines. It could not, and should not, be considered as the basis of a philosophy of nature.

There was debate over the proper role of chemistry. Fabre and de Rochas argued that only chemists could properly comprehend the created world about us. Others, such as Sarcilly, demanded a consistent chemical medicine and refused to compromise with a medicine that added a few chemical remedies to an essentially Galenic system. Riolan and many other Parisian physicians would not have gone even that far; for them chemical methods and remedies should play absolutely no part in either medical theory or *materia medica*.

Regardless of the unyielding position of the Parisian Medical Faculty, the interest in medical chemistry continued to grow. The Medical Faculty at Montpellier had long been known for its interest in chemistry, and French chemical physicians of the seventeenth century were almost invariably graduates of this school. Medical students at Paris who sought chemical knowledge could do so either through independent courses or – after the appointment of the first professor of chemistry, William Davisson, in 1648 – at the Jardin des Plantes. One wonders what would have happened to them if Gui Patin had caught them listening to these lectures. The Jardin des Plantes, founded due to the persistence of Guy de la Brosse, was to become a center for the teaching of chemistry in the late seventeenth and the eighteenth centuries. The failure of the Parisian Medical Faculty to prevent its establishment was a disappointment to many of its members.

A more dangerous rival to the Parisian Medical Faculty, Théophraste Renaudot's Bureau d'Adresse, developed in the 1630s. Available at the bureau were weekly conferences on all manner of scientific and medical questions, free medical consultations for the poor, and a professional welcome to religious and medical heretics. The medical emphasis on chemistry at the bureau was anathema to the medical faculty, and Renaudot's employment of physicians trained elsewhere ran counter to the strict control of the Parisian medical profession claimed by the faculty. A planned expansion of the bureau in 1640 led to a bitter suit against Renaudot, which he lost after the death of his patron, Cardinal Richelieu.

Although the Parisian Medical Faculty was triumphant at the humiliation of Renaudot in 1644, the victory did not last long. The old defenders of Galen led by Jean Riolan the younger and Gui Patin were aging, and the younger members were inclined to accept antimony and other chemical remedies. The cure of Louis XIV in 1658 with *vin émétique* signaled the end of the conflict, and antimony quickly became a fashionable cure among the wealthy. When antimony was proposed as an approved medicine in 1666, only ten percent of the assembled Parisian Medical Faculty opposed the motion.

But if there was a general acceptance of chemistry as an aid to medicine at this time, there remained a question as to its use as an explanation of physiological processes. This was a problem that was to develop in the remaining decades of the century among the followers of the Belgian physician and chemist, Jean Baptiste van Helmont (1579–1644).

4

Chemical continuity and the new philosophy

Le corps de l'animal est comme un de ces merveilleux fourneaux dans lesquels on peut faire à méme temps un grand nombre d'operations diverses. Chaque viscere est un vase dans lequel la Chymie naturelle prepare ses matieres . . .

Si la Chymie est si necessaire à la connoissance du petit monde, elle ne l'est pas moins à celle du grand. Il ne seroit pas mal-aisé de demonstrer qu'elle preside à la production des minereaux, des metaux, des vegetaux, des animaux, & de tous les phaenomenes qui paroissent dans l'Univers. Et si Platon avoit raison de dire que Dieu ne fait rien sans les regles de la Geometrie, on peut ajoûter qu'il ne produit rien sans celles de la Chymie.

Daniel Duncan (1683)[1]

Following the decisive victory of the chemists in the long battle over the internal use of chemically prepared medicines, pharmacopoeias of the late seventeenth century regularly included sections of approved chemicals; in fact, the chemical textbooks authored by the lecturers at the Jardin des Plantes and elsewhere were frequently little more than chemical pharmacopoeias themselves. However, by the middle decades of the seventeenth century a new debate had begun. Although chemistry was now well accepted by most of the members of the medical establishment – at least for its practical contribution to the *materia medica* – it was looked on as a rival philosophy by those mechanists who sought a basis for their new science in mathematics, the physics of motion, and mechanical analogies. Debate between these factions had been anticipated many years earlier in the exchange between Robert Fludd and his adversaries. There is little doubt that many of the members of the new scientific academies found themselves at odds with the chemical philosophers of their day, as did the Aristotelians and Galenists not too many years before.

---

[1] Daniel Duncan (1683), pp. **iv–**iir.

Van Helmont and a "new" chemical philosophy

For many of those interested in a new science during the seventeenth century, the chemical world view of Paracelsus and his immediate followers was unacceptable due to its mysticism. For Mersenne and his correspondents it was a chemistry too closely associated with religion and with an alchemical heritage far removed from the more sober experimental and mathematically oriented science they favored. These authors certainly had no more desire to uphold the authority of Aristotle and Galen than did the Paracelsians, but neither did they sympathize with the natural magic or the Hermeticism of the Renaissance.

Jean Baptiste van Helmont (1579–1644) was a chemical philosopher no less than Paracelsus, but to many of the savants of the middle decades of the seventeenth century his work presented a new philosophy that was comparable to the philosophies of Francis Bacon, René Descartes, and perhaps even Galileo.[2] Van Helmont was in effect the standard-bearer of a renovated chemical philosophy that was, at least temporarily, able to compete with the mechanical philosophy. Mersenne, the implacable foe of Paracelsus, Fludd, and the alchemists, saw in van Helmont a kindred soul who was interested in a rational chemistry that was a servant to medicine.

In the context of van Helmont's own time he was closer to his alchemical heritage than many people would have wished. Born in 1579 to a family that was both rich and influential, he studied classics and philosophy at the University of Louvain before going on to more advanced studies (1594). In his own account of his early life he tells us that he soon realized how little he actually understood. He had studied logic, natural philosophy, mathematics, and astronomy but had found little certainty or truth.

> Therefore having finished my Course, when as I knew nothing that was sound, nothing that was true, I refused the Title of Master of the Arts; being unwilling that Professors should play the fool with me, that they should declare me Master of the seven Arts, who was not yet a Scholar. Therefore I seeking truth, and knowledge, but not their appearance, withdrew my self from the Schooles.[3]

Although he declined taking his degree, van Helmont persevered in his courses. He listened to del Rio on magic and read the works of the ancient stoics as well as the medieval Christian mystics. These authors did not satisfy him, nor did the traditional medical texts.

---

[2] This sketch of the life and work of van Helmont is based primarily on the discussion in Debus (1977), vol. 2, pp. 295–379. I also referred to the more recent work by Walter Pagel (1982) and Robert Halleux (1979).

[3] Jean Baptista van Helmont, "Confessio authoris" (1648), ch. 2, sects. 1–5; reprinted (1966), pp. 11–12; (1662), p. 16.

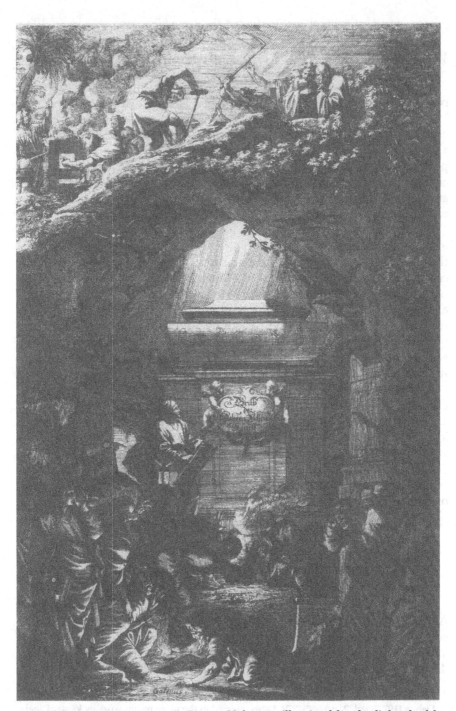

The Chemical Philosopher, J. B. van Helmont, illumined by the light shed by chemical knowledge. Galen, Avicenna, and their followers are left scratching in the dust for medical truths. Compare this illustration with that of medical harmony in the plate from Symphorien Champier (1516), in chapter 1. From J. B. van Helmont, *Aufgang der Artzney-Kunst* (1683). Courtesy of the University of Chicago Libraries.

At length, reading again my collected stuffe, I knew my want, and it grieved me of my pains bestowed, and years: When as indeed I observed, that all Books, as institutions, singing the same Song, did promise nothing of soundness, nothing that might promise the knowledge of truth, or the truth of knowledge.[4]

Nevertheless, at this point he accepted the degree of doctor of medicine (1599).[5]

Like many young men of his time van Helmont traveled and was well received at many courts. After his return to Brussels he married and resumed his studies. It was then that he found the work of Paracelsus, which at first seemed to be more rewarding than the other authors he had read.[6] He himself published nothing until he became involved in a debate over the efficacy of the weapon-salve.

This theory of cure was based on sympathetic action: If a man was wounded, it was argued, a salve or powder containing some of the man's blood would cure the wound if the salve or powder was applied to the weapon that had wounded him. Rudolf Goclenius accepted the cure as valid but ascribed it to purely natural causes in two publications that appeared in 1608 and 1613. A Jesuit, Jean Roberti, rejected the cure and wrote against Goclenius. At the same time Roberti sought support from others including van Helmont. In writing his first work, the *De magnetica vulnerum curatione* (1621), van Helmont found himself opposed to both Goclenius and Roberti. According to van Helmont, Goclenius had oversimplified the phenomenon; and Roberti, who had said that if such a remedy existed it could be nothing but black magic invented by the devil,[7] was a theologian. Theologians should mind their own business and not involve themselves in medicine or natural philosophy.

Nature . . . called not Divines for to be her Interpreters: but desired Physitians only for her Sons; and indeed, such only, who being instructed by the Art of the Fire, doe examine the Properties of things, by separating the impediments of their lurking Powers, to wit, their Crudity, Poysonousnesses, and Dregs, that is the Thistles and Thorns every where implanted into Virgin-Nature from the Curse: For seeing Nature doth dayly Distil, Sublime, Calcine, Ferment, Dissolve, Coagulate, Fix, &c. Certainly we also, who are the only faithful Interpreters of Nature, do by the same helps draw forth the Properties of things from Darkness into Light.[8]

In short, van Helmont told Roberti to "let the Divine inquire concerning God, but the Naturalist concerning Nature."[9] It was not a welcome

---

4 Van Helmont, "Confessio authoris" (ch. 2, sects. 14–15), *Ortus* p. 18; *Oriatrike*, p. 13.
5 Van Helmont, "Promissa authoris" (col. 3, sect. 7), *Ortus*, p. 12; *Oriatrike*, p. 7.
6 Van Helmont, "Promissa authoris" (col. 3, sects. 7–8), *Ortus*, p. 12; *Oriatrike*, p. 7.
7 Van Helmont, "De magnetica vulnerum curatione" (sect. 1), *Ortus*, p. 748; *Oriatrike*, p. 759.
8 Van Helmont, "De magnetica . . ." (sect. 8), *Ortus*, p. 750; *Oriatrike*, p. 761.
9 Van Helmont, "De magnetica . . ." (sect. 8), *Ortus*, p. 750 ("De Deo Theologus, naturalis verò de natura inquirat"); *Oriatrike*, p. 761.

message, neither was van Helmont's rejection of the cure as diabolical, nor his stated acceptance of the macrocosm–microcosm analogy, nor his belief that all substances are composed of salt, sulfur, and mercury. As for Paracelsus, van Helmont said that "he hath . . . snatch'd away the Denomination of the Monarch of Secrets, from all that went before him.[10] In reality, van Helmont felt that the powers attributed to saintly relics acted in a natural way. They were no less miraculous than the action of the weapon-salve.[11]

The *De magnetica vulnerum curatione* set in motion a series of events that were to plague van Helmont for the remainder of his life. The work was denounced by the medical faculty at his own University, Louvain, in 1623,[12] the same year that the Rosicrucian placards had appeared in Paris. And when van Helmont published a new work on the mineral waters at Spa, it seemed an attack on a widely lauded work on the same subject by the influential physician, Henry van Heer.[13] Van Heer responded and the two men met in a personal confrontation. None of van Helmont's actions were destined to win him friends.

His enemies extracted two dozen propositions from his work and submitted them first to a tribunal at Malines-Brussels and then to the Spanish Inquisition.[14] The propositions were shortly condemned for heresy and magic (1625). Van Helmont was interrogated on these propositions and three others taken from Paracelsus (1627). He duly asserted his innocence and submitted to the judgment of the Church, but he was censured by the faculty of theology at Louvain (1628) and by the college of physicians at Lyons (1629). He was forced to acknowledge his errors again in 1630 and in 1634 was arrested and placed first in an ecclesiastical prison and then in a minorite convent at Brussels before being assigned to house arrest for nearly two years.

In the course of his examination by the ecclesiastical court, van Helmont had been accused of departing from the true philosophy and of following the work of Paracelsus and his disciples. It was a charge that could be supported on the basis of his *De magnetica vulnerum curatione*. That he continued to maintain these views can be seen by examining his surviving correspondence with Mersenne (1630–1). Visiting Brussels in June 1630, the French savant consulted van Helmont concerning a se-

---

10 Van Helmont, "De magnetica . . ." (sect. 53), *Ortus*, p. 759; *Oriatrike*, p. 771.
11 Van Helmont, "De magnetica . . ." (sect. 46), *Ortus*, p. 757; *Oriatrike*, p. 769.
12 On van Helmont's troubles with the Church, see R. Halleux (1983); Pagel, *Van Helmont* (1982), pp. 8–13. Older accounts of the prosecution are Paul Nève de Mévergnies (1935), pp. 123–43; C. Broeckx (1849); C. Broeckx, (1856); Willem Rommelaere (1868); and A. J. J. Vandevelde (1929), pt. 1, pp. 453–76; (1929), pt. 2, pp. 715–37; (1929), pt. 3, pp. 857–79; (1932), pt. 4, pp. 109–22; (1936), pt. 5, pp. 339–87.
13 See Henricus van Heer (1614). Van Helmont's *Supplementum de Spadanis fontibus* appeared in 1624 and was reprinted in the Latin *Opera* (1648; 1966 reprint) and the English *Oriatrike* (1662).
14 On these developments, see Nève de Mévergnies (1935), pp. 123–30, and Marin Mersenne (1617–41, 1932–67), vol. 2, pp. 499, 589.

vere case of *herpes mordax*. Some fourteen letters survive, all dated over the following twelve months, which cover a range of topics from mechanics to theology. At the time, Mersenne was involved in his debate with Robert Fludd and must have been delighted with van Helmont's sharp criticism of the views of the English Hermeticist. However, van Helmont refused to accept the far-reaching attacks on Paracelsus that had been made by Goclenius, Erastus, and Libavius. He was convinced that Paracelsus had been a "nonpareil homme" who would in time be numbered among the greatest students of nature.[15]

In his customary fashion Mersenne queried van Helmont on numerous scientific matters relating to muscular fibers and the hardness of bodies,[16] the relationship of air to water,[17] and the force of projectiles.[18] Here van Helmont supported the three principles[19] and gave his observations on the relationship of weight to volume for metals. The letters reveal that ten years after writing the tract on the weapon-salve and in the midst of a potentially dangerous investigation by the Spanish Inquisition, van Helmont still defended Paracelsus and many of his views. When Mersenne asked for his opinion of the barrenness of the French queen and the need for an heir, van Helmont suggested that traditional remedies should be abandoned and replaced by more effective chemical preparations (29 March 1631).[20] Van Helmont was later to say that those who hated him called him a Paracelsian while those who thought highly of his work considered him an adept.[21] Yet, in 1631 when Mersenne addressed him as an adept, he replied, "I pray that you do not give me the title of Adept, because I do not deserve it."[22]

At the time of his death in 1644, van Helmont was still under the cloud of religious suspicion. He had managed to obtain an ecclesiastic imprimatur for his work on fevers (1642) and one other work, a collection of medical works titled *Opuscula medica inaudita* (1644) that appeared shortly before his death.[23] In his final illness he gave his manuscripts to his son, Franciscus Mercurius, asking him to arrange them for publica-

---

[15] Van Helmont (Brussels) to Mersenne (Paris), 19 Dec. 1630 in Mersenne, *Correspondance*, vol. 2 pp. 582–93 (585–6).

[16] Van Helmont (Brussels) to Mersenne (Paris), 11 Jan. 1631 in Mersenne, *Correspondance*, vol. 3, pp. 10–19.

[17] Van Helmont to Mersenne, 15 Jan. 1631 in Mersenne, *Correspondance*, vol. 3, pp. 31–50 (32).

[18] Van Helmont to Mersenne, 6 Feb. 1631 in Mersenne, *Correspondance*, vol. 3, pp. 74–94.

[19] Letter of Jan. 15 cited earlier (note 17), p. 32.

[20] Van Helmont to Mersenne, 29 March 1631 in Mersenne, *Correspondance*, vol. 2, pp. 151–5 (153). Nève de Mévergnies has examined these letters in his "Sur les lettres de J. B. Van Helmont au P. Marin Mersenne" (1948), 61–83.

[21] Van Helmont, "Praefatio" *Ortus*, p. 630; *Oriatrike*, p. 632.

[22] Van Helmont to Mersenne, 14 Feb. 1631 in Mersenne, *Correspondance*, vol. 3, pp. 95–109 (108).

[23] J. B. van Helmont (1642) and (1644). The latter includes (a) *De Lithiasi*, (b) *De febribus*, (c) *Scholarum humoristarum passiva deceptio atque ignorantia*, (d) *Appendix ad tractatum de febribus sive caput XVI et XVII*, and (e) *Tumulus pestis*.

tion.[24] The resultant *Ortus medicinae* (1648) included all of his previously unpublished works along with those few that had appeared during his lifetime. It is a massive volume of over one thousand pages that was published in six Latin editions down to 1707. In addition, there were translations into English (1662, 1664), French (1670, 1671), and German (1683). A Flemish compilation, probably prepared by van Helmont himself, appeared in 1659 and 1660. In addition, numerous tracts and segments from the opera were published separately throughout Europe.

The work of van Helmont appeared at a time when European savants were just beginning to digest the publications of Francis Bacon, René Descartes, and Galileo Galilei. To many, his work seemed to be an updated and more acceptable form of the chemical philosophy. To be sure, the *De magnetica vulnerum curatione* was reprinted in all the editions of the complete works, but with the exception of the *De magnetica* and the work on mineral waters, the texts seem to have been written after his investigation by the Inquisition had begun, and after he had repudiated his errors.[25] As a result, the great bulk of the published *Opera* presents a man who sought to distance himself from some of the dangerous positions he had taken in the tract on the weapon-salve. These later works show him to be critical of Paracelsus even though his influence is still evident. In any case, seventeenth-century chemists found it easy to separate the early from the later texts. Robert Boyle, referring primarily to his specific remedies, wrote that

> . . . I must confess to you once for all, that (always excepting his extravagant piece, *De magnetica vulnerum curatione*) I have not seen cause to disregard many things he delivers, as matters of fact, provided they be rightly understood; having not found him forward to raise remedies without cause, though he seem to do it sometimes without measure . . .[26]

In fact, the work of van Helmont combined elements of both old and new: a statement of the chemical philosophy and at the same time a "nova Philosophia."[27] On the one hand he described alchemical transmutation,[28] and on the other he emphasized quantification in his experimental work.[29] And if he still thought of chemistry as the key to natural

24 F. M. van Helmont, "Amico lectori," *Ortus*, sig. *1ᵛ; *Oriatrike*, sig. b2ᵛ.
25 It has been suggested on the basis of internal evidence that much of the work in the *Ortus medicinae* may date from his period of study at Vilvord (1609–16), but that most of the actual writing dates from the period after 1634 because no relevant manuscripts were found when his house was searched in that year. With the exception of the tract on the weapon-salve, the other works are generally quite critical of Paracelsus.
26 Robert Boyle (1772), vol. 2, p. 149.
27 Van Helmont, "Logica inutilis" (sect. 3); *Ortus*, p. 41; *Oriatrike*, p. 37.
28 Van Helmont, "Vita aeterna," *Ortus*, p. 743; *Oriatrike*, pp. 751–2. "Arbor vitae," *Ortus*, p. 793; *Oriatrike*, p. 807.
29 Debus (1977), vol. 2, pp. 327–9.

philosophy, he insisted that medicine was the proper goal of the sciences.

Above all, the work of van Helmont as arranged by his son seemed to offer a total philosophy of man and nature, which raised numerous questions of significance to those seeking a replacement for Aristotle and Galen. Like other Paracelsians, van Helmont was strongly opposed to the continued dominance of Aristotle and Galen at the universities. It was necessary to "destroy the whole natural Phylosophy of the Antients, and to make new the Doctrines of the Schooles of natural Phylosophy."[30] The ancients had gone wrong primarily in their attempt to apply mathematics to natural philosophy and medicine. Aristotle had "endeavoured to subdue Nature under the Rules of that Science [Mathematics]" and his disciple, Galen, had proceeded to apply this method erroneously to the study of man.[31]

Similarly, they had erred in their emphasis on the study of local motion and in their insistence that a mover is required for every motion. This had improperly encouraged application of mathematics to the study of nature and had led to Aristotle's belief "that in every locall motion, a first unmoveable Mover is of necessity to be appointed."[32] To thus confine the Creator could not be tolerated; it was evident then that the bases of ancient natural philosophy and medicine were fundamentally flawed. For van Helmont these errors could be avoided by accepting the fact that the Creator had placed a motive power in things. How else could we explain the beating of the heart or the motion of the tides?[33]

But if he rejected the application of mathematical method to the study of nature and if he showed little interest in the study of local motion, he spoke just as harshly about the macrocosm–microcosm analogy and astrology. Holy Scripture could not be denied, and the Creation account states that plants had been created prior to the stars.[34] Animals and men had been created later, so it was unthinkable that men should be subject to the stars while plants were not. Thus, except for the passages accepting the macrocosm–microcosm analogy in the early weapon-salve tract and in his letters to Mersenne, there is little in his works to support this concept.

> The name therefore of Microcosm or little World is Poetical, heathenish, and metaphorical, but not natural or true. It is likewise a phantastical, hypochondriacal, and mad thing, to have brought all the properties and

[30] Van Helmont, "Promissa authoris," *Ortus*, p. 6; *Oriatrike*, p. 1.
[31] Van Helmont, "Causae et initia naturalium" (sects. 38, 40), *Ortus*, p. 38; *Oriatrike*, p. 33. "Promissa authoris" (col. 1, sect. 3), *Ortus*, p. 7; *Oriatrike*, p. 2. The views of van Helmont on mathematics and motion are found (with additional points) in two papers: Debus (1968) and (1973).
[32] Van Helmont, "Blas humanum" (sect. 1), *Ortus*, p. 178; *Oriatrike*, p. 176.
[33] See the discussion of van Helmont's "Blas" in Debus (1977), vol. 2, pp. 314–15.
[34] Van Helmont, "Blas humanum" (sect. 5), *Ortus*, p. 180; *Oriatrike*, p. 177.

species of the Universe into man, and the art of healing: But the life of man is too serious, and also the medicine thereof, that they should play their own part of a Parable or Similitude, and metaphor with us.[35]

Although he was willing to admit that there appeared to be a relationship between man and the stars, he insisted that any such correspondence was indirect rather than direct.

By striking at mathematical method, the study of motion, and the macrocosm–microcosm analogy, van Helmont was distancing himself from both the ancients and the more mystical Paracelsians. And what of the elements? *Genesis* does not refer to the creation of fire, so fire must be rejected as an element. There are no "four elements" and "Therefore the fourfold kinde of Elements, Qualities, Temperaments or Complexions, and also the foundation of Diseases, falls to the ground."[36] In short, he said, the whole of ancient philosophy and medicine is based upon the four elements, and if even one of them is not a true element, then the entire superstructure falls.

Van Helmont argued against the elemental nature of earth as well and showed that a five-pound willow tree weighed over 169 pounds after five years, during which time only water had been added to it. "Therefore 164 pounds of Wood, Bark, and Roots, arose out of water onely."[37] Thus, water must be the primal element, a concept that seemed to be sustained by the fact that many earthy substances could be reduced to water.

As for the Paracelsian principles of salt, sulfur, and mercury, van Helmont recognized their usefulness because so many substances could be separated into three fractions; but he argued that heat had transformed the substances and that they did not exist as principles prior to the distillation: "as by a Trans-mutation made by the Fire, they are there generated, as it were new Beings, and there is made that, which was not before."[38] His belief that heat rearranged the components of a substance differed little from the critique of this method of analysis proposed by Thomas Erastus some seven decades earlier, but it also was a rejection of the Aristotelian belief that heat separates bodies into their components.

Fire might not be a proper key for analysis, but chemistry was indeed the key to an understanding of nature.

> I praise my bountiful God, who hath called me into the Art of the fire, out of the dregs of other professions. For truly, Chymistry, hath its principles not

35 Van Helmont, "Scabies & ulcera scholarum" (sect. 33), *Ortus*, p. 328; *Oriatrike*, p. 323.
36 Van Helmont, "Elementa" (sects. 9–10), *Ortus*, p. 53; *Oriatrike*, p. 48.
37 Van Helmont, "Complexionum atque mistionum elementalium figmentum" (sect. 30), *Ortus*, pp. 108–9; *Oriatrike*, p. 109. The experiment was not original with van Helmont. It is to be found in the fifteenth-century *Idiota* of Nicholas Cusanus (fourth book). For an ancient reference, see H. M. Howe (1965).
38 Van Helmont, "Tria prima" (sect. 47), *Ortus*, p. 405; *Oriatrike*, p. 408. I have discussed the history of fire analysis in Debus (1967).

gotten by discourses, but those which are known by nature, and evident by the fire: and it prepares the understanding to pierce the secrets of nature, and causeth a further searching out in nature, than all other sciences being put together: and it pierceth even unto the utmost depths of real truth: Because it sends or lets in the Operator unto the first roots of those things, with a pointing out the operations of nature, and powers of Art: together also, with the ripening of seminal virtues. For the thrice glorious Highest, is also to be praised, who hath freely given this knowledge unto little ones.[39]

Van Helmont believed in alchemical transmutation and gave an account of the transmutation of mercury to gold, which he accomplished with the aid of a sample of the philosopher's stone given to him by an adept.[40] He also presented an alchemical dream sequence as an introduction to his tract "Potestas medicaminum."[41] At the same time he described the *alkahest*, a universal solvent,[42] and he was convinced that there existed a universal remedy capable of curing any illness.

Although chemical tradition may have led him to reject mathematical abstraction in the interpretation of natural phenomena, he did not reject the use of weights and measures in the chemical laboratory. We have already mentioned van Helmont's letter to Mersenne on specific weights; he applied the same method to the comparison of equal volumes of urine, thus applying quantification to medical uroscopy.[43] Van Helmont used the barometer/thermometer of his time to measure heat but demanded a more precise scale than had been used earlier.[44] He also accepted the principles of conservation of weight and the indestructibility of matter.[45] Although his explanation was complex and basically incorrect, he accepted the vacuum – once again in opposition to the Aristotelian position.[46]

Van Helmont's cosmology was traditional, not just because the Copernican system conflicted with the Church system but also because he feared that should it be accepted, it would "ruine all apparitions in the

[39] Van Helmont, "Pharmacopolium ac dispensatorium modernorum" (sect. 32), *Ortus*, p. 463; *Oriatrike*, p. 462.

[40] Van Helmont, "Vita aeterna," *Ortus*, p. 743; *Oriatrike*, pp. 751–2. At the start of the "Arbor vitae" van Helmont stated that he had transmuted mercury to gold "distinctis vicibus." *Ortus*, p. 793; *Oriatrike*, p. 807.

[41] Van Helmont, "Potestas medicaminum" (sect. 3–4), *Ortus*, p. 471; *Oriatrike*, pp. 470–1.

[42] Van Helmont, "Explicatio aliquot verborum artis," *Opuscula*, sig. A4^v; *Oriatrike*, sig. Nnnnn 4^v.

[43] Van Helmont, "Scholarum humoristorum passiva deceptio atque ignorantia" (ch. 4, sect. 31), *Opuscula*, p. 108; *Oriatrike*, p. 1056. In the *Idiota*, Cusanus suggested that a physician might give a more valid judgment of urine "by both weight and colour than by color alone, which may be misleading" (1962), p. 243.

[44] Van Helmont, "Calor efficienter non digerit, sed tantum excitative" (sect. 35), *Ortus*, p. 206; *Oriatrike*, p. 202. Van Helmont's views on the thermoscope and the degrees of heat are discussed by Partington (1962), vol. 2, p. 220.

[45] See the discussion and pertinent references in Debus (1977), vol. 2, p. 329.

[46] Ibid., pp. 329–34.

Heaven, and Predictions."[47] Although he rejected the influence of the stars on earth, he did believe that they contained the knowledge of the future. For this reason they could be "read" for future events.[48] He believed the earth to be an oval or "egg-shaped" body made basically of flint, through which there was a constant circulation of waters.[49] Here he opposed the older concept of a central fire. He thus could not use the distillation analogy as a means of explanation for mountain streams, but his model proved useful for explaining salt deposits and even fossils in the earth.[50]

Van Helmont, no less than any Aristotelian, was a vitalist. For him all things in the universe were living things. The earth was like a womb filled with the seeds of minerals.[51] When a seed found its proper matrix, it would ferment and grow into the appropriate metal or mineral. The process was basically one of watery substance being acted on by a seed containing an archeus through fermentation. It was clearly an adaptation of the older alchemical concept of metallic growth, which he compared with the growth of plants and animals. It is hardly surprising that later Helmontians should seek out examples of immature minerals in mines in support of their position.

Van Helmont believed that he was presenting a new philosophy, but like the Paracelsians before him, he had a special interest in medicine. He too cited *Ecclesiasticus*, chapter 38 to establish the semidivine nature of the physician, created by God.[52] Unfortunately, the medicine of the schools had been developed by Greeks, Arabs, and Jews, men who were not Christians and sought only personal gain. According to van Helmont, these men could not be true physicians because they had not been summoned by God to this profession.[53]

The medicine of the ancients was based on the four humors and the four temperaments, which in turn were based on the four elements. But since the elements did not consist of four entities, van Helmont maintained that the humors and the temperaments could not exist as a

47 Van Helmont, "Astra necessitant; non inclinant, nec significant de vita, corpore vel fortunis nati" (sect. 48), *Ortus*, p. 127; *Oriatrike*, p. 126.
48 Van Helmont, "Astra necessitant" (sect. 13), *Ortus*, p. 120; *Oriatrike*, p. 121.
49 Van Helmont, "Aqua" (sects. 13–15), *Ortus*, pp. 59–60; *Oriatrike*, pp. 55–6.
50 Van Helmont, "Aqua" (sects. 5–9), *Ortus*, p. 55; *Oriatrike*, p. 51. The similar model of Seneca (in the *Naturales quaestiones*) is described in R. J. Forbes (1963), vol. 7, pp. 8–9. Van Helmont discusses the fossil elephant jaw found at "Hingsen, near Scalds" in "Terra" (sect. 17), *Ortus*, p. 56; *Oriatrike*, p. 52.
51 Debus (1977), vol. 2, pp. 339–43.
52 Van Helmont, "De lithiasi" (Philiatro lectori"), *Opuscula*, p. 4; *Oriatrike*, sig. Nnnnn 2ᵛ. This is van Helmont's most thorough treatment of the text of Ecclesiasticus, yet he mentions it throughout the *Opera*. See also the "Tumulus pestis" (Ch. 1), *Opuscula*, pp. 5, 8; *Oriatrike*, pp. 1074, 1076; "Promissa authoris" (col. 2, sect. 6), *Opuscula*, p. 10; *Oriatrike*, p. 6.
53 Van Helmont, "De lithiasi" ("Philiatro lectori"), *Opuscula*, p. 5; *Oriatrike*, sig. Nnnnn 3ʳ.

quaternary either.[54] Van Helmont also rejected the ancient theory of catarrh, which explained that vapors from the stomach condensed in the brain and then flowed down through the inner organs, resulting in pneumonia, consumption, rheumatism, and gout.[55] Van Helmont showed anatomically that no such flow was possible.

He also developed the earlier Paracelsian concept of the archeus, the life force of specific organs. Van Helmont argued that invading disease-semen with their own archei could lodge in an organ and wage battle for control.[56] Depending on the outcome of battle, the result would be health, disease, or death.

Among specific problems of concern to van Helmont was his search for a dissolvent for bladder stones or urinary calculi.[57] Only acids seemed to be effective, but they lost their effect when taken by mouth and were too painful when introduced into the bladder directly through a catheter. Van Helmont did develop a less painful catheter than had been in use before.

Convinced of the importance of the vital spirit, van Helmont, like Fludd and others, sought to isolate it. For him, the answer seemed to lie in the distillation of arterial blood. He noted the similarity of the "salt" obtained from blood and from urine, but he was convinced that the two were different because "the Spirit of the Salt of Venal Blood cureth the Falling-sickness, but the Spirit of the Salt of Urin not so."[58] Van Helmont also opposed bloodletting because of the essential nature of the life spirit.[59]

In writing of the digestive process,[60] van Helmont noted his observations on the effect of acid on a leather glove; he described the process of osmosis, which he then applied to physiological processes in the small intestine. It was also in his consideration of the digestive process that he observed the neutralization that occurs in the small intestine through the action of the bile. Here "the Cream sliding out of the *Pylorus* . . . into the *Duodenum* . . . doth exchange its sourness into Salt . . ."[61]

---

54 Van Helmont, "Scholarum humoristarum passiva deceptio atque ignorantia" (ch. 1, sect. 3), *Opuscula*, p. 70; *Oriatrike*, p. 1017. See also the "Natura contrarium nescia" (sect. 1), *Ortus*, p. 164; *Oriatrike*, p. 161.

55 This is the primary concern of Walter Pagel (1930). See also Pagel (1982) pp. 134–7. The major text is van Helmont, "Catarrhi deliramenta," *Ortus*, pp. 426–47; *Oriatrike*, pp. 429–50. A second English translation is that of Walter Charleton (1650).

56 Van Helmont, "De lithiasi" (ch. 5, sect. 5), *Opuscula*, p. 30; *Oriatrike*, p. 859.

57 Debus (1977), vol. 2, pp. 362–5. The search for a dissolvent for the stone was to remain a high-priority medical goal for many years. It was the reason for the quantitative research by Joseph Black on magnesia alba more than a century later.

58 Van Helmont, "Aura vitalis," *Ortus*, pp. 726–8; *Oriatrike*, pp. 733–4.

59 Van Helmont, "De febribus" (ch. 4), *Opuscula*, pp. 17–25; *Oriatrike*, pp. 949–57. The subject has been covered intensively in P. H. Niebyl (1972), vol. 2, pp. 13–23.

60 Debus (1977), vol. 2, pp. 368–71.

61 Van Helmont, "Sextuplex digestio" (sect. 56), *Ortus*, p. 220; *Oriatrike*, p. 217.

This is, in modern terms, a statement of acid–base neutralization, a concept he was to use elsewhere. Thus, he noted that diuretics are generally alkaline because "in every Wound, a Tartnesse or Acidity . . . doth arise: the which *Alcalies* do easily sup up into themselves, and consume."[62] And again, here writing on the effect of fire in substances, he observed that new things could be produced that were not present originally, either acids or alkalis, while "now and then, the things themselves, together with their adjuncts, are diversly transcharged by the Fire, and become neutral."[63] This acid–base dualism was to prove highly influential among later iatrochemists.

Like the Paracelsians before him, van Helmont rejected the dictum that contraries cure, which was based on the quaternary elements and humors. Health in Galenic medicine was based on the balancing – or, as van Helmont expressed it, the warfare – of opposites to produce a mean. But for him this idea was part of the mathematical error of past theory. Rather we should seek health in harmony and integrity.[64] Neither was van Helmont satisfied by cure by similitude: He rejected the idea that poisons might be overcome by similar poisons, arguing that they were overcome by specific medicinal powers "which do neither bear a contrariety, or character of hostility, mutually toward themselves, nor towards Diseases."[65] He called for a search for the inherent virtues of substances, of which little of value had been discovered so far by physicians, apothecaries, or even by gifted men such as Duchesne who sought the signatures of things.[66] The true virtues would eventually be found through chemistry and the proper use of the fire. He carefully noted the common arguments against the use of chemicals and then refuted them.[67] At the same time he was aware of the danger of chemical medicines and wrote of the need for small dosages,[68] and he wholly dismissed some purgatives such as mercury and antimony as being too violent.[69] However, van Helmont did not compile a list of chemical remedies that could serve as a chemical pharmacopoeia.

The complete works of van Helmont, which appeared first in 1648, were widely read and were influential, but they gave mixed signals to

62 Van Helmont, "De lithiasi" (ch. 5, sect. 17), *Opuscula*, p. 45; *Oriatrike*, p. 863.
63 Van Helmont, "Potestas medicaminum" (sects. 36, 37), *Ortus*, p. 479; *Oriatrike*, pp. 477–8.
64 Van Helmont, "Natura contrarium nescia" (sects. 11 *seq.*), p. 167; *Oriatrike*, pp. 163–4.
65 Van Helmont, "Tria prima chymicorum principia" (sects. 42, 43), *Ortus*, p. 404; *Oriatrike*, p. 407.
66 Van Helmont, "Pharmacopolium ac dispensatorim modernum" (sects. 13, 14), *Ortus*, p. 459; *Oriatrike*, p. 459.
67 Van Helmont, "De febribus" (ch. 15, sects. 1–25), *Opuscula*, pp. 53–8; *Oriatrike*, pp. 989–92 (992 incorrectly numbered as 1002).
68 Van Helmont, "De febribus" (ch. 15, sect. 5), *Opuscula*, p. 55; *Oriatrike*, p. 991 (991 incorrectly numbered as 971).
69 Van Helmont, "De febribus" (ch. 8, sect. 6), *Opuscula*, p. 38; *Oriatrike*, p. 971.

the scholars of the period. Here was to be found a blanket rejection of ancient medicine and natural philosophy coupled with the call for a new philosophy – to this extent he was in agreement with Bacon and Descartes – but though he was critical of Paracelsus, like him van Helmont thought of medicine as the chief science with chemistry as its key. Overall, van Helmont did offer a new philosophy even though he borrowed many ideas from other writers. Some French chemical physicians were influenced by his call for fresh observations and quantification and by his chemical explanations of physiological processes, whereas others turned to specific medical problems that he had addressed; but, always, a few saw his work primarily as a justification for alchemy, pointing to his reported personal experience of transmutation, his description of the universal solvent, and his belief in a universal medicine for all diseases.

Van Helmont and the French

If Mersenne found in van Helmont a kindred soul from whom he sought scientific and medical information, Gui Patin saw in him only a "mechant fripon."[70] Writing on 16 April 1645, shortly after van Helmont's death, Patin called him a wicked Flemish rascal who had never written anything of value. Patin would not retreat on this statement, because having seen all of his work, he found that van Helmont's medicine was based on the secrets of chemists and empirics. Moreover, he had rejected bloodletting and had died raving mad for the lack of it.[71] Learning of a new edition of van Helmont's works in 1654, Patin commented that it was necessary for fools to have their books no less than the wise.[72]

Patin's estimate of van Helmont was seconded by Gabriel Fontaine of the Medical College of Marseilles, the son of Jacques Fontaine (d. 1621) who had written against Paracelsian element theory (1581) and magic (1613). In his lengthy *De Veritate Hippocraticae Medicinae . . . seu Medicina Antihermetica . . . contra Paracelsi . . .* (1657) Fontaine included a detailed refutation of van Helmont. In a short prefatory history of medicine[73] Fontaine spoke of the true medicine of the ancients to which the Arabs had added much useful material. This had been amplified in medieval Europe by discoveries in the application of chemistry to pharmacy. He praised the work of Albertus Magnus, Arnald of Villanova, Ramon Lull, and later authors such as Guinter von Andernach, Johann Hartmann, and others who had confined chemistry to the preparation of medicines. He noted how different those authors were from the avowed Paracelsists such as Joseph Duchesne, Oswald Croll, Claude Dariot, and Jean Bap-

[70] Letter dated 6 April 1661. Gui Patin (1846), vol. 2, p. 461.
[71] Letter dated 16 April 1645. Ibid., vol. 1, p. 355.
[72] Letter dated 20 February 1654. Ibid., vol. 2., p. 114.
[73] D. Gabrielis Fontani (1657), sig. ē iv$^{r.v.}$

tiste van Helmont, whose writings abounded with paradoxes, absurdities, and signs of delirium. Paracelsus had been a damned magician who had added elements of the diabolic art to medicine. His books had been refuted by Erastus and censured by the Roman Church.

In his defense of Hippocratic medicine Fontaine asserted the truth of the Aristotelian elements[74] and discussed the question of cure by contraries,[75] the use of incantations in medicine,[76] and the use of chemistry as a means of preparing medicines.[77] He concluded that chemistry was indeed useful but that antimonial spirits and the sulfur of arsenic were extremely poisonous and should be avoided.[78] Fontaine opposed sympathetic medicine and specifically opposed van Helmont's tract on the magnetic cure of wounds.[79] Noting van Helmont's attack on both the elements and the humors, Fontaine asserted the truth of both before refuting van Helmont on fevers, epilepsy, convulsions, and apoplexy.[80]

It was the Helmontian position on fevers that brought about the first real debate of his medical theories in France.[81] The Galenists believed in a febrile matter that is putrid and hot due to the effect of decay. Van Helmont had not denied the existence of such a matter, but for him it was not putrid. Rather, it was nonvital matter that enters the body and is hostile to the archeus of the body. The archeus expels this matter by means of fever, directing blood to the site of the foreign matter (such as a thorn imbedded in the skin), which therefore becomes overheated. In the case of a high fever or "tremulous rigor," the archeus actually attempts to shake off the unwanted matter. Contractions may occur as well as alternate attacks of fever and chill with sweating. From this, van Helmont said, the physician can recognize the value of sweating and the need for proper medicine to induce it. Van Helmont, opposing the bloodletting used by Galenists as a means of removing putrid matter and cooling, argued that this practice resulted in a diminution of the blood volume and of the vital spirit.[82]

Van Helmont's treatise on fevers was first published separately in 1642 and then reprinted in 1644 as part of the *Opuscula*. Eight years later it was translated into French by Abraham Bauda, a master surgeon of Sedan, as the *Doctrine Novvelle . . . Tovchant les Fievres*. In his introduc-

---

[74] Ibid., pp. 1ff.
[75] Ibid., pp. 149ff.
[76] Ibid., p. 178.
[77] Ibid., pp. 191ff.
[78] Ibid., p. 210.
[79] Ibid., pp. 183–91.
[80] Ibid., pt. 2, beginning p. 245.
[81] Pagel discussed both the ancient and the Helmontian views on fever in his *van Helmont* (1982), pp. 154–9. I have followed his work on this.
[82] Pagel notes that van Helmont had been anticipated in his views on fever by Gomez Pereira (1558) and Tommasso Campanella (1635) who believed that fever itself was not a disease but was a natural cure. See ibid.

tion Bauda attacked Galenic humoral theory and commented that although van Helmont had been born subject to the king of Spain, his work was changing Spanish arrogance to French civility.[83]

Bauda's translation was criticized by J. Didier, a physician of Sedan, who asked why van Helmont should have wanted to overturn the medical teachings of the ancients. For Didier the only answer was the Belgian's vain search for personal glory.[84] He noted that van Helmont had accused Paracelsus of relying on the macrocosm–microcosm analogy. But why then, in his tract on the Blas had van Helmont made comparisons between man and the great world?[85] For instance, van Helmont had compared the sun in the macrocosm with the heart in man, and the earth with "the liver in man which nourishes all parts of the body. And the sea is nothing else than those great vessels which contain a vast quantity of blood which flows through all parts as if they were branches of rivers. In this way the humor (blood) returns finally to the place from which it first departed."[86]

Didier criticized van Helmont also for his application of chemistry to medicine, pointing particularly to the emphasis on mineral and metallic preparations rather than the milder traditional medicines from plants and animals.[87] Didier opposed the use of poisons as cures, even in small quantities. Van Helmont, he said, had sought his medicines from mines, the home of demons who impressed their malignity onto the minerals they lived with.[88] How could van Helmont suggest that when properly prepared these substances would be sweet as sugar? Surely fire did not diminish their corrosive and poisonous nature.

Van Helmont's views were surely known to French physicians in the middle decades of the seventeenth century through the translations of Bauda, the short-lived debate over the theory of fevers, and various other ways. Bernard Joly has clearly established the Paracelsian influences on Pierre-Jean Fabre, but he has also shown that Fabre's later works reflected van Helmont's concept of the archeus, the alkahest, and the theory of the plague. Fabre never referred to van Helmont by name, perhaps because of the Church action against him.[89]

No extensive translation from the work of Van Helmont was made until 1670 when Jean le Conte prepared a French edition of *Les Oevvres*. Of the translator we know very little though he referred to himself as a doctor of medicine.[90] His edition was a severely edited version of the

[83] Jean Baptiste van Helmont (1652), sig. ii[v].
[84] J. Didier (1653) sig. ¢ iii[r].
[85] Ibid., p. 358.
[86] Ibid., p. 359.
[87] Ibid., p. 370.
[88] Ibid., p. 371.
[89] Bernard Joly (1990).
[90] He may be the Joannes Franciscus Le Conte who is listed as the author of a *Clavis*

Ortus medicinae and the *Opuscula*. The original, in most editions more than one thousand pages of Latin, was reduced to some three hundred and fifty pages in French. Although some tracts were followed closely, most were presented in abstract form or rewritten into an entirely new format.

In his introduction le Conte wrote that he had undertaken his work for the benefit of the curious who could read van Helmont better in translation than in Latin, and for surgeons and apothecaries.[91] He asked the Galenists why, if medicine had been in a state of perfection since antiquity, physicians were still unable to cure quartan fevers and other chronic illnesses.[92] He wrote that far too many of the sciences were ruled by presumptious people who blindly believed that they could know no more than they knew already, and by the opinionated who were slaves to their own conceptions. Such people were incapable of learning anything new.[93] Chemistry, he said, is an important new addition to medicine that is not to be feared or rejected, and even if some chemists do indeed recommend dangerous purgatives and violent vomatives, this was not the case with van Helmont, who preferred a class of medicines prepared with the alkahest, a universal solvent by which all solid bodies were purified of their poisons and totally resolved into their first matter.[94]

Le Conte's introduction summarized the Helmontian system, beginning with a rejection of the four elements and turning instead to van Helmont's elemental water and the seminal spirit before going on to a discussion of generation and fermentation.[95] In his praise of van Helmont, le Conte also urged caution. He recognized the importance of chemistry but warned against violent purges.[96] Like van Helmont himself he admitted having once been attracted to the work of Paracelsus, which he now found "remplie d'inconstance, d'obscurité, & de jactance."[97]

Le Conte's translation was reprinted in 1671, but though van Helmont's work was well known in France by that time, few additional translations were made. An exception was the *Avis de Vanhelmont, svr La Composition des Remedes* (1680), prepared by Jacques Massard, Doctor Aggregate at the College of Medicine at Grenoble. Massard thought that the work of van Helmont did indeed conform to the true medical doctrines of Hippocrates,[98] and in his *Avis* he summarized the Helmontian

Hermetica, seu metallorum mineraliumque legitima solutio (1680) and an . . . *opuscula nova medica* (1690) in the British Library catalog.

91 Jean Baptiste van Helmont (1671), p. 5.
92 Ibid., p. 4.
93 Ibid., p. 1.
94 Ibid.
95 Ibid., pp. 5–6.
96 Ibid., p. 29.
97 Ibid., p. 31.
98 Iacqves Massard (1680), pt. 2, p. 65.

treatise *Pharmacopolium ac Dispensatorium modernum*. In the preface to this work he attacked the medicines commonly found in the shops of the apothecaries, complaining that many of these were poisonous, including the regulus of antimony. He thought that physicians should learn how to make their own prescriptions and that the study of medicine should not be separated from pharmacy or chemistry.[99]

The alchemical tradition

Both van Helmont's alkahest and his personal testimony of transmutation appealed to authors who were more interested in traditional alchemy than in medicine, and alchemy remained a subject of intense interest in most of Europe during the seventeenth century.

No less convinced of the truth of transmutation than van Helmont himself was his younger contemporary, Johann Rudolph Glauber (ca. 1603–ca. 1670), a German who lived most of his life in the Netherlands.[100] He was well known for his detailed descriptions of high-temperature furnaces and the chemical substances he distilled and manufactured in his laboratories. Like van Helmont, Glauber rejected the authority of the ancients and stressed the importance of chemistry as the key to natural philosophy. He was contemptuous of the universities and those physicians who graduated from them:

> . . . I never frequented the Universities, nor ever had a mind to do so; for should I have so done, haply I should never have arrived to that knowledge of Nature, which I mention without boasting, as I now possess; neither doth it ever repent me, that I have put my hands to the Coals, and have by the help of them penetrated into the knowledge of the Secrets of Nature . . .[101]

Glauber referred frequently to the traditional alchemists and metallurgists but praised Paracelsus above all others. Along with other Paracelsians he relied on Genesis as a basis for understanding the elements and wholeheartedly embraced the macrocosm–microcosm analogy. A thoroughgoing vitalist, Glauber discussed the generation of metals in the earth, arguing that it was essential to understand this process if one was to perfect them in the laboratory. Indeed, in his *Prosperity of Germany* (1656–61), Glauber proposed a series of schemes that would make Germany self-sufficient in good times and bad.[102] Among these was the suggestion that the country's extensive mines be further exploited for the base metals and minerals because he would be able to teach his countrymen how these could be purified by the judicious use of salt-

---

99 Ibid., pp. 67–70.
100 I have discussed Glauber at greater length in my *Chemical Philosophy* (1977), vol. 2, pp. 425–41.
101 Johann Rudolph Glauber (1689), p. 307.
102 Debus (1977), vol. 2, pp. 434–41.

peter, which eliminated unnecessary volatile sulfur. Thus, it would be possible to prepare the precious metals profitably by alchemical means on a commercial scale. He promised to discuss his processes openly but refused to impart his greatest secrets to the public because he had been betrayed when he had given them away in the past.

In mid-century Glauber was looked upon by many as the equal of van Helmont. His works were available not only in German but also in English, Latin, and French. In 1659 the French translator, Bernard Du Teil, published Glauber's famous work on furnaces and a group of his tracts on alchemy, the universal medicine, and potable gold. Du Teil argued for the importance of chemistry, which he said surpassed all of the work of Aristotle because through it the operator could penetrate into the most hidden places and expose them to view.[103] Aristotle had only analyzed words in his rules of logic, but Glauber showed that chemistry with the philosopher's stone made possible the perfection of the base metals to gold and taught the preparation of chemical oils, spirits, salts, and essences, which were far more effective than the potions of common medicine.[104] Chief among Glauber's medicinal preparations was the universal medicine, the true potable gold.

Among the many alchemical texts of this period was the Paracelsian *Novum inauditum Medicinae Universalis Speculum Cabalisto-Chymicum* by George Figulus, which was printed at Brussels in 1660.[105] Directed less at medicine was D'Atremont's *Le Tombeau de la Pauvreté. Dans lequel il est traité clairement de la transmutation des Metaux* . . . (1681)[106] and Jacobus Tollius' *La chemin du ciel chymique* (1688), in which we read that the cost of the philosopher's stone would be no more than three or four florins, that it could be made in three or four days, and that the work required no more equipment than an earthen pot.[107] Marc-Antonio Crasselame wrote *La Lumiere sortant par soy même des Tenebres* (1687), a work in stanzas.[108] Ludovicus de Comitibus prepared a discourse that dealt with the alkahest and the universal medicine (1669), in which he argued that van Helmont had learned of the alkahest from his study of Paracelsus.[109] Written originally in Latin, this work was to go through many editions into the eighteenth century.

Limojon de Saint Didier (1630–1690) published a *Lettre d'un Philosophe sur le Secret du Grand Oeuvre* in 1686, but he is known best for the collection *Le Triomphe Hermétique*, which appeared posthumously and was written in the form of a dialogue between Gold and the Philoso-

103 Johann Rudolph Glauber (1659), sig. ã ii^r–v.
104 Ibid., sig. ã ii^v – ã iii^r.
105 Georgius Figulus (1660).
106 D'Atremont (1681).
107 Jacobus Tollius (1688), p. 6.
108 Fra Marc-Antonio Crasellame (1687).
109 Ludovicus de Comitibus (1669), p. 5.

phers' Stone (1699).[110] The *Traité Philosophique de la Triple Preparation de l'Or et de l'Argent* and the *De la Droite et Vraie maniere de produire la Pierre Philosophique, ou le sel argentifique & aurifique* were written by Gaston le Doux (De Claves). Here the reader was immediately alerted to the author's goal: "The purpose and the end of Argropée and Chrysopée, that is to say, the Art of Silver and Gold, is to produce Silver and Gold."[111] To help guide the reader through the complexities of the processes it was published with a *Dictionnaire Hermetique, Contenant L'Explication des Termes, Fables, Enigmes, Emblemes & manieres de parler des vrais Philosophes*, in which were over two hundred pages of definitions of alchemical terms.

A collection of alchemical classics including the *Emerald Table of Hermes*, the *Turba philosophorum*, and texts by Nicholas Flamel, Bernard Trevisan, Denis Zachaire, Wenceslaus Lavinius, Philalethes, and others appeared in French translation in 1671, and a second volume appeared seven years later. The compiler/translator is unknown, though the volumes have been ascribed to William Salmon. Two additional volumes were added in a new edition printed in the mid-eighteenth century.

In a lengthy preface to this collection, the reader was told that it was important to make available to the public the works of the alchemical masters because their wisdom led both to legitimate riches and assured health, without which other goods were useless. The author defined chemistry as "an Art, or a practical Science which teaches how to resolve mixed bodies into their natural principles, and by this means to render them more pure and efficacious to serve Medicine or to perfect the imperfect metals."[112] In short, the purpose of alchemy was first to prepare remedies, extracts, salts, and essences from the three kingdoms of nature for medical purposes and second to prepare the philosophers' stone "by means of which the imperfect metals are converted into Silver and Gold."[113] That the latter could be accomplished should not be doubted. Were there not circumstantial accounts of transmutation by trustworthy authors such as Alexander Seton, Jean Baptiste van Helmont, and Nicholas Flamel?

And if it had to be admitted that there were alchemical charlatans, the chemists as a whole could be compared

> to those who seek a passage to the Indies where they hope to enrich themselves with the gold, silver, pearls and precious stones which are there in abundance. But, being led astray in their route, they discovered islands and countries which until now have been unknown to us in Eu-

[110] I have referred to the following two editions: Limojon de Saint-Didier (1971) and (1707).
[111] Gaston le Doux (1979), p. 3 (separate pagination).
[112] Sieur, S. D. E. M. (1672), p. ã vʳ.
[113] Ibid.

rope. And although they did not find what they sought, they have found instead drugs and other goods which had never been seen before and which have proved to be very useful to men.[114]

A more unusual treatise is *Les avantvres dv philosophe inconnv en l'inuention de la Pierre Philosophale* (1646), ascribed to Jean Albert Belin (ca. 1610–1677).[115] In addition to this work, which went through three French editions up to 1709 and a German translation, Belin was the author of a work on the powder of sympathy (1658), a treatise on talismans, and an *Apologie dv grand oevvre* (1659).

The *Adventures of the Unknown Philosopher* was an alchemical picaresque novel in which the hero, having heard of the wonders of the philosophers' stone, leaves his home to search for it. He arrives in a major city, and hearing that an old woman possesses the secret of its preparation, he goes to visit her. She falls in love with him and promises to show him the process if he will marry her. He manages to avoid this fate, but they begin their work nevertheless, only to have it destroyed when the chimney falls on the vessels. After this the philosopher continues his journeys, meeting with numerous adventures and accidents. On his way he encountered false philosophers but eventually meets one who teaches him the true secret of the philosopher's stone. This is an amusing book that clearly attacks the alchemical charlatan.

Critics of alchemy included the Sieur Lussauld, Councillor and Médecin Ordinaire to Louis XIV, who wrote an apology for the physicians against those who accused them of deferring too much to nature (1663). He attacked the weapon-salve and examined van Helmont's account of Tagliacozzi's description of reattaching a nose to a noble's face after it had been cut off in a duel.[116]

Similarly, Pierre Martin de la Martinière, also a physician to the king, wrote on alchemy as the *Tombeau de la Folie* (ca. 1675). Although he had respect for the true chemist, La Martinière attacked the "impossible pretension that one can transmute all metals into gold as it was done by King Midas of Phrygia by contact with an imaginary powder called the powder of Projection."[117] He felt that the transmutation of base metals was impossible, but still there were innumerable cases of alchemical projects and schemes in Europe. Accordingly, he carried out every conceivable type of experiment and showed repeatedly that attempts to transmute base metals failed. Having read that the matter of the philosopher's stone was to be found in human excrement, he distilled fecal matter hoping to isolate an active spirit. He then redistilled his distillate and used the white product he obtained in a trial transmutation without

[114] Ibid., sig. ēē viiᵛ.
[115] [Jean Albert Belin] (1674).
[116] Sieur Lussauld (1663), pp. 142, 145.
[117] Pierre Martin de la Martinière (after 1669), pp. 1–2.

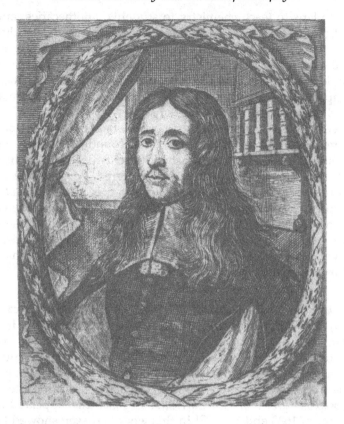

P. M. de la Martinière. From his *Tombeau de la folie* (ca. 1675). Courtesy of the Wellcome Institute Library, London.

success.[118] In another case he gave a good wine to a youth and then collected his urine, which he circulated in the philosopher's egg and separated its quintessence. Once again he tried to transmute metals with this substance and with its salt, but without success.[119]

The teaching of chemistry

Nothing illustrates the popularity of chemistry in the seventeenth century more than the large number of chemical courses and textbooks available. In France these courses were offered mainly outside of the universities due to the persistent opposition of the medical establishment. We have already noted the early rejection by the Parisian Medical

[118] Ibid., p. 108.
[119] Ibid., p. 109.

Faculty of plans to teach chemistry to students, apothecaries, and surgeons. Paulmier had temporarily been expelled from the faculty, and Duchesne and Mayerne had been censured. La Brosse had been opposed initially when he planned a botanical garden with an assistant who would teach chemistry, and Théophraste Renaudot's medical empire collapsed when he sought to expand the Bureau d'Adresse and to prepare chemical medicines at the Bureau.

However, the early chemical course of Jean Beguin had been popular, and his textbook had become the model of countless others published throughout the Continent. As the establishment opposition to chemistry declined, more and more courses were offered. Most of these were taught independently, but there was always a special authority attached to the professors of chemistry at the Jardin des Plantes. In the closing decades of the century chemistry was established even at the major medical schools. To give an indication of what a chemical student was taught, we now discuss a few of the many chemical texts that were printed in the seventeenth century.

William Davisson. At the Jardin des Plantes, William Davisson (ca. 1593– ca. 1669) was appointed the first professor of chemistry in 1648. Davisson, said to have taken a medical degree at Montpellier, taught a private course in chemistry and pharmacy before becoming councillor and physician to Louis XIII.[120] In 1651 he left France to accept a position as physician to John Casimir, the king of Poland. Davisson's textbook, the *Philosophia Pyrotechnia seu Curriculus Chymiatricus*, appeared in four parts between 1633 and 1635.[121] In this work Davisson showed himself to have been strongly influenced by traditional mystical chemistry. It contains long references to Holy Scripture, neo-Platonic authors, Paracelsus, and the Rosicrucians. More than half of it is devoted to a discussion of the universe, both the spiritual and the natural worlds. The fourth part is a dialogue between an Aristotelian and a spagyrist, and the subject is animal, vegetable, and mineral preparations. Davisson accepted the three principles and preferred chemical medicines to the Galenic *materia medica*.

Although the French translation of 1651, *Les Elemens de la Philosophie de l'Art du Feu ou Chemie*,[122] was rearranged and gave more emphasis to purely chemical matters, Davisson's interest in the Paracelsian tradition can be seen in his commentary on Peter Severinus' *Idea medicina philosophicae* published in 1660.[123] With more than seven hundred pages, this

---

120 On Davisson (or Davidson), see J. R. Partington (1962), vol. 3, pp. 4–7, and Héléne Metzger (1923), pp. 45–51.
121 William Davisson (1633, 1635).
122 William Davisson (1651).
123 William Davisson (1660).

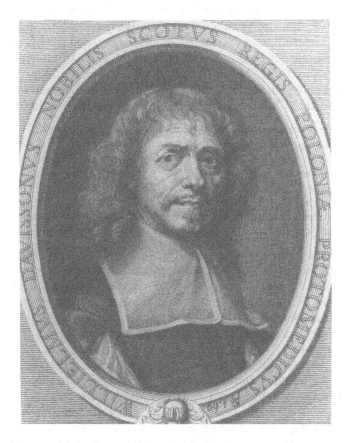

William Davisson (ca. 1593–ca. 1669). Courtesy of the National Library of Medicine, Bethesda.

work dwarfed the original text, which was published along with it in a third edition.

Nicholas Le Fèvre. When Davisson left for Warsaw in 1651, he was replaced by Nicholas Le Fèvre (ca. 1615–1669) who, like Davisson, had offered a private chemical course in Paris prior to his appointment to the Jardin. Le Fèvre remained in this position until 1660 when he became the chemist to Charles II in London.[124] There he was elected a fellow of the Royal Society in 1663.

[124] On Le Fèvre, see Partington, (1962), vol. 3, pp. 17–24, and Metzger, (1923), pp. 62–82. Le Fèvre prepared a short autobiography, which appears in his prefatory piece, "To the Apothecaries of England" in *A Compleat Body of Chemistry* (1670), sig. A4v–av. This English edition is cited here rather than the first French edition of 1660 or the first English edition of 1662.

Le Fèvre's *Cours de chymie* (1660) reflects mystical tradition. He wrote that van Helmont and Glauber were "as the two Beacons and Lights which we are to follow in the Theory of Chymistry, and the best practice of it,"[125] and he referred repeatedly to Paracelsus. Chemistry was a tripartite subject for Le Fèvre: the pharmaceutical preparation of medicines, medical chemistry, and philosophical chemistry. To him there was little doubt that "Chemistry is the true Key of Nature."[126] Indeed,

> Chymistry is nothing else but the Art and Knowledge of Nature it self; that it is by her means we examine the Principles out of which natural bodies do consist and are compounded; and by her are discovered unto us the causes and sources of their generations and corruptions, and of all the changes and alterations to which they are liable: . . . [Further] it is known, that the ancient Sages have taken from Chymistry, the occasions and true motives of reasoning upon natural things, and that their monuments and writings do testifie this Art to be of no fresher date then Nature it self.[127]

Above all, Le Fèvre emphasized the real "evidence and testimony of the senses" derived from the laboratory rather than the "base and naked contemplation" characteristic of the "schoolmen." The latter, he wrote, if asked "What doth make the compound of a body?" resorted to scholastic arguments insisting on the divisibility of matter, saying that although matter is indeed divisible, there must come a time when one reaches an indivisible point. "If it is indeed a point, and consequently without quantity . . . it is impossible it should communicate the same to the body, since divisibility is an essential property to quantity."[128] Nonsense, Le Fèvre concluded. Chemistry rejects "such airy and notional Arguments, to stick close to visible and palpable things." He clearly thought that the concept of atoms or corpuscles was no more firmly supported than the concepts of the Aristotelians or the Galenists. Only the evidence of the chemical laboratory would lead to a proper understanding of nature.

Le Fèvre's chemical principles were the Paracelsian *tria prima* plus phlegm and earth, a typical five-element system for the period.[129] A current question was whether fire was a proper analytic tool for the chemist. He did not doubt that distillation produced five fractions, but there were writers – and here both van Helmont and Boyle come to mind – who argued that the fire produced them through "Composition and Mixture." Although admitting that these substances were obtained by artificial means, he insisted that they were natural "since Art doth contribute nothing else but the Vessels to contain and receive them."[130]

---

125 Ibid., pt. 1, p. 3.
126 Ibid.
127 Ibid., pt. 1, p. 1.
128 Ibid., pt. 1, pp. 9–10.
129 Ibid., pt. 1, pp. 17–29.
130 Ibid., pt. 1, pp. 20–1.

In the end he concluded that the five principles "are not extracted from the Mixt by transmutation, but by a meer natural separation, assisted by the heat of the Vessels and the hand of the Artist: for all things cannot indifferently and immediately be transformed in the like and same things."

Le Fèvre also believed in a universal spirit of life, which circulated around the earth in the atmosphere and was supplied as a necessity to all living things. It was not to be identified simply with common salt-peter but was rather a universal and "Mysterious Salt, which is the soul of all Physical Generations, a Child and Son of Light, and the Father of all Germination and Vegetation."[131] It is a "Divine Salt" and the true vital spirit.

Like other textbook authors Le Fèvre devoted the bulk of his book to practical matters. Furnaces and other chemical equipment were pictured and described in detail, and the expected chemical preparations were divided into their customary animal, vegetable, and mineral origins. Here special interest may be attached to his discussion of antimony. The English translation devotes forty-five pages to the various antimonial preparations.[132] Although the Galenists had traduced antimony "as the vain Idol of Chymistry," the true

> Artists have Antimony in esteem . . . [since] . . . having opened and ana-tomized it, to extract those wonderful Remedies which daily do produce such noble effects, to the great praise and exaltation of Chymistry, and the discredit of those who publickly profess their defaming by Invectives, and ridiculous calumnies against such as daily use it with Skill and Knowl-edge, Order and Method, and consequently with desired success.[133]

The many pages on antimony are a true reflection of seventeenth-century interest in the chemistry of this semimetal. The effects of these preparations seemed truly remarkable. Le Fèvre wrote that

> . . . Diaphoretical Antimony is an unparallel'd Remedy, to resist the cor-ruption which may breed and lurk in the Body, mundifying and rectifying the whole mass of the Blood, and being capable to open the most invete-rate obstructions of the Liver, Spleen, Mesentery, Pancreas, and all other parts besides: it removes the stopping of Courses, cures Green-sickness, Dropsie, Hypochondriacal Melancholy, Pocks, and all the accidents there-of; mundifies and cures inward and outward Ulcers; breaks inward Impostumes without danger: and finally, is singular against malign and Spotted-Feavers, Measels, and small Pocks.[134]

One reason for the value of these preparations was that they partook of the nature of light. Le Fèvre proceeded to show that "the Sun, Father

---

131 Ibid., pt. 2, p. 251; see also pt. 1, p. 38.
132 Ibid., pt. 2, pp. 197–242.
133 Ibid., pt. 2, p. 197.
134 Ibid., pt. 2, p. 210.

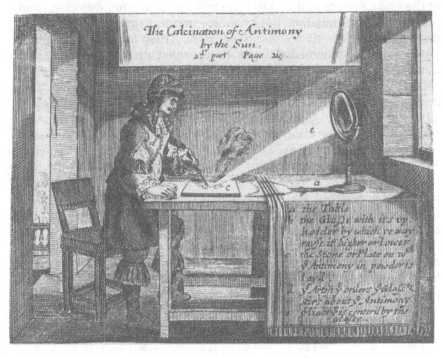

The solar calcination of antimony from Nicasius le Febure [Le Fèvre], *A Compleat Body of Chymistry* (1670). From the collection of the author.

and Spring of the Light" purified and fixed antimony better than any other agent.

> . . . if you calcine . . . [12 grains] . . . of Antimony with a Refracting or Burning-Glass, which doth concentrate the Light of the Sun-beams to make it work upon the matter . . . the Calcination being often reiterated, and the Antimony turned into a white Pouder, you shall find it to weigh xv grains instead of xii that were taken at first . . . but that which is yet more to be admired, and less conceivable, is, that these xv grains of white Pouder are neither vomitive nor purging, but contrariwise Diaphoretical and Cordial. . . . But this wonder shall cease as soon as we begin to apprehend and to know, that Light is that miraculous Fire which constitutes the principle of Antimony, and it is the same now that hath prepared it. By which it appears that this noble Mineral hath a kind of natural Magnes in it self, which makes it capable to attract from the highest Heavens this noble Kin and similar Light, by which it is produced and supplied with its vertue.[135]

Partington has emphasized that Le Fèvre's text is primarily a practical one, but Metzger was surely correct as well in noting the important

[135] Ibid., pt. 2, pp. 215–16.

Paracelso–Helmontian influence on Le Fèvre. In this respect it may be significant to point out that the last edition of Le Fèvre's work was prepared by the Abbé Lenglet du Fresnoy, the eighteenth-century French historian of alchemy.[136]

Christofle Glaser. On the departure of Le Fèvre for London, Christofle Glaser (d. ca. 1670–8) succeeded him at the Jardin des Plantes. Born at Basel, Glaser received his medical degree there and eventually became apothecary to the king and the Duke of Orleans.[137]

Glaser's *Traité de la Chymie* (1663) differed from the works of Davisson and Le Fèvre in its markedly decreased emphasis on theory. To be sure, he discussed the principles, phlegm, and earth, but he criticized those who referred to a more lofty form of chemistry and who claimed to know its grand mysteries. He wrote that these people often appear to want to communicate their knowledge, but they write so obscurely that one could doubt whether their writing represents reality for they seem to present phantasms for substance and thorns for fruits.[138] Some writers did not fly so high but lost themselves in labyrinthine descriptions that others could not follow. And, he said, there are the charlatan alchemists who waste their time and money in the search for riches. So it is little wonder that so many people have declaimed against them and against chemistry itself!

But,

> For myself, I profess to say nothing other than that which I know, and to write nothing other than that which I have done myself. I propose in this small volume to give to the public only a brief and easy method to prepare all the more necessary chemical preparations[139]
> ... I do not give here any preparations which I have not carried out myself and which anyone could not follow after me by adhering to the directions which I have given.[140]

In contrast to other authors, Glaser promised to treat theory very succinctly and did, in fact, do exactly what he promised, devoting only thirteen pages out of nearly four hundred to preliminary matters concerning the definition of chemistry, its object, and the elements and principles. Then he proceeded directly to a description of chemical equipment and operations and after that to the preparations themselves, divided into animal, vegetable, and mineral substances.

In the succession from Davisson to Glaser, we find a gradual shift of emphasis from alchemical mysticism and a universal chemical system of

---

[136] Nicolas Le Fèvre (1751).
[137] On Glaser, see Partington (1962), vol. 3, pp. 24–6; Metzger (1923), pp. 82–6.
[138] Christofle Glaser (1663), sig. ã i^r.
[139] Ibid., sig. ã ii^r.
[140] Ibid., sig. ã ii^v.

the universe to more practical considerations. Davisson was wedded to Paracelsian theory, and the practical preparations he presented filled only a small portion of his book. He was quite ready to use traditional symbolism as a method of expressing chemical truths. Le Fèvre openly acknowledged his debt to Paracelsus and van Helmont and would not accept the more modern mechanical philosophy, but his text was oriented more toward practical preparations than that of his predecessor. Glaser's work pointed more toward the future. Above all, it was a practical work that foreshadowed the immensely popular text of his student, Nicholas Lemery (1645–1715), which we discuss in a later section.

Estienne de Clave. According to Partington, Estienne de Clave, whom we referred to in the previous chapter, taught at the Jardin des Plantes after Davisson. His *Cours de Chimie* (1646) reflects the strong antipathy to Aristotle common to most chemists in the first half of the seventeenth century.[141] De Clave had attacked the views of the ancients earlier in a treatise on the elements (1641), and he had participated in the meeting in Paris on alchemy held in 1624 that had been censured by the Parisian Parlement.

Moyse Charas. Moyse Charas (1619–1698) taught chemistry at the Jardin des Plantes for nine years.[142] His work on the natural history of animals (1668) informs us that he was at that time a demonstrator at the Jardin and apothecary to the Duke of Orleans. At various times he attended Charles II of England and Charles II of Spain, but because of his Calvinist faith he was prosecuted by the Inquisition. He was a well-known figure and elected to the Académie Royale des Sciences in 1692. Best known for his pharmaceutical tract on vipers (1669), he also published a large (more than a thousand pages) *Pharmacopée Royale Galenique et Chymique* (1676), in which the chemical section closely resembled the chemical textbooks of the period. The *Pharmacopée* begins with a hundred-page introduction to ancient (Galenic) and modern (chemical) pharmacy. The remainder of the volume was divided almost evenly between traditional and chemical preparations. He defined "Pharmacie Chymique" as "an Art which teaches how to resolve mixed bodies and by the same means to divide and to study the parts of which they are composed in order to separate the useless components and to keep and to exalt to a higher plane the good components, and to combine them again when necessary."[143] In a long section on the elements he openly took the side of the chemists stating that the four elements were insufficient to explain observations. And like other writers he described three active principles – salt, sulfur, and

---

141 Partington (1962), vol. 3, pp. 7–8; Metzger (1923), pp. 51–9.
142 Partington (1962), vol. 3, p. 27.
143 Moyse Charas (1676), p. 2.

mercury – and the passive phlegm and earth.[144] The chemical section included plates illustrating chemical equipment as well as chemical characters and symbols.

E. R. Arnaud. Among the many writers of chemical textbooks who were not associated with the Jardin des Plantes was E. R. Arnaud, Doctor of Medicine, who published a short *Introduction a la Chymie, ov a la Vraye Physique* (1650). Here we find an author who was acutely aware of the still current medical debate relating to chemistry. Although he discussed the history and definition of chemistry and described chemical equipment and processes prior to giving directions for preparations, he was clearly concerned about the acceptance of chemistry in France. He noted somewhat sadly that it was necessary to go to Germany to see professors of chemistry at the universities and to find a willingness to accept both the old and the new medicines by the establishment.[145] Arnaud was aware that the first state pharmacopoeia to include chemical remedies was German, the Augsburg *Pharmacopoeia Augustana* (1564).[146] He wrote that chemists such as Paracelsus, Mylius, and a hundred others had been physicians to emperors, princes, and electors, and throughout Europe these healers had produced miracles by means of their remedies.[147] Even France has produced Duchesne, Mayerne, and Fabre, he said, and the books of the professors of Montpellier attest to the importance of chemistry; even the pharmacopoeia of Lyon (1627) has a chemical appendix containing approved methods for the preparation of tinctures, extracts, salts, magisteries, flowers, and oils.[148] He continued that even though some writers such as Sennert and Wimpenaeus have tried to reconcile the traditional medicine and the new chemical systems, the medical establishment remains unwilling to accept this new work.[149] Arnaud clearly sought to add chemistry to the required medical training of his day.

Hannibal Barlet. Hannibal Barlet presided over a chemical school in Paris in the 1650s.[150] His *Le Vray et Methodique cours de la Physique Resolutive vulgairement dite chymie* (1653) was lavishly illustrated with full-page plates portraying his view of the universe and the various methods of preparation he employed in his laboratory. For Barlet chemistry was a combination of experiment, metaphysics, and theology or "Theotechnie Ergocosmique," the knowledge of the art of God in the work of the

---

144 Ibid., p. 4.
145 E. R. Arnaud (1650), sig. ã vii^v.
146 Ibid.
147 Ibid., sig. ã viii^{r–v}.
148 Ibid., ẽ i^v.
149 Ibid.
150 Partington (1962), vol. 3, pp. 13–15; Metzger (1923), pp. 61–2.

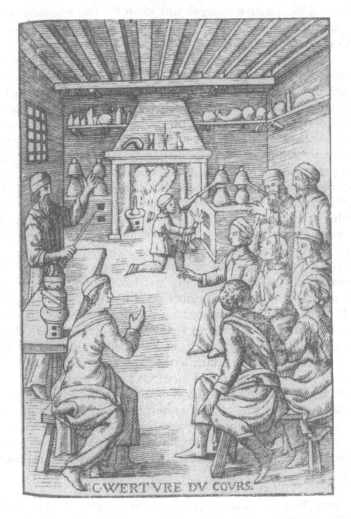

The opening of Hannibal Barlet's course in chemistry. From *Le Vray et Methodique cours de la Physique Resolutive vulgairement dite chymie* . . . (1657). Courtesy of the Wellcome Institute Library, London.

universe.[151] His "Physique Resolutive" refers to the primary job of the chemist, the separation of pure from impure, at the same time a separation of true from false. The true chemist, he said, cannot be a charlatan because the source of his work was divine.[152]

Barlet began his book with nearly one hundred pages about the creation and the cosmos. Although one might expect a chemical description here, one finds instead a rather esoteric mathematical account illus-

[151] Hannibal Barlet (1657), sig. ã viii^r−v.
[152] Ibid., p. 3.

trated by plates. Beginning with a simple universe of concentric spheres, he moves on to the generation of the qualities, elements, and principles, which are developed geometrically through the inscribing of squares and diagonals within a circle. After showing the relationship of the elements to the qualities in a similar fashion, he returns to concentric spheres – now with water and earth in the center – and then proceeds from the outer intelligence to the soul, the spirit, salt, the primum mobile or essence, the stars, the sun, moon, fire, air, water, and earth. There is no void and no plurality of worlds in his system.[153] If indeed Barlet taught the proper chemical preparation of medicines, he did so by means of a world view that was slanted toward Pythagorean symbolism.

Nicholas de Locques. Nicholas de Locques, "Spagyric physician to His Majesty," published his *Les Rvdimens de la Philosophie Natvrelle Tovchant le Systeme dv Corps Mixte* in 1665.[154] This is a "Covrs Theorique" in which he promises to explain clearly the "Precepts and the Principles of Chemistry." He disavows any interest in transmutation[155] and discusses instead the hidden virtues of nature. In fact, he takes up the normal definitions and goes on to discuss the elements, various chemical operations, and chemical symbols. De Locques was convinced of the importance of quantification because "everything has its own weight and measure in a mixture and if this were not the case nothing could be accomplished with this Art, nor engendered in Nature."[156] Thus, each thing has the necessary amount of air to spiritualize itself, enough water for its dissolution, fire for tinging, and earth for fixation. The chemist must determine the amount of water needed to dissolve a substance, the amount of earth for coagulation, and the amount of air and fire needed for rectification and coloring.

De Locques promises his readers that the chemical operations would follow the doctrine of Paracelsus,[157] but his emphasis on fermentation is more reminiscent of van Helmont. He devotes a major section to the magnetic virtues of the blood, expatiating on the spirit in the blood.[158] He refers frequently to Paracelsus, van Helmont, and Glauber, and he accepted sympathetic action in nature, assuring the reader that magnetic virtues exist in the blood that can be employed by the physician as a means of cure.

Marie Meurdrac. In the preface to her *La Chymie Charitable et Facile, En faveur des Dames* (1656), Marie Meurdrac questioned whether a woman should author such a text. Her answer was that

153 Ibid., p. 89.
154 Partington (1962), vol. 3, p. 26; Metzger (1923), pp. 161–2.
155 Nicholas de Locques (1665), sig. ã vii^r.
156 Ibid., p. 159.
157 Ibid., title page, book 2.
158 Nicholas de Locques (1664), p. 8.

Intellects have nothing to do with sex, and if those of women were cultivated as those of men, and if one employed as much time and expense in
their instruction, they would equal them. Our century has seen women
born who yield nothing to the ability and capacity of men in prose, poetry,
languages, philosophy and government, even that of the State. Moreover,
this work is useful in that it contains a quantity of infallible remedies for
the cure of illnesses and the conservation of health, as well as many rare
secrets of value to women.[159]

Much of the volume resembles other chemical texts of the period: the
definition of the subject, the discussion of the chemical principles, and
the various chemical preparations, but a final (sixth) book was written
specifically for women, in which they could find "all those things which
preserve and augment beauty." Here she wisely warned her readers that
some substances, such as mercury, that were then widely used for whit-
ening the skin were dangerous because they "obliterate facial beauty
when used for a long time and they produce very dangerous illnesses
which are sometimes incurable: for this reason women should take care
[in their use]."[160]

Chemical physiology

Chemistry became firmly established as a form of pharmacy in the closing decades of the seventeenth century, but it also became widely accepted as a system for explaining physiological processes. This
acceptance was due partially to the influence of van Helmont, and even
more to that of his younger contemporary at Leiden, Franciscus de la
Boë Sylvius (1614–1672), who advocated chemical explanations. The
work of Sylvius and the chemical "victory" in pharmacy helped to give
many of the new chemical appointments at the European universities an
iatrochemical flavor prior to the concerted opposition of the medical
mechanists or iatrophysicists.

An interesting example of one of these chemical physiologists is Daniel
Duncan (1649–1735), born in Languedoc. His father was a professor of
medicine, and Daniel was sent to Montpellier where he took his medical
degree in 1673. Shortly thereafter he was appointed physician-general to
the army. He moved in high court circles, but being a protestant he left
France at the time of the Revocation of the Edict of Nantes (1685) and
traveled first to Switzerland (1690), then to Cassel (1699), and finally to
England (1714) where he died over twenty years later.

---

159 Marie Meurdrac (1666), sig. ē iv^r. Duveen (1949), p. 401, mentions a first edition of
     1656. Other French editions appeared in 1674 and 1680, and there were translations
     into German (1676) and Italian (1682).
160 Ibid., p. 252.

Duncan's major work on iatrochemistry was completed in France. The first part of his *La Chymie Naturelle ou l'Explication Chymique et Mechanique de la Nourriture de l'Animal* appeared at Paris in 1681, and the second and third parts appeared five years later. Here the author showed little interest in pharmaceutical chemistry. It was not his concern to write another chemical textbook. Rather, he hoped to show "how chemistry is necessary to explain clearly the natural functions of the animal."[161] He wrote of bodily fermentations, filtrations, and circulations: "In a word it is only chemistry which makes it possible to understand how bread becomes flesh, bone etc., and how a lifeless substance is received within a living body."[162]

Duncan wrote against those physicians who thought of chemistry as an art that was contrary to nature. It was his conviction that nature operated chemically. He felt that these physicians would lose their horror of chemical laboratories when they were convinced that their own bodies were nothing but chemical laboratories. How could they help but lose their aversion for chemists "when they have been persuaded by this book that they are chemists themselves without knowing it."[163]

Progressing through Duncan's pages, one finds the internal organs described as chemical vessels, in and through which bodily processes take place chemically. Thus, the structure of the liver permits the passage of the superfluous sulfur of the blood,[164] which in certain circumstances permits one to explain the development of jaundice. But only chemistry permits us to make this discovery. Chemistry also gives us the reason for the reddening of the blood, which is due to the color of the sulfur found in the chyle, which is then transferred to the bile in its own passage.[165]

The heat of the body plays an essential role in this process because, as the fire is the chemists' chief instrument in the artificial conditions of his laboratory, so, too, it is the chief instrument in the natural laboratory of the living body.[166] This can be seen in the digestion of food and the fermentation of the chyle, both of which require heat. The central furnace could be found in the stomach, but each organ is like a chemical vessel, preparing its own materials requisite for the life of the organism.[167]

If the concept of a living chemical laboratory was required for animal life, it was no less necessary for an understanding of the great world about us. How else could we explain the production of minerals, metals,

161 Duncan (1683), sig. *v^v – *vi^r. There are references to a 1681 edition of the first part.
162 Ibid.
163 Ibid., sig. ** ii^v.
164 Ibid., sig. * viii^r.
165 Ibid., sig. * viii^v.
166 Ibid., sig. ** i^r.
167 Ibid.

vegetables, and animals? "If Plato had reason to say that God makes nothing without the rules of Geometry, one can add that He produces nothing without those of Chemistry."[168]

In the second part of the *Chymie Naturelle* (1687) Duncan continued his comparison of the great and small worlds and their chemical processes. In his preface he called the physician the voyager of the microcosm whereas "anatomy is the art of the voyager."[169] The body could be closely compared to the earth, and the physician "in his voyages" regards

> the solid parts as terra firma, the humors which moisten them as the sea of the small world, the large vessels as the rivers and streams and the small ones as the brooks. There are even certain currents which merit the name of torrents or floods because they flow only during a short space of time.[170]

These periodic torrents were analogous to menstruation. In his search for the course of this rush of blood the anatomist found the vagina to be similar to a great canal in the macrocosm.[171]

In his search for an explanation of this occurrence in women Duncan turned both to chemistry and to theology. There was a fermentation that occurs in the blood, but the blood of men was less impure than that of women. Though the impurities of masculine blood could be eliminated satisfactorily through the pores, this did not suffice for the greater mass that must be expelled from a woman's body.[172] Duncan digressed for a moment to ask whether Eve had been created with blood as pure as Adam. Surely she had been, but the fruit she ate had corrupted her humors, and it was divine justice that had altered her blood from its earlier harmony to violence and disorder.[173] Thus there was a ready cause for the monthly evacuation. And this explanation could be extended to the pain of childbirth:

> One can only prove by divine authority that this evacuation followed the rebellion of the first woman since she did not give birth in a state of innocence, seen through the lack of menstrual blood which prepares the womb for generation. "You will give birth with pain" is a judgment that the Judge of the world pronounced without doubt against a criminal Eve, and the Justice of God does not permit him to condemn to this punishment an innocent person.[174]

Duncan's prolific work shows the extent to which a dedicated iatrochemist could apply chemistry as a model in physiological explana-

---

[168] Ibid., sig. ** ii.
[169] Daniel Duncan (1687), sig. A iiii^r.
[170] Ibid.
[171] Ibid., sig. ** ii^v.
[172] Ibid., sig. B ii^{r-v}.
[173] Ibid., sig. B iii^v.
[174] Ibid., sig. C i^v.

tions. However, the works of Thomas Willis (1621–1675) and Franciscus de la Boë Sylvius (1614–1672) were more influential.[175] Both were skilled anatomists and chemists.

Willis was educated at Oxford where he received the degree, bachelor of medicine, in 1646. During the Interregnum, Oxford became the center of English science with the presence of John Wallis, Robert Boyle, John Wilkins, Seth Ward, and many others. Willis himself was a major figure in this illustrious group, and at the restoration of the monarchy in 1660 he was appointed Sedleian Professor of Natural Philosophy. He later moved to London where he became a prominent member of the Royal Society. Although he is known best as an anatomist, Willis' first publication was on a typical chemical subject, fermentation. The *De fermentatione* (1659) began with a discussion of the elements. He found the Aristotelian elements of little value. Atomism was more helpful, but he preferred the five principles of the chemists (spirit, sulfur, salt, water, and earth) which were determined by distillation analysis.[176]

Willis attributed change in natural phenomena primarily to fermentation, of which he gave examples from the animal, vegetable, and mineral kingdoms. The earth, he said, is a "pregnant womb" in which metals and minerals grow due to local ferments, which free saline particles in the form of vapor. When this vapor is mixed with earthy matter or moistened with water, the result is fountains and spa waters.[177]

In vegetable life, Willis identified the fermentation process with the growth of seeds, whereas his description of animal life centered on man. The life spirit resulted from a fermentation in the heart and was distributed throughout the body by the circulation of the blood.[178] He associated other sources of fermentation with the bowels, the genitals, and the spleen; and said that both disease and its cure involved fermentation.[179] Willis did not refer to van Helmont's local archei, but there seems little doubt that his concept of the ferment was inspired by the work of the Belgian.[180]

Willis often used chemical analogies. Disease was due to fermentation, the action of the muscles resulted from the reaction of nitrous and sulfurous spirits,[181] and he used distillation as a means of analysis and as a model for explanation. Thus, the body itself was likened to a distillation unit: Blood, heated in the heart, rose to the colder brain where the

[175] On Willis and Sylvius I have followed my previous discussion in Debus (1977), vol. 2, pp. 520–31. The standard biographies are Hansruedi Isler (1968) and E. D. Baumann (1949). See also Partington (1962), vol. 2, pp. 281–90, 304–10.

[176] Thomas Willis (1681), pp. 2–3.

[177] Ibid., pp. 8–11.

[178] Ibid., p. 13.

[179] Ibid., pp. 14–16.

[180] Here I agree with Isler (1968), p. 61.

[181] Ibid., Willis, "Of Convulsive Diseases," p. 2 (separate pagination).

animal spirits were separated from the cruder blood and passed on to the nerves.[182]

Willis' persistent use of chemical analogies is similar to that of his contemporary, Franciscus de la Boë Sylvius.[183] Educated at Leiden and Basel (M.D., 1637), Sylvius practiced medicine at Amsterdam (1641) where he became the friend of the chemists Otto Sperling and Johann Rudolph Glauber. In 1658 he was appointed professor of medicine at Leiden where he remained until his death fourteen years later.

The work of Sylvius reflects a Galenic training in his discussion of the pulmonary circulation and in his interest in the animal spirits.[184] Like Willis, he was an able anatomist, and was keenly aware of the mechanistic views of Descartes, whom he knew personally. While at Leiden (1638–41) he had been one of the first to teach the Harveyan circulation.[185]

For Sylvius, chemistry was essential for a proper understanding of nature and therefore for medicine. To those persons who charged that he was dependent on van Helmont, Sylvius answered that his chemical views had been presented in 1641, prior to the publication of van Helmont's *Ortus medicinae*.[186] Nevertheless, Sylvius stressed fermentation as had van Helmont and his English contemporary Willis. He was convinced that all physiological processes could be explained chemically – primarily through fermentation, effervescence, and putrefaction. Though van Helmont had pointed to acid, alkali, and neutralization as important factors in physiological phenomena, they became much more fundamental with Sylvius.

Thus, he believed that the pancreatic juice was acid and that it effervesced with an alkaline gall in the duodenum. Like van Helmont, Sylvius had a special interest in digestion,[187] arguing that mastication prepares food for the necessary fermentation process in the stomach and that saliva, which contains the required fermentative forces (water, salt, and spirit), is a necessary preparatory agent. The stomach contributes a moderate heat (fire), which originates in the heart and is communicated by means of the blood. A chemical process of separation then follows in the intestines as a result of the bile and the pancreatic juices (alkaline and acid). The resultant chyle contains the volatile spirit of food plus small amounts of alkaline salt and acid spirit, and in this form it enters the bloodstream. On reaching the left ventricle of the heart, the still

---

[182] Ibid., Willis, "Of Fermentation," pp. 14–15.

[183] In addition to the references cited in note 173 on Sylvius, see Lester S. King (1970), pp. 93–112.

[184] José Maria López Piñero (1973), vol. 4, p. 281.

[185] Ibid., p. 284.

[186] Franciscus de la Boë Sylvius (1680), p. 10.

[187] Sylvius's views on digestion are well treated by King in his *Road to Medical Enlightenment* (1970), pp. 98–104. His discussion is the basis of the present account.

imperfect blood is further heated and rarified before going on to the lungs and to the right ventricle where it is rarefied again and made ready for circulation. The circularity provides a continuous nourishment of the internal fire of the heart and at the same time maintains vitality throughout the body.[188]

An admirer of the work of Glauber, Sylvius was influenced by that chemist's belief in the dual nature of salt (acid–alkali).[189] Salt was to become an essential part of this concept of fermentation, and the result was an explanation of disease in terms of excess acid or base. Acrimonius influences were ascribed to fluids such as the lymph, the saliva, the pancreatic juice, and the bile, and characteristic diseases resulted from their acidic or alkaline natures.

Although Sylvius's use of chemistry as a means of explanation seems to reflect the work of van Helmont, it may be best to interpret both Willis and Sylvius as men who logically extended a chemical tradition that can be traced to Paracelsus. An important distinction between them and earlier authors is their lesser interest in chemistry as a total philosophy of nature. Both men surely subscribed to such a view in general, but the thrust of their work centered on physiological problems. And although they were deeply interested in chemistry, theirs was a chemistry that differed from that of chemists who confined themselves primarily to the preparation of chemical remedies. It is with these authors that we see the full development of a new phase of iatrochemistry. The many students of Sylvius in particular promoted his chemical interpretations throughout Europe after his death.

Perhaps the chief French exponent of this iatrochemical school was Raymond Vieussens (ca. 1635–1715), who took his medical degree at Montpellier in 1670, never held an academic position, but served as a physician at the chief hospital in Montpellier, the Hôtel Dieu St. Éloi, where he was eventually promoted to chief physician. His earliest books, on the nervous system (1684) and fermentation (1688), attracted widespread attention, and he was rewarded by the king with an annual pension of 1,000 livres.[190] He was later elected to the academy of sciences (1699) and named as a councillor of state (1707).

Like Sylvius, Vieussens's work reflects Cartesian mechanism and late seventeenth-century iatrochemistry. The *Neurographia universalis* (1684) consciously follows Willis; but Vieussens considered his work on the blood to be his most important contribution, and in that, his concern with fermentation is clearly evident. Writing of his own research, he said that he began his anatomical studies in 1671 but went on to write a

---

[188] Like others in the Paracelsian tradition Sylvius noted the similarity between life and combustion and gave a significant role to the aerial niter in the respiratory process. Ibid., pp. 104–5.

[189] Ibid., pp. 111–12; López Piñero (1973), pp. 282, 285.

[190] Raymond Vieussens (1698), sig. ã i^r.

treatise applying the principles of chemistry to the human body, to which he added a treatise on fermentation.[191]

The *Traité Nouveau des Liqueurs du Corps Humain* began with a section on element theory in which there was no reference to the familiar chemical principles. Rather, he turned to the three Cartesian elements: the first, very small bodies of varied shapes moving at great speed; the second, spherical bodies of medium size and speed; and the third, larger bodies, irregularly shaped and nearly without movement. The first of these corresponded to the fire of the ancients, the soul of the world of the Platonists, the igneous matter of Hippocrates, and the central fire of the chemists. The second was simply ethereal matter; the third was earth.[192]

Vieussens was spurred on to his study of the blood by his reading of Robert Boyle.[193] He hoped first to determine the particular nature and qualities of the parts, and second to determine their proportions and quantities.[194] He underscored the importance of quantification by noting that without a knowledge of proportions one cannot know the true nature of a substance, its causes, differences, signs, or changes of temperament.[195]

From his chemical analysis of the blood Vieussens concluded that it is composed of four principles that are essentially different from one another: "I understand that all the bodies of which blood is naturally composed may be reduced to four substances, which are phlegm, salt, sulfur, and earth."[196] The salt could further be divided into volatile and fixed fractions. He was convinced that he had found an acid salt in the blood and proceeded to discuss its formation through a fermentation process in the heart.[197]

Describing the passage of the blood from the right to the left ventricles, Vieussens tells us that the blood loses heat as it passes through the lungs, where it is impregnated with the aerial niter, and then regains the lost heat on its return to the left chamber.[198] The blood contains both passive and active principles, the latter, which is nothing else but a spiritous substance impregnated with volatile saline-acid particles, is requisite for the natural fermentation of the blood. "I wish to say that the vital spirit is united to the animal spirit . . . And by vital spirit I understand a very fine liquor diffused throughout all the mass of the blood, and principally composed of a very subtle air, charged with entirely volatile nitrous particles and united to the volatile acid salt of food."

191　Raymond Vieussens (1715), vol. 1, sig. ē iii^v.
192　Vieussens, ibid., vol. 2, (titled *Traité Nouveau des Liqueurs du Corps Humain*), pp. 1–2.
193　Vieussens (1698), sig. ã2^r.
194　Ibid., sig. ã 3^r.
195　Ibid.
196　Ibid.
197　Vieussens (1715), vol. 2, pp. 122–3.
198　Ibid., vol. 1, pp. 120–2.

A marginal note tells us that "L'esprit animal n'est autre chose que l'esprit vital, filtré & rectifié dans le cerveau."[199] It is little wonder that Vieussens considered his work on blood his most important achievement. Here he stood at the end of a century-long quest for the material vital spirit.[200] Robert Fludd thought that he had found this spirit in his repeated distillations of wheat grains, and van Helmont had turned to human blood, which had to contain the spirit, and identified a substance with remarkable healing properties. Robert Boyle had gone on to a more thorough analysis of the ingredients of blood, which had inspired Vieussens to his own work. Through all of this ran the Paracelsian tradition of an aerial life spirit that was requisite for all forms of life. Vieussens referred not only to Boyle but also to John Mayow and Thomas Willis; and if he reflected some strains of Cartesian mechanism, at the same time he formed part of this very prominent iatrochemical tradition.

Chemistry and the universities

Although many of the followers of Paracelsus had claimed that chemistry was the fundamental science for the study of man and nature and had demanded the reform of the educational establishment to conform to their convictions, they had been met with firm opposition by those entrenched in the venerable seats of learning. Nowhere had this opposition been more formidable than in France where chemical physicians had been repeatedly censured or banished from the Medical Faculty of Paris. The efforts of Théophraste Renaudot had met with such opposition that he was left a ruined man. The medical school at Paris remained a bastion of tradition in this field until much later than most universities, and even Montpellier did not appoint a professor of chemistry until relatively late.

Those chemists who sought a total reform of the European universities saw little to encourage them, but nevertheless, chemistry became widely accepted in medical schools during the seventeenth century.[201] The first such appointment was that of Johann Hartmann at Marburg in 1609.[202] This appointment was specifically in the medical faculty, and it was to set the pattern for future appointments elsewhere. Hartmann was a Paracelsian, but his job was to teach the preparation of chemical medicines. He was a prolific author and an effective teacher. His students found positions at other institutions and his books – both his original texts and his editions of Beguin, Croll, and others – were widely used and influential throughout Europe.

---

[199] Ibid., p. 122.
[200] On the history of this search, see Debus, "Chemistry and the Quest" (1984).
[201] This section is based on my paper "Chemistry and the Universities in the Seventeenth Century" (1986). See also Wlodzimierz Hubicki (1968), vol. 4, pp. 41–5.
[202] On Hartmann, see Lynn Thorndike (1923–58), vol. 8, pp. 116–17. Partington (1962), vol. 2, p. 177.

Not long after Hartmann's appointment, Zacharias Brendel offered a course in chemistry at Jena (1612) in the medical faculty.[203] His son, also named Zacharias, continued in this tradition and was followed by Werner Rolfinck, who was named the first professor of chemistry at Jena (1641). Over the next fifty years chemistry became established at Wittenberg, Helmstedt, Erfurt, Leipzig, and Halle. In almost all of these universities the initiative was taken by the medical faculties.

At the University of Leiden, which was to become the center of chemical teaching in Europe in the eighteenth century because of Hermann Boerhaave (1668–1738), the chair in chemistry was established primarily due to the influence of Sylvius who had been appointed professor of clinical medicine in 1658.[204] When Anton Deusing was being considered for an appointment to the Leiden medical faculty in 1666, Sylvius threatened to resign unless given a chemical laboratory and a professorship in chemistry. These were promised to him by the board, but nothing came of the promise initially. Only three years later did the board confirm its earlier decision, noting that "nothing was lacking to make the distinction of the Medical Faculty complete but the preparation of medicaments in a chemical manner and the performance of experiments in the field of chemistry."

The first appointment by the University at Leiden was Carel de Maets (1640–1690) who had been trained by Glauber in Amsterdam and then had gone on to the University of Utrecht as an unsalaried docent. But there he had no laboratory, so he was attracted to the new position at Leiden where the chemical laboratory opened in 1669. He was appointed without salary, but by 1672 he was an ordinary professor in the faculty of philosophy, and seven years later he was given the same appointment in the medical faculty. De Maets had some competition from Jacob Le Mort (1650–1718) and Christian Margraaf (1626–1687). Le Mort had worked in Glauber's laboratory before setting up his own laboratory in Leiden; he had also gone to Utrecht for a medical degree (1678). Margraaf's doctorate had been taken at the University of Franeker in 1659. He then moved to Leiden where he gave chemical lessons to students, much to the annoyance of Sylvius, De Maets, and Le Mort. At the death of De Maets in 1690, Le Mort was given the management of the chemical laboratory at Leiden, but other recognition was slow to come. Approval of his promotion to professor was obtained in 1697, but the appointment was not made official until 1702. At his death, Boerhaave added the chair of chemistry to his chairs in medicine and botany.

The professorship in chemistry at Leiden had been established because of the recognized need of this subject for medical students. De

203　Ernest Giese and Benno Von Hagen (1958), pp. 96–121.
204　J. W. Van Spronsen (1975), pp. 329–43 (335).

Maets' two chemical textbooks, the one by Le Mort, and the *Collectanea chymica Leydensia* compiled by Christopher Love Morley, an English student, all testify to the fact that the chemistry being taught had nothing to do with the new chemical theories in physiology. Rather, they reflected the practical preparations of pharmaceutical products and the long tradition of chemical textbooks that had originated with Jean Beguin.

The last quarter of the century was active in the establishment of chemistry as an integral part of the medical curriculum. Adrien Regnault became the first professor of chemistry at Louvain in 1685,[205] and regular lectures in chemistry began with Robert Plot at Oxford and John Francis Vigani at Cambridge in 1683.[206]

Much of the formal teaching in France had been carried on at the Jardin des Plantes and in private courses, as we have seen. The opposition to chemistry was so strong in Paris that a formal appointment was delayed longer than elsewhere. At the opening of the sixteenth century there were only two professors at the University of Paris, one who taught "choses naturelles et non naturelles" (including anatomy) and another who taught "choses contre nature," which included pathology and *material medica*.[207] It was only during the seventeenth century that some reforms were made. A chair of surgery was established in 1634 and twelve years later a chair in botany. The statutes were revised in 1696, and two years later a fifth chair was established to teach a course in chemical and Galenic pharmacy for medical students. It was not until 1756 that a demand was made for nine professors for (1) anatomy, (2) physiology and hygiene, (3) pathology, (4) *materia medica*, (5) therapeutics, (6) *histoire des maladies* and therapeutic practice, (7) surgery, (8) legal medicine, and (9) theoretical and practical chemistry. With the time lag it is little wonder that chemical progress came not from the medical school in Paris, but from elsewhere.

Even at Montpellier the move toward an appointment in chemistry was far from rapid.[208] Montpellier had had a long connection with medical chemistry, and almost all of the most prominent French chemists

---

205 Annette Felix (1986).

206 R. T. Gunther (1922–1967), vol. 1, pp. 39–51; (1937), pp. 221–2.

207 On the development of the Medical Faculty at Paris, see Dr. August Corleiu (1877), pp. 124–43. The recent research of L. W. B. Brockliss (1978, 1981, 1987) discusses the teaching of medicine and natural philosophy in the seventeenth and early eighteenth centuries. With few exceptions he notes that theses oriented toward chemical medicine are not to be found before 1665. In natural philosophy, Brockliss found that chemistry was seldom mentioned during the seventeenth century with the exception of the case of element theory. Here the Paracelsian principles were uniformly rejected. A single exception is to be found in Jean Cecil Frey's discussion of Aristotle's *Meteorologica* (1633) in which he spoke of the influence of the stars, the doctrine of signatures, and referred his students to the works of Oswald Croll and Joseph Duchesne [(1981), 42].

208 Jean Astruc (1767), pp. 268–70.

had taken their degrees there; but there was no actual appointment until relatively late. Antoine d'Aquin, doctor of the medical faculty at Montpellier and first physician to Louis XIV, became convinced that the study of this science should be established at Montpellier. In 1673 he arranged for the official appointment of a demonstrator in chemistry. The position was given to Sebastian Matte, called La Faveur, who had been giving lectures on the subject at Montpellier for some years and whose *Pratique de Chymie* had been published two years earlier. His lettres-patentes of 1675 permitted him to give a public lecture course every year in the faculty of medicine. However, he was given a salary commensurate with that of a full professor, with similar rights, prerogatives, exemptions, and immunities. These privileges came as a shock to the members of the medical faculty, who had no wish to see a chemical operator, whom they considered to be illiterate, raised to their own status. Arguing that this was a medical subject, they recommended that a new chair in chemistry be established and given to a medical doctor who would then be set over and above the chemical demonstrator. This suggestion was approved, and Arnaldus Fonsorbe (d. 1695), Doctor Aggregé of the faculty since 1665, was appointed the first professor of chemistry at Montpellier. There is no evidence that he published anything of significance in the field, but there is no evidence of any undue friction between him and Matte.

Matte's *Pratique de Chymie* gives a good indication of his teaching of the subject. He defined chemistry in its relation to medicine. It was "the Art of separating the parts of a natural body, purifying them, and reuniting them for their use in Medicine."[209] His elementary substances were phlegm, spirit, sulfur, salt, and "terre morte," the most commonly accepted group from this period.[210] After a description of chemical operations and equipment he devoted the remainder of his book to chemical preparations, which he divided into the customary categories of mineral, vegetable, and animal. Perhaps the most novel aspect of the book is in the author's preface where he asked why another chemical text was needed at all. He cited the excellent texts of Beguin, Hartmann, Crollius, Duchesne, Schroeder, Davisson, Le Fèvre, and Glaser, which (he said) some might argue "leave nothing further to be said on this matter."[211] His only defense was that he would add some preparations not to be found in the other authors and that occasionally he would present the subject matter in a different fashion.

Montpellier continued to be in the forefront of the teaching of chemistry in the eighteenth century. After the death of Fonsorbe in 1695, Antoine Deidier (d. 1746) was appointed professor of chemistry in 1697,

209 S. Matte La Faveur (1671), p. 1.
210 Ibid., p. 9.
211 Ibid., sig. ã 2ᵛ.

a position he held until his retirement to Marseilles in 1732.[212] Deidier, who had taken his medical degree at Montpellier in 1691, wrote on many medical subjects over the course of a long life. His views on chemistry can be illustrated by two of his books, the *Chimie Raisonnée* (1715) and the *Institutiones Medicinae Theoricae* (1711).

Deidier's chemical text was based on his Latin lectures presented at Montpellier but was translated into French to be more useful "for young physicians, surgeons, and pharmacists in the more remote Provinces . . ."[213] In his introductory letter to the volume Dr. Pestalossi of Lyon noted the lingering public suspicion of chemistry due to the prevalence of charlatans and imposters who promised cures for all illnesses with a single universal remedy. However, he added, true medicinal chemistry is an art of which the utility is known to all people of learning and good sense.[214] Deidier wrote in the tradition of seventeenth-century medical chemistry. His text differed from those of his predecessors primarily in that he spent no time on the history and definition of the subject, nor did his book present the reader with the familiar descriptions of chemical equipment and operations, topics that were standard in most other accounts. Deidier turned first to the chemical principles: water, earth, salt, sulfur, and spirit.[215] He made the point that these elements, which he defined as the simple bodies of which all things are composed, were not the same as the elements of Descartes.[216] The latter formed the basis of Cartesian cosmology but were of little value to the chemist who sought his elements through laboratory separations and distillations. This preliminary material completed, Deidier then turned to the heart of the book, the chemical preparation of substances of medicinal value. Most of these were prepared from inorganic substances.

As a member of the Montpellier Medical Faculty, Deidier did not hesitate to publish on purely medical subjects. His *Institutiones Medicinae Theoricae* is divided into discussions of physiology, pathology, and therapeutics. In the section on physiology he notes that this subject had been altered due to the modern discoveries in physics, chemistry, and anatomy. This new information has "led to the more perfect knowledge of the nature and structure of the human body."[217] Deidier divided the

---

212 Lester S. King [(1978), pp. 914] drew attention to Deidier when he compared Deidier's *Institutiones Medicinae Theoricae* (1711) with Nicholas Lemery's *Cours de chymie* (here he used the English translations of 1677 and 1720). However, although the *Institutes* shows the interest of the author in chemistry, it was essentially a medical textbook. It would have been better to have compared Lemery's chemical textbook with Deidier's *Chimie raisonnée* (1715).

213 Antoine Deidier (1715), sig. *v[r].

214 Ibid., sig. *ix[v]–*x[r] (dated Lyon, 23 November 1714).

215 Ibid., pp. 1–9.

216 Ibid., pp. 9–11.

217 Antoine Deidier (1711), sig. ã 2[r].

subject into three parts: the principles, the fluids, and the solids.[218]
Again he presented the Cartesian position on the three sizes of elementary particles and their cosmological significance,[219] but he turned to
chemical tradition when he stated that all substances were mineral,
vegetable, or animal in origin. These, he assured his readers, are composed of the five chemical principles.[220]

Deidier's long tenure at Montpellier helped to assure the continued
influence of chemical medicine at that institution. And if it is evident that
he was aware of Cartesian philosophy, it is also clear that his work
reflected the French chemical textbook tradition. The history of chemistry
at Montpellier deserves detailed research because of the development of
vitalistic medicine there in the eighteenth century,[221] but the roots of this
school may be based in the continued influence of seventeenth-century
iatrochemistry at a time when that medical philosophy was being supplanted elsewhere by a more mechanistic approach to medicine.

Chemistry and the new philosophy

Van Helmont wrote of his concept of the chemical philosophy as the
"new philosophy" that was to replace the philosophy and medicine of
the ancients, but for the twentieth-century historian the term *new philosophy* is more likely to refer to the changes that occurred in the physical
sciences in the course of the seventeenth century. Today we normally
associate the scientific revolution primarily with mechanical analogies
and atomism, the use of mathematical abstraction, the developing experimental method, and above all, an avoidance of mysticism and occult
explanations. The chemical and medical developments of the period
seldom play a major part in these presentations. The mechanical philosophy is the philosophy of Galileo and Newton. In England the new
philosophy was initially associated with the inductive methodology of
Francis Bacon and in France with the deductive methodology of René
Descartes, but the latter was to be an interpretation of Descartes from
which his earlier mystical views had been removed or forgotten. What
remained was Descartes the mathematician, the atomist, and the philosopher who sought to overturn the ancients.

Thus, in the very decades when chemistry was finally being accepted
by the medical establishment, there was to be a new reaction against it.
No longer were physicians opposed to the use of chemically prepared
medicines, but the success of the mechanical philosophy in the physical

218　Ibid., sig. ã 2^{r-v}.
219　Ibid., pp. 4–6.
220　Ibid., pp. 8–14.
221　Elizabeth Haigh (1984), pp. 15–46.

sciences had medical overtones, causing an iatrophysical school to arise in opposition to the iatrochemists.

This new science is reflected in the textbook tradition, in which we have seen a decreasing interest in the Paracelsian chemical world view as we progressed from Beguin, Hartmann, and Davisson to the work of Glaser. Le Fèvre even praised the universal spirit and the principles of the chemists in comparison with the "airy" speculations of those who argued about atomism. This differed considerably from the most popular of the chemical textbooks, the *Cours de chymie* of Nicholas Lemery (1645–1715), which went through many editions in French, Latin, German, English, and Spanish between 1675 and 1757.[222] Lemery studied chemistry at the Jardin des Plantes under Glaser and lectured on chemistry at Montpellier. A respected scientist, he was elected a member of the Paris Academy of Sciences in 1699.

One would expect Lemery's chemical text to reflect that of his predecessors; and indeed, it does present similarities: an introduction discussing the principles of the art, a long section devoted to chemical preparations, and the division into mineral, vegetable, and animal substances.

For Lemery no less than Le Fèvre there is a universal spirit, diffused everywhere, that produces the

> different things according to the different Matrixes, or Pores of the earth in which it settles. But because this *Principle* is a little *Metaphysical* and falls not under our senses, it will be fit to establish some sensible ones . . .[223]

At this point he turned to the customary chemical agent: fire, which reduces substances to water, spirit, oil, salt, and earth. These are "Principles" in a practical sense because they "are only Principles in respect of us" because one can advance no farther in the division of bodies.[224] In contrast with the doubts of van Helmont and Boyle, Lemery remained convinced that fire analysis was a valid tool of the chemist in his quest for the elements.[225]

It is in Lemery's constant use of atomic or corpuscular explanations that we find a break with chemical tradition. Like Robert Boyle, and in the tradition of Pierre Gassendi, he relied on the characteristic shapes of atoms to explain chemical reactions. Thus, acids were described as spiked and alkalis as porous. Their reaction was mechanical and accompanied by heat and effervescence. Lemery explained that alkalis were recognized

> by pouring an *acid* upon them, for presently or soon after, there rises a violent *Ebullition*, which remains until the *acid* finds no more bodies to

---

[222] Partington (1962), vol. 3, pp. 28–42; Metzger (1923), pp. 281–340.
[223] Nicholas Lemery (1686), p. 3.
[224] Ibid., p. 5.
[225] Ibid., pp. 6–9.

rarifie. This effect may make us reasonably conjecture that an *Alkali* is a terrestrious and solid matter, whose *pores* are figures after such a manner that the *acid* points entring into them do strike and divide whatsoever opposes their motion; and according as the parts of which the *Alkali* is compounded, are more or less solid, the *acids* finding more or less resistance, do cause a stronger or weaker *Ebullition*. So we see the *Effervescency* that happens in the dissolution of *Coral* is very much milder than that in the dissolution of *Silver*.[226]

Lemery's interest in acids and alkalis is symptomatic of a significant theme in seventeenth-century chemistry. We have already noted van Helmont's emphasis on the role of acids and alkalis in the digestive process, which had led him to recognize the phenomenon of neutralization; he also believed that this process took place in the healing of wounds. Similarly, Franciscus de la Boë Sylvius explained disease and illness in terms of acids and alkalis. The subject was further developed by Otto Tachenius (d. after 1699), whose *Hippocrates chimicus* ascribed the acid–alkali theory to Hippocrates and Galen.

A corpuscular development of the acid–alkali theory was described in France by François de Saint André, "Docteur en Medecine de la Faculté de Caen." In his *Entretiens sur l'Acide et sur l'Alkali* (1672), André pointed to the importance of the recent work of anatomists and chemists, which had brought forth a new basis of medicine.[227] Turning to the five elements and principles, he noted that these were generally divided into three active and two passive principles. This dichotomy, he felt, could further be understood as a fundamental acid and alkali division of matter.[228] For André, therefore, the concept of acids and alkalis could be extended from questions of digestion and disease to the fundamental elements of nature. He was opposed by Robert Boyle who felt that his theory went against the mechanical philosophy in its insistence that "chemical reactions depended on an acid–alkali 'strife'."[229] Still, André, no less than Boyle, used pointed and porous particles as a means of describing chemical reactions.

The relationship of the chemical philosophy to the mechanical philosophy occasionally resulted in rather unusual works. Theodore Barin's *Le Monde Naissant ou La Création du Monde* (1686) claimed to demonstrate the principles according to the account of Moses. Here the author attempted to unite the corpuscular views of Descartes with the creation account in Genesis.[230] He pictured a universe of Cartesian *tourbillons* complete with an angelic region beyond the fixed sphere of the stars.

---

226 Ibid., p. 25.
227 François de Saint André (2nd ed. 1677), pp. 5–6. The first edition appeared in 1672 and a third edition was published in 1680.
228 Ibid., pp. 8–10.
229 Marie Boas discussed the debate in some detail (1956).
230 Theodore Barin (1686), pp. 19–23.

Barin did describe the cardiovascular system and other scientific phenomena, but other aspects of his work were more reminiscent of the alchemical cosmology of Fludd than of the mechanical philosophy.

An interesting comparison of the old and new philosophies was published by Jean-Baptiste Duhamel (1624–1706), a noted mathematician and the first secretary of the Académie Royale des Sciences (1666–97). In his *De Consensv Veteris et Novae Philosophiae* (1663) he discussed the confused state of philosophy.[231] Each sect seemed determined not to borrow from any other because each of them was convinced that it alone was right, and each centered its philosophy around the area in which it excelled. In fact, Duhamel said,

> Aristotle surpassed the others in logic and metaphysics whereas the chemists have gone further than Aristotle in discovering the principles that comprise natural bodies.
> Descartes excelled in his description of motion.
> The chemists reject the general notions and terms of the Aristotelians and have invented instead a new vocabulary.
> The Aristotelians accept nothing unless they find it in the writings of their master.
> The Cartesians want nothing from any other philosophers, having made an entirely new physics and metaphysics of their own.
> The Platonists have turned to natural theology and the explanation of universal causes, insisting that the basis of true philosophy consists in the contemplation of God.
> The disciples of Democritus and Epicurus turn to atomism and dismiss every other consideration.
> The Aristotelians accommodate their natural science to their metaphysical speculations.
> The Cartesians reduce everything to their geometry and mathematics.

For Duhamel the only satisfactory solution was to borrow the best from all of these philosophical groups. Thus, he divided his book into two parts: the first on the views of the Platonists, Aristotelians, Epicureans, and Cartesians on the principles of natural bodies; and the second on the elements and principles of the chemists, which he hoped to bring into agreement with the other sects. In Duhamel's text, chemistry is presented as the chief philosophical rival of all other sects. It is treated as a philosophy of nature, not just a subdivision of medicine useful for the preparation of remedies.

The ever-increasing interest in mechanical explanation in the sciences brought new opposition to the physiological iatrochemistry of the turn of the century as can be seen in the case of Philippe Hecquet (1661–

---

[231] Jean-Baptiste Duhamel (1663), sigs. ē iii^r – ē v^r ("Ratio operis").

1737).[232] Educated first at Abbeville, he took his medical degree at Paris in 1697. Thoroughly opposed to chemical explanations, Hecquet sought an understanding of organic action in the vibration of fibers and internal trituration. Reacting specifically to the fermentation theories of Vieussens, Hecquet prepared his *De Digestion, et des Maladies de l'Estomac suivant le Systême de la Trituration & du Broyement, sans l'aide des Levains on fait voir l'impossibilité en santé & en maladie* (1712). Comparing his mechanical system with that of the iatrochemists, Hecquet wrote that trituration explained phenomena more simply, with more certainty, and more understandably. The chemists spoke of degrees of heat, concentrations, coagulations, fermentations, effervescences, humors, and juices. The mechanists, however, had simpler explanations related to the oscillation of fibers, relative diameters, and forces. The chemists discussed bile, phlegm, blood, melancholy, acid, alkali, volatility, and fixity and spoke of the aqueous, sulfurous, spiritous, and phlegmatic nature of substances when in fact it was necessary to speak only of solids and fluids. And when the chemists wrote of faculties, qualities, and flavors, they should have limited themselves to resistances and forces. "In short, and because we do not wish to repeat ourselves too much, all these names and qualifications [used by the chemists] are in their imaginations while solids and liquids are in nature."[233]

For Hecquet the promises and attractions of chemistry had tarnished the reputations of otherwise great physicians. Surely, this was true of Willis and Sylvius, both of whom devoted themselves too much to the dreams of Paracelsus and van Helmont. Hecquet continued that even the present physicians of France are too devoted to Paracelsian secrets and chemical delusions[234]; if this continues, he said, medicine will degenerate to a monstrous science.

Chemistry, the Parisian Academy, and the Journal des Sçavans

France had a long history of short-lived groups interested in the sciences, such as the Paracelsian meetings organized by Jacques Gohory in the sixteenth century and the weekly discussions on scientific and medical matters at the Bureau d'Adresse under Théophraste Renaudot. Also

---

[232] L. W. B. Brockliss (1989) has examined the relation of Hecquet's iatrophysical views with his Jansenist beliefs. Hecquet was a convinced mechanist who debated in print with the iatrochemist Andry de Boisregard (1658–1745) in 1710. Throughout his life he became increasingly suspect of chemically prepared medicines; but like earlier Paracelsians, he was convinced that God expected man to learn to read the book of nature and that a true physician must be a pious person like a priest. Indeed, he thought that medical cure occurred only in cooperation with the Holy Spirit.

[233] Philippe Hecquet (1730; 1st ed. 1712), vol. 2, pp. xliv–xlv.

[234] Ibid., vol. 1, pp. 564–5.

during the second quarter of the century Father Marin Mersenne gathered friends at his moñastic cell in Paris for scientific discussions, and he corresponded regularly with scientists throughout Europe, gathering and diffusing information. These meetings declined after Mersenne's death, but in 1666 Jean Baptiste Colbert, intendant and chief councillor to Louis XIV, founded the Académie Royale des Sciences, which he hoped would encourage the sciences and benefit the state. Duhamel was the first secretary, and the other members were Huyghens, Roberval, Picard, Perrault, and the chemists Claude Bourdelin (1621–1699) and Samuel Cottereau Duclos. From the start this group was physically rather than medically oriented.

Surely Duclos was the most active chemist. He was a physician to the king, though he retired to a Capuchin convent in 1685 where he survived another thirty years.[235] Duclos is perhaps best known for his comprehensive study of the mineral waters of France; but Alice Stroup, who has examined the manuscript account of his presentations at the Académie, has shown that most of these relate to the chemical analysis of plants.[236] Between 1675 and 1685 he presented only four proposals for future work, a fact that Stroup has attributed to a falling off of his own scientific work and to "a somewhat diminished interest on the part of his fellows in recording what Duclos had to say on the various topics he spoke about."[237]

In fact, Duclos was interested in traditional chemical themes. On 8 August 1668 he presented to his fellows of the académie a lengthy paper on "Le sel circulée de Paracelse," which referred frequently to van Helmont as well.[238] In a *Dissertation sur les Principes de Mixtes Naturels* (1680) he discussed the difficulty of chemical analysis and suggested a range of elements from the corporeal and sensible to the incorporeal and solely intelligible. He argued that bodies are able to interact without physical contact because of the universal spirit, which surrounds and penetrates them. Through this spirit, or ether, nature can impress specific characteristics on bodies.[239]

Although the académie did not have a regular journal until 1699 when the *Histoire* and *Mémoires* began publication, news of the académie and reviews of new scientific books were available from 1665 in the pages of the *Journal des Sçavans*. The following year a lengthy article appeared in the *Journal* on the hundred-year debate about the internal use of anti-

---

[235] Partington (1962), vol. 3, pp. 11–13.
[236] I am indebted to Professor Stroup for the information she has given me in a number of private communications, including photocopies of manuscript accounts of Duclos's presentations at the Académie. She also prepared in typescript a useful "bibliographical note" on the "Memoires" of Duclos in the Procés-Verbaux.
[237] Alice Stroup, "Implications of the Bibliographical Record" (pri. comm. typescript), p. 8e.
[238] Manuscript photocopied by Alice Stroup, AdS, Reg., 4:134r–166r.
[239] Sr. Duclos (1680), p. 101.

mony, which had culminated in the approval of this substance by the assembled members of the Parisian Medical Faculty.[240]

Still, reviews of chemical works were relatively uncommon in the early years of the *Journal*. Johann Joachim Becher's introductory *Oedipus Chimicus* was reviewed in 1666,[241] and the second edition of Duhamel's *De Consensv Veteris et Novae Philosophicae* was discussed three years later.[242] Books reviewed in the 1670s included John Mayow's *Tractatus quinque* on the aerial niter (1676),[243] Moyse Charas's *Pharmacopée Royale* (1676)[244] (the reviewer noted that Charas believed that both Galenic and chemical medicines were needed by the physician), Johann Kunckel's *Observationes* (1678),[245] John Webster's *Metallographia* (1678),[246] and Nicholas Lemery's *Cours de chymie* (1679).[247]

It is interesting that this scholarly journal did not neglect new publications in traditional transmutatory alchemy. Thus, a reviewer attempted to explain chemically the most mystical of alchemical picture books, the *Mutus Liber*, in 1677,[248] and Pantaleon's critical *Examen Alchymisticum* was discussed the following year.[249] An interesting oddity was a book titled *Utis Udenii*, which was devoted to chemical operations that could not be accomplished, such as the transmutation of metals and the resuscitation of plants from their ashes (1697).[250] Note was taken the same year of Glauber's *Dissertatio de Tinctura Universali, vulgo Lapis Philosophorum dicta*, in which he asserted that the philosopher's stone could be made and that transmutation could be accomplished; the reviewer suggested drily that "Nous laissons à ces Messieurs à éprouver la verité des experiences qu'il rapporte."[251]

Chemical medicine was represented by reviews of a work on aurum potabile by Albertus Othon (1679)[252] and the *Medicina Magnetica* (1679) of Anthony Maxwell, which dealt with sympathetic medicine.[253] Maxwell's book was barely mentioned in the *Journal*, but a century later it was to be seen as an important predecessor to the work of Mesmer.

The 1680s saw an increased number of chemical reviews in the *Journal*. The short chemical textbook of Vigani, the *Medulla Chymiae*, was noted

240 *Journal des Sçavans*, 1666 (Nouvelle edition, Paris: Pierre Witte, 1723), pp. 164–7.
241 Ibid., p. 11.
242 *Journal des Sçavans*, 1668 (Amsterdam: Pierre le Grand, 1685), pp. 563–6.
243 *Journal des Sçavans*, 1676 (Amsterdam: Pierre le Grand, 1685), pp. 32–6.
244 Ibid., pp. 271–3.
245 *Journal des Sçavans*, 1678 (Amsterdam, 1683), pp. 435–7.
246 Ibid., pp. 301–4.
247 *Journal des Sçavans*, 1679 (Amsterdam, 1683), pp. 206–8.
248 *Journal des Sçavans*, 1677 (Amsterdam), pp. 242–5.
249 *Journal des Sçavans*, 1678 (Amsterdam), pp. 55–6.
250 *Journal des Sçavans*, 1679 (Amsterdam), pp. 165–6.
251 Ibid., p. 132.
252 Ibid., pp. 220–2.
253 Ibid., p. 230.

in the 1681 volume as well as the major text by Becher, his *Physica subterraneae*.[254] Here the reviewer commented that the scope of the work was similar to that of Athanasius Kircher's *Mundus subterraneus*, but that Becher's work was limited to chemical explanations whereas Kircher drew from all fields.

In the same year Daniel Duncan's *La Chymie Naturelle* was discussed in some depth because, as the reviewer understood, he had attempted to show that all nature follows chemical rules.[255] Raymond Vieussen's *Tractatus duo* received a long review in 1687 because he had renounced the medicine of the ancients and was beginning to build a new system based on a study of bodily fluids and the process of fermentation.[256]

Also in 1687 Fouët's *Nouveau Systéme de bains & eaux minerals de Vichy* permitted the reviewer to discuss the progress of the acid–alkali system,[257] the origin of which he attributed to Otto Tachenius and to note Bertrand's *Reflexions* of 1683, which had been written in opposition to the theory. In his *Systéme*, Fouët had replied to Bertrand.

New editions of Lemery, Charas, Helmont, and Juncken were reviewed, as well as purely alchemical texts such as the *Hermes curiosus* by Adolph Baldwin[258] and an anonymous *Magni Philosophorum Arcani Revelator* printed in 1688.[259] Here the author promised to reveal the secret work, and the reviewer followed his presentation, expressing no personal opinion.

The final decade of the seventeenth century witnessed very few chemical reviews in the *Journal*. Passing reference is made to the *La Pratique de Medecine* by Theodore de Mayerne[260] and the fact that he used mineral-based remedies only when herbal remedies proved to be too weak (1693). Pierre Pomet's *Histoire generale des drogues* received an eight-page review in 1694,[261] and four years later there was a review of a letter "sur l'impossibilité de operations sympathetiques."[262]

Conclusion

The closing decades of the seventeenth century witnessed the final acceptance of chemistry as a necessary branch of medicine. Throughout the universities of Europe, chairs of chemistry were established, almost always through the incentive of medical faculties. It was finally under-

254 *Journal des Sçavans*, 1681 (Amsterdam), p. 32.
255 Ibid., p. 355.
256 *Journal des Sçavans*, 1687 (Amsterdam), pp. 509–15.
257 Ibid., p. 222.
258 *Journal des Sçavans*, 1681 (Amsterdam), p. 367.
259 *Journal des Sçavans*, 1688 (Amsterdam), p. 369–71.
260 *Journal des Sçavans*, 1693 (Amsterdam), pp. 309–10.
261 *Journal des Sçavans*, 1694 (Amsterdam), pp. 239–47.
262 *Journal des Sçavans*, 1698 (Amsterdam), p. 30.

stood that the use of chemically prepared remedies did not conflict with Galenic theory nor did it imply the user's endorsement of a mystical Paracelsian universe. If chemical purgatives were sometimes more violent than the old-fashioned herbal mixtures, it seemed that on occasion they were necessary. Accordingly, Sebastian Matte was appointed demonstrator in chemistry through the Medical Faculty of Montpellier in 1673, and Arnaldus Fonsorbe was named its first professor of chemistry. The Medical Faculty of Paris, even more reluctant to approve of the art of the fire, yielded only to an appointment for the teaching of chemical and Galenic pharmacy in 1698.

Students willing to go beyond the academic halls had a variety of courses to choose from. Surely the most famous teachers were those who taught chemistry at the Jardin des Plantes. Davisson, Le Fèvre, Glaser, and Charas all wrote textbooks for their courses that went through many editions in French and other languages. Nicholas Lemery, who studied at the Jardin des Plantes, wrote the most popular text of all, one that went into its final edition in 1757. And as we have seen, there were others that one could turn to for instruction, such as Clave, Arnaud, Barlet, Locques, and Meurdac.

These authors were concerned primarily with pharmaceutical chemistry, which had been the chief cause of debate relating to chemistry from the mid-sixteenth century onward, and chemistry had been triumphant. But there was a second major theme in the debate about Paracelsian medicine: Paracelsus had explained disease and some physiological processes in chemical terms. This aspect of iatrochemistry was developed by many of his followers and became a subject of special interest to van Helmont in the early seventeenth century. For van Helmont, Sylvius, Vieussens, and many others, the special interest of chemistry lay in its ability to explain bodily processes either through analogy or chemical experimentation. Thus, just when chemical remedies were being accepted as additions to the traditional *materia medica*, chemistry seemed to promise new answers for medical theory. The *Opera* of van Helmont went through numerous editions into the early eighteenth century, as did the works of Sylvius and Willis, and Vieussens was widely recognized as one of the chief figures of European medicine.

Van Helmont called his chemical medicine a "nova Philosophica," but it was not the new philosophy we associate with the mechanists. The iatrochemistry of the late seventeenth century attracted many members of the medical establishment, but it did so at a time when the mechanical philosophy was dominating the newly founded academies of London and Paris. Accordingly, it is not unexpected that the medical chemistry of van Helmont, Willis, and Sylvius was questioned by those who sought to make medical physiology a physical rather than a chemical discipline. The iatrophysics of Borelli and Baglivi was in conflict with the iatrochemistry of Sylvius by the closing years of the seventeenth century. We have noted this debate in France in the case of Philippe Hecquet, who demanded physical explanations of physiological phenomena rather than the chemical explanations of Vieussens.

A final theme that persisted in the Paracelsian tradition was that of transmutational alchemy and miraculous cures. These topics were of little interest to the textbook authors or the chemical physiologists, but an historian cannot simply dismiss these authors as nonscientific and ignore them. In fact, van Helmont claimed to have carried out the transmutation of mercury to gold with the aid of one quarter grain of the philosophers' stone, which had been given to him. As we have seen, a great number of alchemical texts continued to be published throughout the seventeenth century. The most unexpected aspect of this activity is the fact that many of these works were mentioned or reviewed in the pages of the *Journal des Sçavans*. This persistent interest is a cause for a sudden increase in the number of such publications in the early years of the eighteenth century. This and the continued activity of French Paracelsians is the subject of the next chapter.

5

Alchemy in an Age of Reason: the chemical philosophers in early eighteenth-century France

> Je dirai donc que parmi les Modernes, Paracelse semble avoir surpassé tous ses Prédécesseurs; & qu'avec raison il s'est attribué le titre, de *Monarque des Arcanes*.
> François Marie Pompée Colonne (1724)[1]

Étienne François Geoffroy and the alchemical charlatans

In 1722, readers of the *Mémoires* of the Académie Royale des Sciences of Paris may have been more than a little surprised to find a paper on the deceits practiced by alchemists.[2] The author was Étienne François Geoffroy (1672–1731), one of the earliest of the French Newtonians and the author of the first table of affinity (1718). His name is usually associated with a few others in a pantheon of eighteenth-century chemists whose work formed the background of the chemical revolution.[3]

This paper by Geoffroy is seldom referred to because it reflects a literature that stems back to the Middle Ages rather than the Enlightenment. Here Geoffroy warned those who sought quick wealth not to be duped by alchemists. Such people were ready prey for alchemists who claimed to have made the elixir of life or the philosophers' stone because of the widespread belief in this art.[4] He described the many tricks of these charlatans: their double-bottomed cupels and hollow stirring rods,

This chapter is a version of a paper first presented at the conference "Hermeticism and the Renaissance," which was held in March 1982 at the Institute for Renaissance and Eighteenth-Century Studies in the Folger Shakespeare Library in Washington, D.C. Titled "Alchemy in an Age of Reason: The Chemical Philosophers in Early Eighteenth-Century France," this paper has since appeared in *Hermeticism and the Renaissance: Intellectual History and the Occult in Early Modern Europe*, edited by Ingrid Merkel and Allen G. Debus (Folger Books: Washington: The Folger Shakespeare Library; London and Toronto: Associated University Presses, 1988), pp. 231–50.

1 François Marie Pompée Colonne (1724), sig. *iiiᵛ–*iiiiʳ.
2 E. F. Geoffroy, Académie Royale *Memoirs* (1722) (Amsterdam, 1727, pp. 81–93).
3 On Geoffroy's life and work, see the article by W. A. Smeaton (1972), pp. 352–4 (with a good bibliography), and J. R. Partington (1962), pp. 49ff.
4 Geoffroy (1722), 61–2.

their amalgams with concealed precious metals, their acids with dissolved gold and silver, and even filtration papers prepared with minute amounts of gold that could be recovered by combustion.[5] The charlatans were a clever lot, and their ingredients and equipment had to be carefully checked because they had frequently deceived even skilled chemists. Geoffroy himself had been part of a committee named by the Académie to investigate a process of the Abbé Bignon, which supposedly destroyed gold. This, too, had proved to be a clever trick.[6]

Bernard Fontenelle (1657–1757), perpetual secretary to the Académie from 1697 to 1739, gave prominent attention to Geoffroy's paper in the *Histoire*.[7] He declined to take a firm stand on the theoretical possibility of transmutation, but he did warn his readers against the pretended "adepts, Infants in the Art, Hermetic Philosophers, Cosmopolites, Rosicrucians, and others, people whose mysterious language, fanatic conduct, and exorbitant promises must render them highly suspect. . .TH." These people spoke of a powder of projection, a few atoms of which could produce great masses of gold; but what rational system of physics could possibly accommodate such a concept?

Geoffroy's attack on alchemy is a very late example of a genre that we have traced in France from the mid-sixteenth century, one that can be traced back in European literature at least to Chaucer's "Canon's Yeoman's Tale." But more important is the fact that here we are given clear evidence of the concern felt by members of the Académie for the widespread contemporary interest in alchemy and transmutation.

Alchemy and the chemical philosophy beyond the establishment

The French literary works of the early eighteenth century leave little doubt that alchemy and the supernatural continued to attract widespread interest, and it is true that some intellectual historians have pointed to the prevalence of magic, alchemy, and other occult arts in the eighteenth century.[8] We see this in works as well known as Montesquieu's *Lettres persanes* (1721)[9] and Bordelon's *Historie de M. Oufle* (1710).[10] In his *Voyages* (1712), Paul Lucas described a visit to Central Asia where he learned that the fourteenth-century French alchemist Nicholas Flamel was still alive and at work on the secrets of the world, a story that

---

[5] Ibid., 62–3.
[6] Ibid., 68–9.
[7] Académie Royale, *Histoire* (1722) (Amsterdam, 1727, pp. 52–5).
[8] A short but useful survey of this literature is to be found in Constantin Bila (1925). A far more exhaustive account of the end of the eighteenth century is in August Viatte (1969, 1st ed. 1927).
[9] Charles Louis de Secondat Montesquieu (n.d.). See Letter 58, vol. 1, pp. 151–2.
[10] Laurent Bordelon (1711), pp. 223–5.

excited numerous other authors throughout the century who had an interest in alchemy and the prolongation of life.[11]

If we turn from literary to occult texts, it would be difficult to ignore the many editions of the *Secrets* of Albertus Magnus that appeared throughout the century,[12] or the new French translation of Agrippa's *De occulta philosophia* (1727),[13] or the Abbé Villars de Montfaucon's best seller, the *Comte de Gabalis*, which appeared first in 1670 and frequently thereafter.[14] Indeed, booksellers supplied their clientele with a broad spectrum of titles on black and white magic, the divining rod, witchcraft, astrology, and all forms of occultism.

But Geoffroy was not concerned with witchcraft and magic, only with the alchemists of his day. Had he wished, he could have pointed to a seemingly unending publication of alchemical texts. Still popular were traditional texts dating from the past century or earlier, such as Jean Collesson's *L'Idée parfaite de la philosophie hermétique* (1630)[15] and Limojon de Saint Didier's *Le triomphe hermétique* (1689).[16] The seventeenth-century classic by Michael Sendivogius, the *Novum Lumen Chymicum,* was translated into French in 1723; this edition was highly sought by alchemists and chemists alike.[17] The copy at the Cornell University Library bears the bookplate of Antoine Lavoisier.

There were new works as well. A *Traité de la poudre de projection* (1707) by D. L. B. sought a new key to alchemy through a novel interpretation of the story of Abraham, Sarah, and Lot in Genesis.[18] In 1719 an anonymous *Lettre a un ami* deplored current attacks on alchemists when they should be honored because of the wonderful metallic remedies they had discovered,[19] which was highly productive work compared with the useless work done by the members of the Académie.[20] In truth, said the letter, we should return to the problems posed by the alchemists and recognize that the search for the determination of longitudes among mathematicians is no more important than the search for a potable gold among chemists and physicians.[21]

[11]   See the long account by Claude and Sabine Stuart Chevalier (1765), pp. 84ff. The Chevaliers cite Paul Lucas, *Voyages* (1712), p. 102.

[12]   Editions referred to in the course of this research include the *Secrets Merveilleux* (1743) and *Les admirables Secrets d'Albert le Grand* (1758).

[13]   Henri Cornelius Agrippa (1727).

[14]   Nicholas Pierre Henri de Montfaucon Villars (1742). There are at least three eighteenth-century editions prior to the publication of Geoffroy's paper (1700, 1715, 1718).

[15]   Jean Collesson (1630, 1631, 1719).

[16]   [Limojon de Saint Didier] (1699). This work was translated into German and English.

[17]   Michael Sendivogius (1723).

[18]   D. L. B. (1707).

[19]   Anon. (1719), pp. 3–4.

[20]   Bernard Fontenelle, secrétaire perpétuel of the Académie Royale, was the editor of the *Histoire* and *Memoires* of that society. He was characterized by the author of the *Lettre* as the creator of dialogues of the dead. Ibid., p. 8.

[21]   Ibid., sig. A2^r.

So well known was this literature that it resulted in several warnings in the decades prior to Geoffroy's 1722 paper. An anonymous *Explication de quelques doutes touchant la medecine* (1700) turned specifically to the alchemical claims of the wonders of potable gold and the conviction that there is a universal remedy for illnesses. The reader was told that the hope of a soluble gold is only an illusion. False chemists had adopted astrology, and they were little more than charlatans who hid their shame and ignorance in an enigmatic language and allegorical emblems.[22] In 1711 François Pousse produced a stinging *Examen des principes des alchymistes sur la pierre philosophale*, in which the possibility of the multiplication of the metals was flatly denied. Moreover, the long search for the elixir of life had been a waste of time, gold and silver are practically useless as metals. Rather, lowly iron is the metal used to make the instruments necessary for life. Why then is there no learned attack on alchemy, especially in France where it is most needed?

> The Germans and the English apply themselves to alchemy. The Dutch are not so curious. (One might say that commerce takes them away from the sciences.) But of all the nations, the French are the most ardent and the most intoxicated by it: It is for this reason that I have written this small *Examen* in French, so that it might be examined by all the world.[23]

However, the scope of alchemy was not limited to transmutation. Over the centuries many alchemists had adopted a far-reaching philosophy of nature that served as a basis for the explanation of natural phenomena. These authors argued for a vitalistic universe, in which all parts of the macrocosm and the microcosm are interconnected. Confirmation of these concepts was avidly sought through laboratory observations. One example is the Tree of Diana.[24] The method of production was simple. An ounce of silver was dissolved in a few ounces of nitric acid, and then the solution was evaporated to half its volume, poured into a container with twenty ounces of water, and allowed to stand for forty days. At the end of that time the silver "will have formed a sort of Tree, with Branches and little Balls at the end of them, which represent the Fruit." Well known by the mid-seventeenth century, this demonstration was used by chemical philosophers to show that "Art mimicks what Nature does, when she produces Silver in the Mines; and some have pretended that this Artificial Vegetation is like the Vegetation of Plants." Nicholas Lemery described the process in his popular *Cours de Chymie* (1677) and then proceeded to note that "this Operation may be fitly compared with the manner of Generation and Nourishment of Plants in

---

22 Anon. (ca. 1700).
23 [François Pousse] (1711), sig. a viii.
24 Pierre Le Lorrain, Abbé de Vallemont (1707), pp. 302–7. The first French edition appeared as the *Curiositez de la Nature et de l'Art sur la Vegetation: Ou l'Agriculture, et le Jardinage dans leur Perfection* (1705).

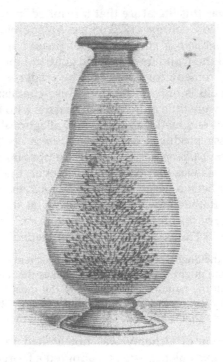

The Tree of Diana. From Pierre Le Lorrain, the Abbé de Vallemont, *Curiositez de la Nature et de l'Art sur la Vegetation: ou l'Agriculture, et le Jardinage* . . . (1711). From the collection of the author.

the Earth."[25] In short, the Tree of Diana seemed to offer chemical philosophers proof of life in the mineral kingdom. Here, too, was experimental evidence of metallic growth that confirmed the belief that ores would replenish themselves in mines if allowed to stand fallow, a belief that persisted to our own century in certain parts of Europe. This was an important discovery for chemical philosophers because it upheld a significant part of their world view.

The Tree of Diana was also of interest to chemists of the Académie Royale des Sciences. Guillaume Homberg (1652–1715) examined this experiment in detail in 1693 and rejected the vitalist explanation, arguing that the formation was simply crystallization.[26] Nevertheless, papers on this observation and similar metallic formations were described in the pages of the *Mémoires* for the next forty years.

For Pierre Le Lorrain, Abbé de Vallemont (1649–1721), the Tree of Diana was an important subject for discussion in his *Curiositez de la*

[25] Nicholas Lemery (1686), pp. 89–91.
[26] Le Lorrain (1707), pp. 305–6.

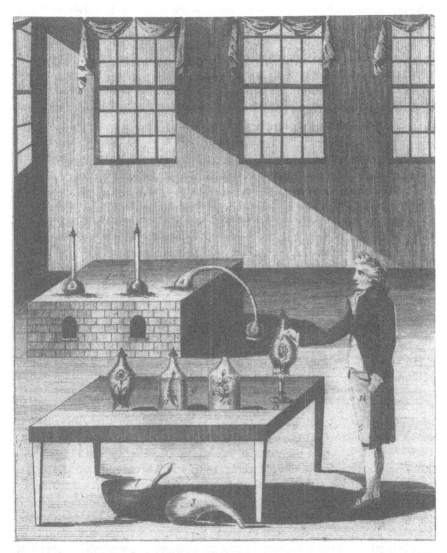

Palingenesis in an eighteenth-century laboratory. From Ebenezer Sibley, *A New and Complete Illustration of Astrology* (1792). From the collection of the author.

nature et de l'art sur la Vegetation . . . , which went through at least eight editions between 1705 and 1715. On this subject the Abbé sided with Homberg in his belief that the formation was due to crystallization, but on other matters Vallemont reflected his alchemical heritage. He wrote another popular monograph on the divining rod, and closed his *Curiosities* with a forty-page discussion of one of the greatest miracles of the age, palingenesis. Since the late sixteenth century it had been widely believed among chemists that if plants were calcined to ashes and the ashes heated in an hermetically sealed flask, the form of the original plant would appear in the flask.[27] Vallemont cited accounts by Paracelsus, Joseph Duchesne, Sir Kenelm Digby, Athanasius Kircher, and other prominent authors to prove that "there is no longer room for incredulity."[28] However, he added, even greater wonders are possible than the reproduction of plants. Martin Kergerus attests to the fact that

> in the substance of Salts, the specifick Forms of the Bodies, from whence they are extracted, are contain'd: and tho' the Body, it self be destroy'd, we may preserve this exterior Form, and see it under the Figure of a Shade, or of a subtil Cloud, compos'd of Vapours and Exhalations, almost in the same manner as we believe the bodies of the Dead to be when they appear in Church-yards. He adds: I am assured that this Reproduction has been effected, not only upon Plants, but also upon Animals. Particularly they speak of a little Sparrow, that was made to appear in that manner, in a Vial where its Ashes were kept. . . . Thus we have a Sparrow rais'd to Life, like a Phoenix from the midst of its Ashes. . . . *Digby* has done more than this. From Animals that were dead, and pounded to Dust, he has drawn living Animals of the same Kind.[29]

In this observation was to be found experimental evidence of divine truth. "There is not in the World a more faithful Image of the Resurrection of the Dead, and I am persuaded that Nature and Art can never offer to our Eyes a More divine Spectacle."[30]

Vallemont's interest in alchemy and traditional chemical philosophy reappears in Harcouet de Longeville's monograph on the lives of people who had lived for many centuries.[31] Here the author drew heavily on the alchemical dream of the prolongation of human life, and he referred to a newly discovered manuscript of Arnald of Villanova in the possession of the Abbé de Vallemont. Because this text seemed to be an important key to rejuvenation, he asked for financial support to make it available in print.

De Longeville's work underscores the close connection between medicine and alchemy, which had existed in Western Europe since the thirteenth century. This traditional alchemical medicine was still current in early eighteenth-century France. Books on the universal remedy and

27 Recent papers on palingenesis include Jacques Marx (1971); Allen G. Debus, "A Further Note on Palingenesis: The Account of Ebenezer Sibley in the Illustration of Astrology" (1973); and François Secret (1979).
28 Le Lorrain (1707), p. 327.
29 Ibid., pp. 348–9.
30 Ibid., pp. 327–8. A discussion of the Resurrection as a chemical process is to be found in Joseph Chambon (1714), pp. 367–70.
31 Harcouet de Longeville (1715).

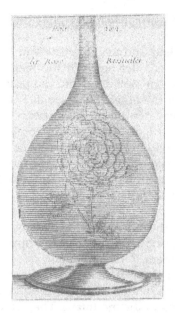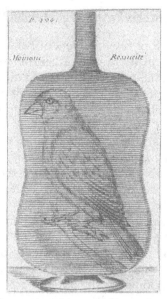

The phenomena of palingenesis: a rose and a sparrow resuscitated. From Pierre
Le Lorrain, the Abbé de Vallemont, *Curiositez de la Nature et de l'Art sur la Vegetation: ou l'Agriculture, et le Jardinage. . .* (1711). From the collection of the author.

chemical elixirs were common,[32] but the complex interrelation of alchemy and medicine in this period can best be illustrated by three small
books published by Charles Le Breton, a "Medecin de la Faculté de
Paris." His first publication (1716) was a very general collection of herbal
and chemical preparations.[33] Six years later we find him preparing a
French translation of the *De statica medicina* (1614) of Sanctorius (1561–
1636), a landmark work that introduced quantification to medicine
through a study of variation of weight due to ingestion and excretion.[34]
But Le Breton had other interests as well. In the same year he published
a work on *Les clefs de la philosophie spagyrique*.[35] Here are to be found a
series of alchemical aphorisms. The first part concentrates on chemical
operations and the second on preparation of the mineral elixir for transmutation. In short, we find here a member of the medical establishment
who was aware of the significance of the work of Sanctorius, but who
could at the same time see fundamental truths in the mystical texts of
the alchemists.

[32] As examples, see Domenico Auda (1711) and D. J. B. D. F. Y. C. (1722).
[33] Charles Le Breton (1716).
[34] Sanctorius Sanctorius (1722).
[35] M. Le Breton (1722).

The eighteenth-century French Paracelso-Helmontians

The work of the followers of Paracelsus and Jean Baptiste van Helmont resulted in more than a century of conflict between the medical and educational establishments of Europe on one hand and the proponents of a chemical approach to nature on the other. Evidence in France that this familiar late seventeenth-century "battle of the ancients and the moderns" was much more than a struggle between Aristotelians and mechanists can be found in an anonymous text of 1697, *Le Parnasse assiégé ou la guerre declarée entre les philosophes anciens & modernes*. In the preface the reader is told that the author plans to "demonstrate the reality of Hermetic science and the truth of the Medicine of Paracelsus."[36]

The plot is simple. Apollo, god of the sun and of the healing arts, has died on Mount Parnassus. Each philosopher takes this as an opportunity to assert his primacy over all the others.[37] The mountain need only be climbed and the throne seized. But the lack of success of any one of them to dominate the others leads to abandonment of this civil war, and the philosophers join together to assault the mountain. The author then lists the various philosophers and their places in this unusual army. At one side are the academicians commanded by Plato and his disciples. Closer to the mountain are the followers of Gassendi and Descartes, who discover roads that lead to the top. Even Confucius and other Chinese philosophers are present and demand a proper place for the attack.[38]

Dissension arises when Aristotle is appointed the Prince of Philosophers, but this does not delay the continuing preparations for the assault.[39] Galileo is placed in charge of the cavalry, Cardan and Porta are to lead the artillery, and Parmenides, Heraclitus, and Democritus are given command of the infantry.[40] Descartes commands the dragoons, and his lieutenants include a group of his disciples and other seventeenth-century corpuscularians. Surprisingly we find that the chemical physicians, Daniel Sennert and van Helmont, have been placed in charge of the baggage.[41]

But now four spies – all important alchemists – inform the assembled army that the mountain is nearly inaccessible and is open only to philosophers of the school of Hermes. The officers of Hermes carry a standard

[36] Anon. (1697), sig. Aii[v].
[37] Ibid., p. 1.
[38] Ibid., pp. 4–6.
[39] Ibid., p. 11.
[40] Ibid., p. 12.
[41] Ibid., p. 13.

marked *FRC* (Fraternity of the Rosy Cross). After a lengthy discussion these spies disappear.[42]

In the new strategem various groups unsuccessfully try to penetrate the mists leading to the summit. Among a group of vivandiers we have a glimpse of "Harvée porta des oeufs"[43] while a group of chemists (including Libavius and Glauber) are forced to return to camp after losing their way.[44] Then another spy is caught, the alchemist Geber, who informs the besiegers that the mountain is defended by many philosophers who are guided by reason and truth, men who have been taught by Hermes, the father of all knowledge.[45] Galen explodes in rage,[46] but he is stilled by the announcement that an important prisoner has been captured. This is no less than Paracelsus who has already injured the members of his escort and is using such strong language that some are calling for his death. But instead, Aristotle calls for his interrogation and permits Paracelsus to defend himself.[47]

It is from the prisoner that the leaders of the attacking army learn the names of the principal defenders of the summit: Moses, Solomon, Roger Bacon, Nicholas Flamel, Hippocrates, Basil Valentine, Ramon Lull, and Arnald of Villanova in the first rank – with others behind them, including Joseph Duchesne, Gerhard Dorn, Roch le Baillif, Agrippa von Nettesheym, Oswald Crollius, Robert Fludd, Heinrich Khunrath, and Michael Maier.[48]

Unexpectedly a copy of Paracelsus' *Archidoxes magica* is found and condemned to the fire. Paracelsus is given a reprieve from his fate only if he agrees to show the philosopher-warriors the road by which they might avoid the mists and clouds that shield the summit from those below. He agrees to this and begins to lead a physician (Andreas Laurentius or du Laurens) up the slope by hand. But the latter is not worthy of his charge and he falls to the ground in darkness, an event that symbolizes his ignorance. Paracelsus, the true champion of truth, continues on to join his comrades at the top, leaving behind the bickering philosophers, who represent every modern and ancient philosophical sect except the true one.[49]

The view of Paracelsus as the ultimate alchemist that we see in *Le Parnasse* is even more explicit in the work of François Pompée Colonne (ca. 1649–1726), an author who published very little until late in life.

[42] Ibid., pp. 14–15.
[43] Ibid., p. 100.
[44] Ibid., p. 103.
[45] Ibid., pp. 109–10.
[46] Ibid., p. 115.
[47] Ibid., p. 116.
[48] Ibid., pp. 127–8.
[49] Ibid., pp. 136–8.

Beginning in 1718 and continuing after his death, a number of alchemical texts appeared under his name or his pseudonyms that clearly
establish Colonne as a man interested in the more mystical interpretations of nature: geomancy, astrology, and above all, alchemy.[50] "The
Seed of the Chemical Philosophers" is a defense of this art against a
critic. He followed alchemical tradition in quoting earlier authors at great
length, mostly medieval figures, though there are several references to
"the Great Paracelsus"[51] and to the specific remedies of Robert Boyle.
Colonne defended the fact that the alchemists did not publish the method of making gold:

> What will you says Cosmopolite at the end of his work, that they should
> teach you to make cheese with Milk, would you that they should make
> their Philosophy contemplable to good women in publishing this great
> secret that they should render it, not only useless, but that they should
> over throw the usual order of things, letting all the World know how to
> make Gold & Silver.[52]

Elsewhere he taught the theory of metallic growth, the means of extract-
ing quintessences, and the secrets of transmutation. Colonne defended
the alchemists' secrecy and tried to explain their enigmas and paradoxes
to his perplexed readers; but it would be wrong to dismiss him as a
popularizer of the occult. He was well aware of the work of Boyle and
Descartes,[53] and he accepted the corpuscular philosophy, which he ascribed to the work of the chemists. Indeed, he wrote, the true elements
of bodies are not common earth, water, air, and fire, but rather, the
essences or qualities of these bodies,

> which one can imagine being the smallest particles of the afore mentioned
> visible and corporeal four elements which we call Water, Earth, Air and
> Fire. Of these the invisible particles which one calls Qualities, amassed in
> large quantity, form the visible water or earth.[54]

50 We know little of the life of this author beyond the fact that he died in the flames of his
   house and that a student (Gosmond) prepared several of his manuscripts for the press
   and answered one of his master's critics, the Reverend Father Castel. His first publication was an *Introduction à la philosophie des anciens, par un amateur de la verité*, which
   appeared in 1698, but then there was complete silence for a quarter century. His *Les
   Secrets les plus cachés* (1722, reprinted 1762), *Les Principes de la nature* (1725), *Suite des
   Expériences utiles* (1725), a work on geomancy (1726), and possibly a few additional texts
   appearing under the name of Le Crom were published shortly prior to his death. There
   appeared posthumously his *Principes de la nature où de la génération* (1732) and a multi-
   volume *Histoire naturelle de l'univers* (1734). In addition, a mid-nineteenth-century copy
   of an English translation of one of his works, "The Seed of the Chemical Philosophers,"
   exists at the Wellcome Historical Medical Library.
51 Colonne (1737), pp. 35, 84.
52 Ibid., pp., 91–2.
53 François Marie Pompée Colonne (1724), pp. vii–viii.
54 M. Colonne (1731), pp. 26–7.

Colonne's understanding of generation was based largely on his reading of Harvey and Malpighi, both of whom he quoted at length.[55]

Although Colonne read widely, it is clear from his *Abregé de la doctrine de la Paracelse et de ses Archidoxes* (1724) that he thought that one author should be consulted above all others. In this substantial volume of five hundred pages he is unequivocal in his praise: "I will say then that among the Moderns, Paracelsus seems to have surpassed all his predecessors, and with reason he has been given the title, *Monarch of Arcana*."[56] Paracelsus had established his doctrine on physical reasons rather than on unintelligible enigmas[57] and was a true physician who presented to his readers the rules for the preparation of all sorts of remedies for the cure of mankind and for the perfection of metals.[58] The key to Paracelsus's great accomplishment was to be found in his *Archidoxes*, which Colonne prepared for the reader in an abridgment that reflected his own interpretation.

Colonne begins with his own introductory explanation of the principles of chemistry, describing chemistry as the art of resolving mixed substances and of separating the pure from the impure.[59] In his discussion of the principles, Colonne accepts the five principles most commonly accepted in the late seventeenth century: the Paracelsian salt, sulfur, and mercury, plus phlegm (water) and *caput mortuum* (earth), derived from the four elements of Aristotle. These elements, he argues, are true and certain because they are based on laboratory experience.[60]

Colonne proceeds to discuss the traditional four qualities: heat, dryness, cold, and humidity. However, for him these differ from the visible elements, rather, they are the small invisible parts of them. Thus, water from a river

> is not properly called "la qualité humide"; but it is necessary to understand that this which one calls a quality is the most subtile vapor, or, if you wish, the smallest particle of it, of which an innumerable number of them joined together from the drops of sensible water . . . [61]

Similarly fiery flame is very different from the pure quality of heat, which consists of most subtle and mobile ethereal particles.[62]

It did not seem useless to Colonne to speculate on the shapes of the elementary particles. One might even consider that the three elements of the Cartesians could be replaced by four because each of the Cartesian

---

[55] Ibid., pp. ca. 70–200.
[56] Colonne (1724), pp. iii^v–iiii^r.
[57] Ibid., sig. iiii^r.
[58] Ibid., sig. iiii^v.
[59] Ibid., sig. i.
[60] Ibid., sig. i–v.
[61] Ibid., sig. iv.
[62] Ibid., sig. v.

three "is not absolutely equal either in substance, shape, or motion."[63] However, Colonne did not seek to ascribe size, shape, and motion to particles: He argued that the chemists' approach to the corpuscularian philosophy was based on experience and was far superior to that of other philosophers.[64]

Having prepared the reader, he discusses the *Archidoxes*, presented in the form of a "commentary-abridgment," with the addition of two works on alchemy. For Colonne, as for earlier alchemists, the true chemist should be able to apply his knowledge not only to the imperfect metals but to the ills of man. The macrocosm–microcosm universe assured the operator that a cure for one would cure the other. Colonne also discussed at length the growth process of metals from the seed,[65] and he was clearly convinced of the possibility of transmutation in the laboratory.

Colonne's interest in Paracelsus was associated primarily with his belief in transmutational alchemy. But authors whose concerns were mainly medical referred more often to the great Flemish iatrochemist, van Helmont, interest in whom also continued well into the eighteenth century. There were several reasons for this, one of which was his stirring call for a new understanding of the great world and of man based on chemistry. Another reason, not to be overlooked, was the fact that van Helmont believed in the transmutation of the base metals into gold and in a universal medicine. His alkahest was the universal solvent, sought by generations of chemists and alchemists. So, we also find a number of eighteenth-century Helmontian texts reflecting alchemical themes.

It is interesting to note that Joachim Polemann's *Novum lumen Medicum* (1647) was translated into French in 1719. The anonymous translator paid tribute to the achievements of Paracelsus and van Helmont and then added that "de tous ceux qui ont travaillé sur Vanhelmont, Joachim Poleman est le Maître le plus assûré, que nous ayons pour l'intelligence de la profonde doctrine de ce Philosophe."[66] Polemann's interest in van Helmont was due to the mysteries he presented to the reader. Solid medical advice was of far less interest than obscure passages that could be interpreted with the aid of even more mystical alchemical texts.

The same kind of interest in van Helmont is found in Jean Le Pelletier's *L'Alkaest ou le Dissolvant universel de Van-Helmont* (1704, reprinted 1706) for which the author combed the entire alchemical corpus to locate references to the alkahest. He concludes that van Helmont was the first to write of it[67] but that he was not the most open in his description. Pointing to the importance of the writings of George Starkey, Le Pelletier

63 Ibid., sig. vii–viii.
64 Ibid., sig. ix.
65 Crosset de la Haumerie (F. M. P. Colonne) (1722).
66 Joachim Polemann (1721), Preface.
67 Jean Le Pelletier (1704), p. 25.

proceeded to translate much of his *Pyrotechny* for the benefit of French readers.

More ambitious was a work titled *Le chimiste physicien* (1704). Here, J. Mongin, "Docteur en Medecin," lauded the modern discoveries that had overturned the sterile ancient philosophy.[68] Chief among the moderns were van Helmont, "who dared cry out against the errors of the ancient school, and M. Descartes to whom the learned have a special obligation for having struck out on a new path."[69] He went on to say that the discoveries of these two pathfinders have excited others and deeply influenced them; indeed, the scholars of the Académie Royale have recently uncovered so much new material that the concept of nature is now very different from that of the ancients. In the shade for so many centuries, the sciences have finally blossomed in the reign of our "Louis the Great."[70]

Mongin agreed with van Helmont that the greatest hope for advance was through chemistry,[71] a field in which there had been a special interest in France. French chemists had done much to overturn the elements of the ancients and to establish salt, sulfur, water, and earth in their place. Still, anatomists have not paid enough attention to this work; much of the future of medicine would rest on a chemical examination of the body, the "nature and uses of the liquors which revolve there without ceasing."[72] This work would lead to a determination of how the functions of the body are sustained, and it would be in the tradition of other discoveries that already have produced a clear and distinct idea of the dissolution of foods, of the change in the chyle and the blood, of the nourishment and growth of the bodily parts, and of the various filtrations that occur in the body.

After these wonderful discoveries it might seem that there was nothing more to discover. But, Mongin insists, there still remains an infinity of wonders to be found. The more we learn, the more we stand in awe and adoration of the first cause, God.[73] It was, then, Mongin's intent to address himself to the most fundamental subject of all, the true elements of nature.

Mongin's book is less a chemical investigation of physiology than a comparison of the rival schemes of the elements, in the tradition of Boyle's *Sceptical Chymist*. It was not enough for a chemist to know his way about the laboratory, he also had to be an expert analyst, able to separate the principles of bodies, to know their nature, to distinguish

[68] Mons. J. Mongin (1704), sig. ãiiiᵛ.
[69] Ibid., sig. ã iiiiᵛ.
[70] Ibid.
[71] Ibid., sig. ã iiiiᵛ–ã vʳ.
[72] Ibid., sig. ã vᵛ.
[73] Ibid., sig. ã vᵛ–ã viʳ.

one from another, and, as a physician, to know how to prescribe them.[74] Like Boyle, he rejected the Paracelsian principles and Aristotelian elements before going on to discuss van Helmont's single-element theory. He devoted the third section of his book to van Helmont's tree experiment and concluded that salt, sulfur, and earth are not produced by water.[75] Thus, although van Helmont was one of the two chief founders of the new science, he had erred in his concept of the primal nature of water.

The Paracelsian and Helmontian medical influence is best seen in the lengthy texts of Joseph Chambon (1656–1732).[76] Here we can clearly see a continuation of the chemical philosophy into the mid-eighteenth century. Born at Grignon, Chambon studied medicine at Aix where he received his doctorate. He began practice at Marseilles, but a quarrel forced him to leave the city, so he traveled to Italy, Germany, and Poland where he became the physician to the king, Jan Sobieski. At the seige of Vienna (1683) Chambon left the royal service to confer with Paracelsian and Helmontian physicians in the Low Countries. From there he traveled to Paris where he was well received by Fagon, physician to Louis XIV, but not by the Parisian Faculty of Medicine. Hoping to bypass the medical establishment, Chambon sought a special sanction and managed to continue his practice until his involvement in politics resulted in his imprisonment in the Bastille for two years. After his release he returned to Grignon for the remainder of his long life.

Chambon's reputation ultimately rested on two publications, *Principes de physique* (1st ed.?, 1711, 1714, 1750) and *Traité des metaux* (1714, 1750), in which he pointed to the relatively slow progress of medicine compared with other sciences – all the more evident in a period when astronomy and mathematics were rapidly changing.[77] Why, even the basic principles of medicine had not yet been discovered!

The rules of mathematics are infallible and those of medicine should be no less so.[78] But how should one proceed? The ancients had said that one must travel to learn, and Chambon agreed. He had no desire to rest on book-learning alone, so for "eight years I went to study medicine in foreign countries."[79] The result was his belief that the advance of medicine depended on chemistry and that Paracelsus was the greatest of all

[74] Ibid., p. 5.
[75] Ibid., pp. 195–223.
[76] On Chambon's life I have followed the accounts in the *Nouvelle Biographie Général* and the *Dictionnaire de Biographie Française*. His earliest work (which I have not seen) is Cl. Guiron and Joseph Chambon, *E. sanitas a calidi, frigidi, humidi & sicci moderatione* (Paris, 1696).
[77] Joseph Chambon (1711), Preface, pp. a v^v–a vi^v.
[78] Joseph Chambon (1714), pp. á iv^v–á v^v.
[79] Chambon (1711), p. ē iv^v.

men.[80] Medicine would have been much better if people believed that he had spoken seriously.

True religion, a knowledge of nature, and the healing art are interrelated. This truth is unknown to the academic physicians who follow the books of Galen and Hippocrates and their commentators. Therefore it is necessary to renounce Hippocrates and Galen and the speculative philosophers who have acquired their title by sophisms and arguments. Their imaginary speculations have caused us to deviate from the true path.[81] The true physician should not depend on the books of the ancients but rather should know that

> Prudence and simplicity are the true guides for discovering the mysteries of nature; it is through them that we should allow ourselves to be led: it is only with their help that we will arrive at the knowledge of nature, and it is through nature that we will become professed in Medicine.[82]

For Chambon the study of chemistry had a special importance:

> I am devoted to these [medical] sciences, but principally to Chemistry. If Anatomy teaches us to understand the parts of the machine which is the object of Medicine, Chemistry sheds much light on the liquors which nourish the parts. Besides, and this Anatomy can not do, Chemistry allows us to administer remedies which are alone capable of curing an infinity of illnesses.[83]

Even van Helmont would have applauded Chambon's insistence that to properly "penetrate into the true knowledge of nature, the Philosopher and the good Physician only have need of the fire; they begin with the fire, they perfect themselves with the fire, and they practice with fire: In *igne, cum igne, & per ignem.*"[84] We need not be surprised to find that Chambon explained physiological processes in chemical terms. Thus, "digestion, or the transmutation which is made in the stomach, is the first of the works of the small world."[85]

Chambon's deep convictions led him to open his *Principes de physique* with a chemical catechism so essential that no student should proceed in his medical studies without having mastered it. The chemical orientation is evident from the start.

> Nature accomplishes all of its works in dissolving and coagulating.
> When it dissolves it returns substances to their natural or undigested
>   state, and when it coagulates it cooks and ripens them.
> There is a spirit or a hidden fire in every body in nature.

---

80 Chambon (1714), p. 321.
81 Ibid., p. 459.
82 Ibid., pp. 459–60.
83 Chambon (1711), p. ï ii^r.
84 Joseph Chambon (1750), p. 478.
85 Chambon (1714), p. 209.

> This spirit or this fire is, so to say, the soul of each body and is always in
> motion.[86]

He also wrote that the spiritual cause of movement tends either to formation or destruction, and this is fermentation, a process that leads to
the separation of the pure from the impure.[87] The reader is reminded of
van Helmont again in Chambon's belief that each body perfects its seed
and that this is required for its own generation. This is as true for the
mineral world as it is for animals and vegetables.[88]

Above all Chambon insisted on the essential nature of the three Paracelsian principles – salt, sulfur, and mercury – of which all bodies are
composed.[89] Each of the principles operates differently in the matter in
which it resides. The chemist is directed to the properties of color, odor,
taste, liquidity, solidity, and weight because these are signs by which the
principles can be distinguished.[90] For the physician it is essential to
know that because there are only three principles there can be only three
fundamental illnesses: an "illness of salt, of sulphur, and of mercury."
How different this is from the teachings of the schools; "What a blow to
the Medical Libraries . . ."[91]

Beyond the principles, Chambon believed in a fundamental *prima
materia*. With van Helmont he was convinced that this was water. I
believe

> with some Philosophers that water is the principle of all things, and that
> all things are made of water; that the sun is the source and the center of
> waters, and that the whole world is composed of this material; the motion
> and the brilliance which appear within the matter of which the sun is
> composed, strongly resemble purified gold, which a [our] Philosophy has
> considered as gold in a cupel, and the parts which compose the sun, or
> this same matter in its totality, as a sealing wax which sets in place all the
> different works of nature which differ among themselves only in that the
> parts of one are at rest and the others are in motion . . .[92]

An essential unity is to be found in nature: "Man, heaven and earth are
the same thing and it would be a surprise if there were not an accord
between them: *Coelum est moderator omnis sanitatis, morbi, veneni, boni &
mali usque ad mortem.*"[93]

The books of Chambon are lengthy, but they read well. His frequent
digressions often recount personal experiences. Thus, the story of his

---

[86] Chambon (1711), p. 1.
[87] Ibid., p. 2.
[88] Ibid.
[89] Ibid., pp. 4–6.
[90] Ibid., p. 6.
[91] Chambon (1714), p. ë iv[v].
[92] Chambon (1711), p. 23.
[93] Chambon (1714), p. 390.

meeting with a group of Spanish monks leads to a discussion of the differences between true religion and superstition.[94] Again, his critique of Descartes sheds light on the way in which a Paracelsian viewed the then dominant form of the mechanical philosophy.[95] And, again as a Paracelsian, Chambon discusses and compares at length the growth of metals with the growth of the stony deposits in the body that result from "tartaric" diseases.[96] In the tradition of the alchemists he discourses on the similarity between the calcination of metals and their subsequent recovery by reduction and the death and Resurrection of Jesus Christ.[97] Above all, Joseph Chambon was presenting to a new century an approach to chemical medicine that differed little from that proposed by the followers of van Helmont nearly a century earlier. The fact that these works were reprinted as late as 1750 attests to the interest in this approach in the midst of the Enlightenment.

Alchemy and the scholarly world: the Académie Royale des Sciences

The eighteenth-century authors in the alchemical and Paracelsian traditions mentioned so far have been outside the scientific and medical mainstream. What do we find if we turn to the medical schools, the Académie, and the learned journals? In fact, we find some of the same issues being debated. The University of Montpellier continued to be identified with chemical medicine. The Paracelsian influence there can be traced back to the sixteenth century, and we have already noted that throughout the seventeenth century French Paracelsists and Helmontians were associated with Montpellier. The chemical and many of the medical texts printed there in the first half of the eighteenth century clearly show this influence.

If we look at the activities of the members of the Académie in the first decades of the century, we find that the academicians were keenly aware of problems related to their alchemical heritage. True, they were opposed to alchemy, but the subject remained current and was frequently brought to the fore.

The *Histoire* and *Mémoires* of the Académie, beginning in 1699, seem at first glance to reflect a world far removed from that of the authors we have been discussing. The prefatory essay to the first volume is a hymn of praise to mathematics and the physical sciences.

> The geometric spirit is not so elusively attached to Geometry that it could not be drawn upon or transported to other areas of knowledge. A work on

[94] Chambon (1711), p. 170.
[95] Chambon (1750), pp. 492ff.
[96] Chambon (1714), pp. 210ff.
[97] Ibid., pp. 367–70.

morals, on politics, on criticism, perhaps even eloquence, will be better, all other things being equal, if it is prepared with the hand of Geometry.[98]

If we look to the biological sciences, we note that only anatomy equals astronomy for the person who seeks truth of his Creator.

> Above all, Astronomy and Anatomy are the two sciences which offer us most visibly two grand characteristics of the Creator; the first, his Immensity which may be seen by the distances, the grandeur and the number of celestial bodies, the other, his infinite Intelligence, by the mechanics of animals. True natural philosophy rises to the level of becoming a type of Theology.[99]

And what of chemistry? This subject leads to a knowledge of mineral remedies valuable for the physician, but the mystical concepts of traditional alchemy are to be avoided.[100] This theme reappears frequently in the early volumes of the *Mémoires*. It is true that Nicholas Lemery reported observations from various alchemists, but his explanations varied considerably from theirs.[101] And note was taken of a "cure" by De Fronville using "potable gold," which he advertised as a universal cure.[102] The Académie delegated Lemery and Guillaume Homberg (1652–1715) to examine De Fronville's much vaunted preparation, and they concluded that it had been made with aqua regia. Thus, although it had been called the universal solvent or alkahest of Paracelsus and van Helmont, the preparation was now separated from its previous mystery.

As for the Tree of Diana, Homberg reported to the Académie in 1693 that although the tree seemed to grow as a plant, in fact it was a form of metallic crystallization.[103] Nevertheless, this preparation was to remain a subject of special interest to academicians for years as they sought to identify "trees" of other metals.

One senses a conscious attempt to renew chemistry as an acceptable part of the new philosophy by stripping away the mysticism of the past. When Fontenelle noted in the *Histoire* for 1701 that "Chemistry has departed at last from the mysterious shadows in which the false Philosophers have enveloped it on purpose, but it still retains a part of its natural obscurity," he was referring not to the work of the medieval alchemists but rather to Homberg's attack on the proponents of the late seventeenth-century acid–base theory, which purported to explain all physiological phenomena.[104] But Homberg was not so sure. His chem-

---

98 L'Académie Royale des Sciences (Paris) (2nd ed., Amsterdam, 1734, Preface, p. xvii).
99 Ibid., p. xxi.
100 Ibid., p. xii and L'Académie Royale, *Histoire* (1699) (2nd ed., Amsterdam, 1734, p. 71).
101 Ibid., p. 76.
102 See the discussion of the investigation of M. De Fronville's potable gold by Homberg and Lemery, L'Académie Royale, *Histoire* (1701) (2nd ed., Amsterdam, 1735, pp. 95–6).
103 Le Lorrain, *Curiosities*, pp. 305–6.
104 L'Académie Royale, *Histoire* (1701) (2nd ed., Amsterdam, 1735, p. 86).

ical essays, which appeared in the *Mémoires* from 1702 to 1709, were written to serve as a new foundation for chemistry.

> The old Chemists, most of whom were at least partly visionaries, enveloped this science with an affected obscurity, or we might say, a pious enormity; the time has come for more sensible Chemists of better faith to dissipate these artificial shadows; but the natural obscurity has partly remained and this is more difficult to dispel.[105]

In traditional fashion Homberg began with a discussion of the elements and the principles. However, as a mechanist he argued that the chemical principles must be those of physics because chemistry is but part of physics.[106] This was far from the approach of Colonne or Chambon.

Homberg was concerned about the lingering influence of alchemy, but in fact, the Académie had as one of its members a distinguished Italian iatrochemist. Martino Poli (1662–1714)[107] was born in Lucca and established a chemical laboratory in Rome in 1691, where he was granted pontifical letters patent as apothecary in 1700. Not long after, he discovered a secret of war that he offered to Louis XIV. This was declined because of its destructive potential; but the king conferred on Poli a pension as engineer to the king, and he was made an extra foreign associate of the Académie in 1702. Poli returned to Italy two years later but decided to return to France permanently in 1713, where he died only a few months after his arrival.

Poli wrote several articles that appeared in the *Mémoires* and one book, *Il Trionfo degli Acidi vendicati dalle calunnie di molti Moderni . . .* (1702).[108] Here he complained of the many abuses by physicians who adhered to the use of the mechanical principles. Indeed, a major purpose of his work was to demonstrate the absurdity of the mechanical philosophy, especially as it was described by the followers of Descartes and Gassendi.

He began with a discussion of fermentation and the elements. Like many of the earlier Paracelsians he did not discard the four elements of the Aristotelians but criticized the acid–base system of Otto Tachenius and the five principles of Thomas Willis (spirit, salt, oil, and water). Far better were the three principles of the Paracelsians, the true Hermetic chemists: salt, sulfur, and mercury. These three had been "confirmed by experience." The others had not.[109]

The second part of Poli's book contained his refutation of the mecha-

---

[105] L'Académie Royale, *Histoire* (1702) (2nd ed., Amsterdam, 1737, p. 60).

[106] Guillaume Homberg, L'Académie Royale, *Mémoires* (1702) (Amsterdam, 1737, p. 44).

[107] On the life of Martino Poli, see Fontenelle's éloge in the L'Académie Royale, *Histoire* (1714) (Amsterdam, 1729, pp. 165–72).

[108] Martino Poli (1706). I was not able to examine the book in detail, and the present account is based primarily on the long review in the *Journal des Sçavans*, vol. 38, (1707), pp. 328–47.

[109] Ibid., p. 333.

nists. The hope of the Cartesians that the universe could be explained in terms of the motion, rest, shape, and place of particles was rejected as a hopeless dream.[110] More specifically, Poli argued that living bodies could not be discussed in terms of inert ones. Why then did the mechanists continue to use gross mechanics and analogies taken from machines when these were meaningless? They might speak of filters transmitting some liquors and excluding others, but the passage of the chyle in the lacteal veins is not the result of filtration or of any purely mechanical cause nor are the separations of urine in the reins or the bile in the liver. Rather, these operations are due to fermentation, dissolution, sublimation, "and other similar operations which occur in the body of an animal as in the laboratory of a chemist."[111]

It short, Poli bitterly opposed the medicine and physiology of contemporary iatrophysicists such as Baglivi.[112] His views expressed the doubts of a number of physicians who questioned the attempt to reduce life processes to mechanical analogies. Fontenelle was not pleased, and in his éloge he noted that Poli had attacked the corpuscular philosophy but that "one need not be surprised to find this kind of thought in an Italian since it is a country where the ancient Philosophy still is dominant . . ."[113] Fontenelle was wrong. The Paracelsian chemical philosophy was far removed from the philosophy of the ancients in many key areas, and interest in alchemy remained widespread through the eighteenth century.

We consider one last example of the continuance of Paracelsian thought from the pages of the *Mémoires*. In 1704 Geoffroy noted that, on combustion, a mixture of a sulfur (here an inflammable oil of vegetable origin), a vitriolic salt, and an earth always result in an ash that contains iron, which seemed to be synthesis of a metal. He wrote also that iron particles are always found in the ashes of plants and can be detected with a magnet. He questioned in print whether any plant ash is devoid of iron.[114]

Louis Lemery (1677–1743) replied to Geoffroy in a denial that iron could be synthesized as he claimed.[115] The iron in plants is there because of the growth process, during which it is drawn into the roots and elevated through the vessels of the plant by its life force. The pattern is similar to that of a Tree of Diana. In fact, he had discovered a Tree of Mars, its iron analog.[116] Over the next four years a series of attacks and

[110] Ibid., p. 335.
[111] Ibid., pp. 336–8.
[112] Ibid., pp. 338–9.
[113] L'Académie Royale, *Histoire* (1714) (Amsterdam, 1729, pp. 165–72 [169]).
[114] E. F. Geoffroy, L'Académie Royale, *Mémoires* (1705) (2nd ed., Amsterdam, 1746, pp. 478ff).
[115] L. Lemery, L'Académie Royale, *Mémoires* (1706) (2nd ed., Amsterdam, 1747, pp. 529ff).
[116] L. Lemery, L'Académie Royale, *Mémoires* (1707) (2nd ed., Amsterdam, 1747, pp. 388–425).

counterattacks were printed in which Geoffroy insisted that both analysis and synthesis upheld his conclusion and Lemery argued that the iron exists in the plants from the beginning.

The final paper in this exchange was by Lemery (1708).[117] Not only was Geoffroy wrong, he was not even original. His methods and conclusions were to be found in J. J. Becher's *Actorum laboratorii Chimici Monacensis* (1671). And who was Becher? No one but a "medical chemist, and known as such by his many writings given to the public which seek to reanimate the courage of those who work at metallification and defend alchemy against its injuries to the public . . ."[118] This was an attempt at guilt by association since the purpose of Becher's work had been to prove that it was easier to make metals than most authors would admit. At the very least Geoffroy was being tagged a fellow traveler of the alchemists. Harsh words, indeed, from the man who was to condemn the deceits of the alchemists not too many years later.

The Journal des Sçavans

We can supplement these notes from the *Mémoires* with references to reviews in the *Journal des Sçavans* in the early decades of the eighteenth century. Surely the most recent publications on alchemy were well covered in the pages of the *Journal*. Manget's massive folio compilation of alchemical texts appeared in 1702 and was discussed in an eight-page review the following year.[119] A review of this scholarly work might have been expected, but texts of lesser importance were reviewed as well. A new edition of D'Espagnet's seventeenth-century mystical *Enchiridion Physica Restituta* was reviewed in the *Journal* in 1720,[120] and Emmanuel Konig's *Regnum minerale generale & Speciale* (1703) was singled out because it included a hitherto unpublished treatise by Arnald of Villanova that seemed to teach clearly how to make gold.[121] Nor were living alchemists ignored. The 1719 volume includes a review of François Marie Pompée Colonne's *Plusiers Experiences utiles & curieuses . . .* , a text openly devoted to transmutation and to preparation of the essences, oils, and salts of the adepts.[122]

Other volumes were devoted to topics that were closely associated with alchemy. In 1705 Jonas Conrad Schramm's *Introductio in Dialecticam*

---

117 L. Lemery, L'Académie Royale *Memoires* (1708) (2nd ed., Amsterdam, 1747, pp. 482–515).

118 Ibid., p. 484.

119 *Journal des Sçavans, 31* (1703) (Amsterdam: Waesberge, Boom & Goethals, 1703), pp. 834–41.

120 *Journal des Sçavans, 67* (1720) (Amsterdam: Janssons à Waesberge, 1720), pp. 303–7.

121 *Journal des Sçavans, 31* (1703) (Amsterdam: Waesberge, Boom & Goethals, 1704), pp. 1028–44.

122 *Journal des Sçavans, 66* (1719) (Amsterdam: Janssons à Waesberge, 1719), pp. 83–9.

Cabbalaeorum (1703) was discussed at length, but it was noted that this subject was far removed from the spirit of the times.

> It is amazing that in a century as enlightened as ours that one finds scholars who esteem the Kabbala of the Jews so much as to apply it seriously to this study; one should be less surprised to learn that these scholars are Germans and Peripaticians. . . As for Aristotelianism, what philosophy accommodates itself better to the obscure sciences and places within them the most happy spirit of progress? A Cartesian is incapable of these sciences; he knows nothing without light. It is the Peripatician, accustomed to see as clearly in the darkness as in the light of day, to make profound mysteries of Astrology, Alchemy, Kabbala, and all the other sciences of this nature.[123]

This anonymous reviewer could not have been the same person who soberly discussed the context of Jean Henri Cohausen's *Ossilegium historico-physicum* (1714), in which the concept of palingenesis was extended to man.[124] Do sparks of life and seeds of immortality remain in the ashes after death? Cohausen offered many accounts by chemists to indicate that this was so. One of the most convincing was by Robert Fludd, who had calcined the skull of an executed criminal and then dissolved the ashes in water. Within the solution was seen the figure of the hanged criminal! The close connection of longevity and rejuvenation with alchemy was evident in the review of Harcouet de Longeville's history of those who had lived for many centuries (1715).[125] Again, special emphasis was placed on the work of Arnald of Villanova, and a plea was made for the publication of his newly discovered manuscripts on this subject.

Showing no bias, the editors also reviewed works attacking alchemy, such as the *Examen des principes des Alchymistes* (1711).[126] Here it was pointed out that there was no real basis for a belief in transmutation. Indeed, gold and silver are not the final products of nature, and they are far less useful to man than iron. The reviewer rejected the arguments for metallic generation and bolstered his arguments with biblical and laboratory evidence.

The disciple of antimechanistic medical systems was even better served than the devotee of alchemy. The books reviewed clearly illustrated the rivalry of the various medical sects of the early eighteenth century. Bernhard Albinus' sixty-page *Oratio* on the progress and state of medicine in the seventeenth century (1711) was given a twelve-page review the following year. Here much space was devoted to the debate over the priority of the discovery of the circulation of the blood, but full credit was given to Paracelsian and Helmontian physicians for their attempt to reform medicine. And if their writings were often obscure,

123 *Journal des Sçavans*, 33 (1705) (Amsterdam: Janssons à Waesberge, 1707), pp. 167–9.
124 *Journal des Sçavans*, 59 (1716) (Amsterdam: Janssons à Waesberge, 1716), pp. 71–9.
125 *Journal des Sçavans*, 58 (1715) (Amsterdam: Janssons à Waesberge, 1715), pp. 383–98.
126 *Journal des Sçavans*, 49 (1711) (Amsterdam: Janssons à Waesberge, 1711), pp. 179–86.

nevertheless, "Medicine has taken from the inexhaustible source of Chemistry an infinite number of remedies which have enriched it."[127] The reviewer of Johann J. Waldschmidt's *Opera Medico-practica* (1707) also described contemporary medical sects. Although a Cartesian, Waldschmidt discussed the chemical physicians, whom he divided into two main branches: the Spagyrists, Hermeticists, and alchemists on the one hand, and the more sober, "dogmatic chemists" on the other.[128]

Far more detailed treatment was given to a Spanish work by Miguel Marcelino Boix, *Hippocrates defendio* (1711), which was given a thirty-six page review in two consecutive issues of the *Journal* in 1712.[129] Here the author painted a scene in which physicians of each major medical sect sought to cure a patient. The Galenists suggested frequent bleedings and the followers of Paracelsus and van Helmont "spoke only of elixirs, quintessences, and other mysterious remedies." A disciple of Willis suggested a variety of medicines and bleeding, as did a follower of Sylvius. The Cartesian suggested nothing specific but rambled on about the proportions of the particles in the blood. The follower of Baglivi spoke of the equilibrium of solids and fluids, the correction of contractions, and the wrinkling and shriveling of the bodily fibers. Having thus established the foolishness of current medical theory, Boix allowed Hippocrates to lead these doctors to truth.[130]

It is clear from this review, and from a number of others from the same period, that chemical medicine remained influential in the early decades of the eighteenth century. It is surely for this reason that so much space was devoted to new works on Paracelsian and Helmontian medicine. It is interesting that Poli's *Trionfo degli acidi vendicati* was given a twenty-page lead review in the November 1707 issue.[131] Here his objections to the mechanical philosophy were presented in great detail. Four years later there was an account of Chambon's *Principes de physique* that showed the reviewer's considerable understanding of the chemical and alchemical bases of the author's medical system.[132] The final collected edition of van Helmont's *Opera omnia* (1707), edited by Michael Valentini, was reviewed in 1708.[133] The prefatory material was singled out for comment, noting that Valentini compared the persecution of van Helmont in his lifetime with that of Bacon and Descartes. Indeed, his reforms in medicine were as important as those of Luther and Zwingli in religion.

127 *Journal des Sçavans*, 52 (1712) (Amsterdam: Janssons à Waesberge, 1712), pp. 659–70 (668).
128 *Journal des Sçavans*, 39 (1708) (Amsterdam: Janssons à Waesberge, 1708), pp. 278–82.
129 *Journal des Sçavans*, 52 (1712) (Amsterdam: Janssons à Waesberge, 1712), pp. 212–28.
130 Ibid., pp. 276–83.
131 *Journal des Sçavans*, 38 (1707) (Amsterdam: Janssons à Waesberge, 1707), pp. 328–47.
132 *Journal des Sçavans*, 50 (1711) (Amsterdam: Janssons à Waesberge, 1711), pp. 132–6.
133 *Journal des Sçavans*, 41 (1708) (Amsterdam: Janssons à Waesberge, 1709), pp. 123–9.

Many monographic studies related to the chemical philosophy were also reviewed in the pages of the *Journal des Sçavans*. We have already noted a number of the divergent views on the elements that were expressed by chemists. This debate was also reflected in reviews in the *Journal*. In 1704 we find a review of Mongin's *Chemical Physician* detailing this author's theory of four elements and his rejection of van Helmont's primal water.[134] But the same volume contained a review of a book by David Van der Becke (1703) supporting the Helmontian view that water is the material principle of all things.[135]

Le Pelletier's book on van Helmont's alkahest (1706) was discussed in its alchemical context, and keen interest was shown in the Helmontian archeus.[136] This interest is seen also in a review of Martinus Heer's *Introductio in archivum Archei vitale & fermentale viri magnifici Joannis Baptistae Van-Helmont* (1703), which provides a survey of the physiological importance of this life force in the body.[137] Also deriving from iatrochemical tradition was the interest in fermentation. Henri Louis de Rouviere's book on fermentation (1708) was discussed by pointing out the connection of fermentation with health – and through a sharp criticism of Cartesian mechanistic explanations.[138] Even Charles Musitano's old defense of Helmontian medicine (1683), when it appeared in a new edition (1701), received a lengthy review emphasizing the role of fermentation in disease theory.[139]

Other aspects of nonmechanistic medicine were also reflected in the pages of the *Journal*. The early years of the century witnessed a running debate about digestion. Iatrophysicists argued for a mechanical cause, trituration, whereas chemical physicians (Vieussens, Astruc, and Gastaldi) were certain that the result was due to fermentation.[140] No less controversial was the acid–base theory that had been developed late in the seventeenth century by chemists.[141] Although rejected by mechanists as insufficient for the explanation of bodily processes, others found it essential for medical theory and practice. These debates, which had their roots in the seventeenth-century conflict between the chemists and the mechanists, were well covered in *Journal* reviews.

134 *Journal des Sçavans*, 32 (1704) (Amsterdam: Waesberge, Boom & Goethals, 1705), pp. 476–9.
135 Ibid., pp. 174–89.
136 *Journal des Sçavans*, 34 (1706) (Amsterdam: Janssons à Waesberge, 1707), pp. 831–8.
137 *Journal des Sçavans*, 32 (1704) (Amsterdam: Waesberge, Boom Goethals, 1705), pp. 47–9.
138 *Journal des Sçavans*, 39 (1708) (Amsterdam: Janssons à Waesberge, 1708), pp. 317–23.
139 *Journal des Sçavans*, 37 (1707) (Amsterdam: Janssons à Waesberge, 1707), pp. 23–5.
140 As an example, both sides of the debate are discussed in the review of Jean Baptist Gastaldi, *Quaestio proposita . . . An alimentorum coctio seu digestio à fermentatione vel à tritu fiat* (1713) [*Journal des Sçavans*, 55 (1714) (Amsterdam: à Waesberge, 1714), pp. 24–32].
141 See the review of Gastaldi's *Institutiones Medicae . . .* (1712) [*Journal des Sçavans*, 54 (1713) (Amsterdam: Janssons à Waesberge, 1713), pp. 200–6] in which the reviews concentrated on the author's views on acid–base theory.

Conclusion

The first quarter of the eighteenth century did not see an end to the interest in alchemy or in the often mystical medicochemical world of the Paracelsians. Many people remained active in these fields, and book publishers continued to find their writings lucrative. No other reason satisfactorily explains the many alchemical books published at this time.

Nevertheless, the fierce debate between the mechanical and the chemical philosophers in the seventeenth century had resulted in a scientific establishment that favored mechanistic explanations. Geoffroy's 1722 paper against the alchemical cheats and tricksters surely supports this establishment view. Yet, at the same time, it gives solid evidence of the extent of contemporary interest in alchemy. It was a time when sincere alchemists could defend their beliefs with new experimental evidence such as the discovery of metallic "trees," which grew in chemical flasks and seemed to offer proof that the life force was present in the inorganic as well as the organic world; and the phenomenon of palingenesis seemed to offer hope for the resurrection of the body.

All of these ideas were intertwined with the tradition of the chemical philosophy of the physicians. The medicochemical world view of Paracelsus and van Helmont was meaningless without an understanding of macrocosmic influences and chemical analogies as they related to man. They had believed in alchemy, and alchemical concepts played a crucial role in their views of nature. Their French disciples of the eighteenth century did as well. Colonne's Paracelsian text of 1724 was an alchemical work, and Chambon's treatise on medicine and metallic remedies clearly reflected its Paracelsian and alchemical origins.

Even in the Académie Royale des Sciences alchemy was not entirely a thing of the past. To be sure, mechanical explanations were dominant, and for most of the members, chemistry had only a practical value as the source of new medicine. Still, alchemy remained so widespread that the academicians could not ignore it. Homberg wrote his lengthy chemical essays as a replacement for the outmoded mysticism of the alchemists and the Paracelsians. It must have distressed him sorely to have as a foreign associate Martino Poli, one of the most prominent opponents of the mechanical philosophy, a man who sought to establish the Paracelsian principles as the basis of physics and medicine. Even debates within the Académie occasionally had alchemical overtones. We noted Geoffroy's belief that artificial iron could be produced from plant substances and that he was attacked for reviving an alchemical view originally proposed by Becher.

But more interesting is the broad coverage of alchemical and antimechanical science and medicine in the *Journal des Sçavans*. From this source we can see that alchemy remained a subject of considerable interest to French scholars. As for the chemically oriented medicine of the

Paracelso-Helmontians, it is obvious that they were still treated as members of a major medical sect in this period.

There seems little doubt that Geoffroy had good reason to be concerned about the activities of the alchemists when he presented his paper to the Académie in 1722. And yet, although French chemistry in 1725 reflected its stormy development over the past century and a half, it was about to change drastically. To be sure, the deep-seated interest in alchemical transmutation was not about to die, and the application of chemistry to medical remedies had by this time been thoroughly established. But the development of a new vitalistic medicine and phlogiston chemistry had deep roots in an iatrochemical past and with them came a theoretical divorce of these subjects. The chemistry of most interest to Lavoisier, Priestley, and Black was not the medicinal chemistry that had still been dominant at the beginning of the century. It is of interest then that the same Étienne François Geoffroy who had attacked the alchemists was one of the first French disciples of the phlogiston theory.

6

Postscript

[Chemistry] chassera mille questions oiseuses, qui
amusèrent trop nos pères sur l'acide, l'alkali et ces acri-
monies supposées: ces êtres, la plupart imaginaires,
n'approchent point des principes vraiment chimiques
du corps vivant; ils n'en sont pas les élémens nécessaires
on utiles ou méme possibles à manier.

Théophile de Bordeu (1764)[1]

It is difficult to assign opening and closing dates to most subjects of
intellectual history because all periods are transitional. However, the
early years of the sixteenth century and the end of the first quarter of the
eighteenth century in France define a reasonably satisfactory interval for
this study. We have been concerned with a two-hundred-year period
that witnessed the introduction and eventual acceptance of chemistry by
French physicians. This acceptance, which was a practical one, was
largely limited to the chemical preparation of medicinal substances. Debate still raged in the early eighteenth century between iatrochemists
and iatrophysicists over chemical and mechanical explanations of physiological processes.

In addition to the general acceptance of chemistry as an academic
subject, there is another reason for the choice of ca. 1725 as the closing
date of this period. Having attained recognition from the medical faculties of Europe, chemistry was on the verge of becoming independent
from medicine. Georg Ernst Stahl (1660–1734), who lectured on both
chemistry and medicine at Halle, developed the phlogiston theory in
chemistry but at the same time rejected chemical interpretations of
bodily functions. And even though Hermann Boerhaave (1668–1738)
held the chairs of both medicine and chemistry at Leiden, he was to
separate the two fields decisively. Both authors were highly influential,
and their authority surely furthered the move toward a chemistry that
was no longer chained to medicine.

---

[1] Théophile de Bordeu, "Recherches sur l'Histoire de la Médecine" (1764) in *Oeuvres
complètes de Bordeu* (1818), vol. 2, p. 670.

These developments can be seen in context with a concurrent move toward a new school of vitalistic medicine at Montpellier. This school, though rooted in seventeenth-century vitalism, was to discard the connection with chemistry that had been so evident earlier in the work of van Helmont and his followers. But before we briefly touch on these subjects (they should properly form the subject of another book), we shall summarize the intertwined roles of chemistry and medicine in the two-hundred-year period that we have covered.

Two centuries of medical chemistry: the results

The intensity of the chemical debates in France is best viewed in relation to the then recent revival of interest in Galenic medicine. The end of the fifteenth century and the early years of the sixteenth century saw a new interest in the search for ancient medical texts that could be translated properly from the Greek and that hopefully would be more accurate and complete than the "barbarous" translations available to Western scholars since the thirteenth century. In some cases entirely new texts were discovered. These brought about a new veneration for the ancient physicians, especially for Galen. For many scholars this led to contempt for the works of the Moslem physicians, which had served as the basis of medical teaching until then. The Medical Faculty at Paris became a center for this activity. If the authority of the Islamic physicians was not immediately overthrown, surely by the mid-sixteenth century Galen was looked on as the prince of physicians and held a position among academics comparable to that of Aristotle in natural philosophy.

This medical humanism was accompanied by another kind of humanistic revival, which was connected with the *Corpus Hermeticum*, neo-Platonism, and other mystical writings of late antiquity. Texts on these subjects fostered an interest in natural magic and the world of cosmic harmonies that were thought to envelope man and the world about him. Paracelsus (1493–1541), influenced by natural magic, the religious reformation of his lifetime, and the alchemical and medical pursuits of his father, called for a new medicine, which would in fact be the chief pursuit of the natural philosopher. For him this would be a synthesis of true religion, which would accept only God's Revelation as seen in the Holy Scriptures and created nature. These two would be the unimpeachable authorities. Man was urged to investigate nature on his own and apply the result to the cure of the illness in man. Because of the truth of the macrocosm–microcosm analogy, this seemed reasonable, and the medical implications were enormous. But the question remained as to just how these observations were to be made applicable to man. Although the answers are unconvincing today, Paracelsus and his followers were convinced that the answer was to be found in the proper use of chemistry, which should serve both as the means to prepare new medicines and as the basis of understanding physiological processes. Chemistry, Paracelsus argued, was the key to man and nature.

It is little wonder that the medical views of Paracelsus seemed radical to the Medical Faculty of Paris, which was one of the great European bastions of Galenism. The first printed references to Paracelsus in French seem to have been in the section on antimony in the translation of Mattioli's *Commentaires sur Dioscorides* (1561). This was noted by Loys de Launay, an otherwise obscure physician of La Rochelle, who wrote a tract on the value of antimony as a purgative (1564). He was answered by Jacques Grévin who argued that antimony was not a medicine at all but a dangerous poison (1566). A member of the Medical Faculty of Paris, he was largely responsible for the decree of 1566 condemning antimony as a poison and forbidding its use.

For the next century there was heated debate over the use of antimony, but within the next twelve months it became evident that the question involved more than the medical use of a single substance. Galenic medicine had cured by contraries whereas Paracelsians argued that like cures like. For a Paracelsian a poisonous disease should be cured with a similar poison that had been properly altered chemically. It was perhaps inevitable that the debate should spread to a confrontation between Galenic and Paracelsian medical theory. In 1567 Pierre Hassard published his translation of Paracelsus' *Grossen Wundartznei*, and in the same year Jacques Gohory prepared a short *Compendium* of Paracelsian philosophy.

Galenists found it convenient to damn Paracelsus as an evil magician. Of special concern to them was the new sect's insistence on the importance of chemistry for medicine. This was a subject that seemed beneath the dignity of a learned doctor of medicine. But although the members of the Medical Faculty of Paris tried to rid themselves of the chemists, they were unable to do so. The alchemical tradition had been very strong in France for centuries, and to the Galenists the new chemical physicians seemed quite similar. Perhaps they were not obsessed with the search for transmutation of the base metals, but their belief in a universal medicine, the elixir of life, and an *aurum potabile* seemed too similar. Both groups shared the belief that chemistry was the key to great secrets.

The Medical Faculty of Paris seemed to find the detested combination of alchemist, Paracelsian, and medical empiric personified in Roch le Baillif who promoted Paracelsian chemical medicine and alchemy in his *Le demosterion* (1578). In the same year he arrived in Paris, where he was appointed médecin ordinaire at the court and began a series of lectures on the new medicine. The Parisian Medical Faculty demanded his expulsion, citing their privileges of limiting medical practitioners in the City to their own graduates. Le Baillif was brought to trial and ordered to leave

Paris. It was a significant victory for the medical establishment on paper, but it seemed to have little effect on the growth of the number of alchemical and Paracelsian publications issuing from the French presses. Typical of these was Claude Dariot's new translation of the *Grossen Wundartznei* (1588) and his tracts on gout and on chemical medicines, which went through three editions into the next century to the despair of the Parisian doctors.

Divisions between Galenists and Paracelsians existed not only over the value of chemistry and the ancient authors, but also in regard to religion. Most chemists were Protestants whereas the Galenists – and surely those from Paris – were Roman Catholic. Even though Henry of Navarre converted to Roman Catholicism when he took Paris in 1593, he continued to favor chemical physicians at his court. For the most part these men had had their medical training at Montpellier, an added offense to the Medical Faculty of Paris. Henry's chief physician, Jean Ribit, was a proponent of chemical medicine, and he was to appoint Joseph Duchesne and Theodore Turquet de Mayerne as royal physicians. The former had supported chemistry in print as early as 1575 and would begin a heated debate that affected physicians in all parts of Europe with his *De priscorum philosophorum verae medicinae materia* (1603). This work went beyond a simple support of chemically prepared medicines to discuss the question of the elements and the Paracelsian cosmology with its system of myriad correspondences and sympathetic influences. The work resulted in a sharp debate, not only with the members of the Medical Faculty in Paris, but with physicians and chemists throughout Europe. Mayerne, who had written in Duchesne's defense, was eventually to leave Paris for London where he became first physician to James I and was instrumental in including chemicals in the *Pharmacopoeia* of the Royal College of Physicians (1618).

Within the Parisian Medical Faculty the Jean Riolans, father and son, were most active in opposing the views set forth by Duchesne and the chemists. They were instrumental in preparing the decree against Mayerne (1603), and the continued debate was to result in a further decree forbidding the sale of all chemical medicines (1615).

Duchesne was a physician who enthusiastically supported a chemically oriented medicine, but his work, more than that of others, had placed this medicine in its Hermetic and Paracelsian context. With the publication of the Rosicrucian texts in 1614 and 1615 the broader implications of the Paracelsian call for a new science became more evident. Here was a call for a new learning to replace that of the universities. Chemistry and medicine were to play major parts in this educational reform. To many people this was an appealing suggestion, and there is some evidence that Descartes may have been influenced by these texts. And surely Mersenne, who saw the future of the sciences in mathematics and quantification, looked with alarm on the claim of the chemists that theirs was the true answer to the outmoded natural philosophy of Aristotle and the medicine of Galen. When a Hermetic and alchemical conference was held in Paris in August 1624, it was dispersed on order of the Parlement. The fourteen alchemical theses that had been discussed were condemned by the doctors of the Sorbonne the following month. Mersenne applauded this action.

Of special interest for the development of chemistry at this time was the work of Guy de la Brosse and Théophraste Renaudot. The first, in spite of the opposition of the members of the Parisian Medical Faculty, promoted the establishment of the botanical garden in Paris. This was to include teaching facilities and a chemical laboratory. The Jardin des Plantes was not officially established until 1635 but it would become the center of chemical teaching in Paris after the appointment of William Davisson as the first professor of chemistry in 1648. He was followed by a series of prominent chemists, many of whom wrote their own texts. These became the best-known guides to chemical preparations for nearly a century.

Simultaneously Renaudot was establishing a medical center in Paris that he hoped would be independent of the medical faculty. He too was a graduate of Montpellier (1606) and was an early supporter of Richelieu, who saw to it that Renaudot received the title of royal physician and who helped him to found his Bureau d'Adresse (ca. 1630). Among the Bureau's many activities were its weekly conferences, at which many scientific and medical subjects were discussed, and its medical activities, which included free advice to the poor. Renaudot favored chemical medicines and frequently recommended the use of antimony and its compounds. Furthermore, he employed other chemical physicians at the Bureau, many of which had been trained at Montpellier.

The Parisian Medical Faculty saw in Renaudot's far-flung interests the basis of a second medical center in Paris, one that was anti-Galenist and included teaching facilities through its regular conferences and a clinic through its advice to the poor. The final straw was his plan to install furnaces at the Bureau so that he could manufacture his own chemical remedies. The privileges of the Parisian medical establishment were threatened, and they rose as a whole to defend them. Not only did they attack the use of antimony and chemical methods in medicine, they used this confrontation to attack their rival medical school at Montpellier, the source of so many of these chemical physicians. Unfortunately for Renaudot, both Richelieu and Louis XIII, his benefactors, died. No longer able to count on their protection, he lost his case. He was stripped of his titles, and the Bureau d'Adresse was disbanded (1644).

The legal victory of the Parisian Medical Faculty might have seemed complete, but it was not. The older Galenists were gradually being supplanted by younger physicians who found chemical medicines and especially antimony useful in their practices. In 1658 Louis XIV was cured in the field with an antimony purge, and in 1666 the Parisian Medical Faculty met in full session and approved the use of *vin emétique* in the list of approved purgatives, thus reversing the condemnation of exactly one hundred years earlier.

The middle decades of the century witnessed the growth of a new interest in chemical explanations of physiological processes. Ultimately, this derived from the works of Paracelsus, but there was a sense of modernity to this topic in the seventeenth century, when chemistry was looked upon as an alternative to the mechanical world view. Instrumental in shaping this new iatrochemistry was the *Opera omnia* of van Helmont. Here he dealt less with chemical preparations than with chemical theory, which he applied universally. Because he attacked Paracelsus on many counts, his work seemed to present a more acceptable account of the chemical philosophy. Mersenne looked on him as an ally in his debate with Fludd, and Boyle also expressed an appreciation of his work. Van Helmont had been motivated by his religious views, as had his chemist forebears, but this religious motivation was to decline later in the century as iatrochemistry took on some aspects of the mechanistic world view with Thomas Willis and Franciscus de la Boë Sylvius.

Van Helmont's works were surely known in France in the 1640s when they were attacked by Gui Patin, and within a few years there was a debate over the Helmontian explanation of fevers. In succeeding years a number of French physicians sought to develop the concept of a total chemical philosophy. Jean le Conte prepared a partial translation of van Helmont's *Opera* in 1670, and Daniel Duncan sought to develop a total understanding of animal chemistry in a three-part *Chymie Naturelle* (1681–6). More important was Raymond Vieussens, who took his degree at Montpellier and was to attain prominence both in the Académie des Sciences and as a councillor of state. He admitted his debt to Willis and sought to apply chemistry to an understanding of bodily processes. In his study of body fluids Vieussens examined blood by chemical analysis and was convinced that he had reached an understanding of the chemical nature of the vital spirit.

The final acceptance of antimony by the Medical Faculty of Paris (1666) coupled with the increasing interest in a new iatrochemistry reflect a more general European phenomenon. Following the appointment of Johann Hartmann to teach chemical preparations to medical students at Marburg (1609), many other universities made similar appointments. By the fourth quarter of the seventeenth century most European universities had either appointed or were discussing such chairs in chemistry. Montpellier established a chair in chemistry in 1675, and even Paris made an appointment in chemical and Galenic pharmacy in 1698. In both cases the purpose was to teach the preparation of medicinal substances, not the new chemical physiology. It is important to note that the subject of chemistry became academically acceptable through medicine, not through natural philosophy.

With the new prominence of chemistry it is not surprising that interest in new publications should have been reflected in the most important French scholarly review periodical, the *Journal des Sçavans*. Here we find a continuous stream of reviews of all types of chemical publications, ranging from traditional alchemy and the chemical textbooks to the latest works on acid–alkali theory and the research of Raymond Vieussens.

The Académie des Sciences in Paris showed concern with the continued interest in undesirable areas of chemistry. The early volumes of its *Histoire* and *Mémoires* placed a high premium on studies in mathematical physics and astronomy. Chemistry was considered a lesser science with a shady past, and the paper by Geoffroy in the 1722 volume indicates the far-flung activities of contemporary French alchemists. Other members such as Homberg tried to establish a chemistry that was devoid of traditional mysticism. Nevertheless, interest in subjects such as palingenesis continued, and a long debate in the pages of the *Mémoires* centered on the Tree of Diana and its metallic analogs because of the underlying question of the possible existence of the life principle in inorganic matter.

An interest in the older systems of Paracelsus and van Helmont remained, and F. P. Colonne prepared an *Abrégé de la doctrine de la Paracelse* . . . (1724) whereas J. Mongin's *Le chimiste physicien* (1704) was essentially a text of Helmontian chemistry. Joseph Chambon's *Principes de physique* and his *Traité de metaux* (both saw four editions up to 1750) also presented a traditional Paracelso-Helmontian approach to chemical medicine. One of the foreign associate members of the Académie, Martino Poli, defended the Paracelsian tradition against the mechanists (1706). There is every reason to believe that interest in all aspects of alchemy and chemistry increased rather than declined in the opening decades of the eighteenth century, a conclusion one can reach by noting the large numbers of reviews of these subjects in the pages of the *Journal des Sçavans*.

The development of a nonmedical chemistry and a nonchemical medicine

Our two centuries witnessed the gradual acceptance of chemistry by the medical establishment. It was not a smooth development, and the "harmony" of the ancient physicians had in the end been shattered by debates over the new chemical medicines and new chemical theories. Although Paracelsus, Duchesne, van Helmont, and others saw their chemical philosophy as a total replacement for Aristotelian natural philosophy and Galenic medicine, the main battle was fought in the field of medicine. In the end, chemistry was first accepted academically by medical faculties. The new texts of natural philosophy of the late seventeenth century reflected recent developments in the mechanical philosophy rather than chemistry, which was considered to be a branch of medicine. However, this was to change rapidly in the half century after 1725. By the time of Lavoisier it was not necessary to deal with this medicochemical tradition. In the third quarter of the century, chemistry was no longer tied to medicine. To give a hint of this development we can turn briefly to the work of Stahl and Boerhaave and the rise of a new school of vitalistic medicine at Montpellier.

Herman Boerhaave (1668–1738) was one of the most influential teachers of the eighteenth century.[2] Students flocked to his courses at Leiden from all parts of Europe and even from North America. His textbooks of chemistry and medicine were considered the very best of their kind and were printed and reprinted throughout the century.

Born in 1668, Boerhaave could not help but have been exposed to both the iatrochemical and the iatrophysical schools of thought as a student, but like so many others of his generation, he leaned toward the work of the mechanists. Even though he had been a student at Leiden, he took his medical degree at the Academy of Harderwijk in 1693. The breadth of his reading in chemistry can be judged from his dissertation, in which he referred to Paracelsus, van Helmont, Boyle, Tachenius, and Sylvius.[3] He then established his practice in Leiden and in 1701 was appointed there as a lecturer in medicine. His talent as a teacher was soon noted, and two years later (1703) he was offered a professorship at the University of Groningen. To keep him, the governors at Leiden promised him the first professorship that fell vacant; but he was to wait six years for this promise to be fulfilled when he was appointed to the recently vacated chair in botany and medicine (1709). In 1703 Boerhaave was granted permission to present an academic oration. This lecture, the *De usu ratiocinii mechanici in medicina*, was given in that year. Here we find Boerhaave to be a strong proponent of a mechanistic medicine.[4] Clearly impressed with the achievements of the new philosophy in physics and astronomy, he felt that it was only in medicine that the science of mechanics was ignored. Surely, he thought, the same laws of physics applied to man as they did to inorganic objects.

In his own explanations he discarded contemporary iatrochemical thought and turned to hydraulic and mechanical principles, referring to

---

[2] The standard treatment remains G. A. Lindeboom, M.D. (1968). Lindeboom also prepared an abstracted version of his research for the *Dictionary of Scientific Biography* (1973), vol. 2, pp. 224–8. Of special importance for chemistry is the chapter in J. R. Partington, *A History of Chemistry* (1961), vol. 2, pp. 736–68 and the article by F. W. Gibbs (1958).

[3] Partington, vol. 2, p. 741.

[4] Discussed by Lindeboom (1968), pp. 66–7. See also Lester S. King, M.D. (1978), pp. 121–3.

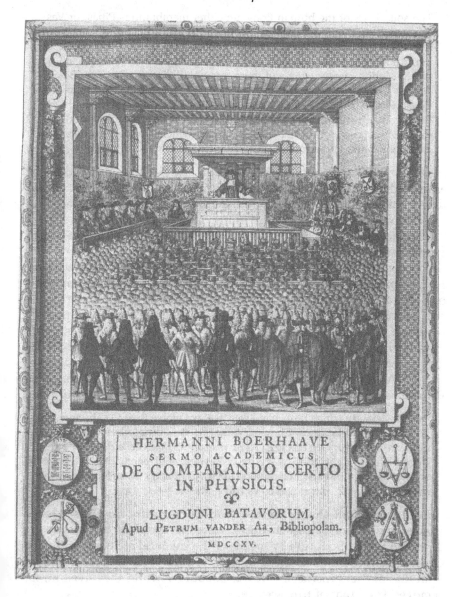

Boerhaave lecturing at Leiden. From Hermann Boerhaave, *Sermo Academicus De Comparando certo in Physicis* (1715). Courtesy of the University of Chicago Libraries.

the velocity of the blood, the diameter of the blood vessels, and the sizes and shapes of particles.[5] In regard to the structure of the body he told his students that

[5] Lindeboom (1973), vol. 2, p. 226.

The solid Parts of the human Body are either membranous Pipes, or Vessels including the Fluids, or else *Instruments* made up of these, and more solid Fibres, so formed and connected, that each of them is capable of performing a particular Action by the Structure, whenever they shall be put in Motion; we find some of them resemble *Pillars, Props, Cross-Beams, Fences,* Coverings, some like *Axes, Wedges, Leavers,* and *Pullies,* others like *Cords, Presses* or *Bellows;* and others again like *Sieves, Strainers, Pipes, Conduits,* and *Receivers;* and the Faculty of performing various Motions by these Instruments, is called their *Functions;* which are all performed by *mechanical Laws,* and by them only are intelligible.[6]

In short, Boerhaave argued that vital processes could and should be examined with the aid of the new mathematical physics.[7] But he did urge caution because "they who think that all physical appearances are to be explained mechanically are in my opinion misled."[8]

Boerhaave was also appointed to the chair of practical medicine five years later (1714), and finally – on the death of Jacobus Le Mort in 1718 – he became professor of chemistry. His lectures on medicine were famous, and he began them with a history that gives us insight into his opinion of chemistry. He considered the work of Paracelsus to be for the most part useless.[9] It is true, he said, that Paracelsus could practice medicine as well as most of his contemporaries, and he did know the medicinal use of opium, mercury, and some metals, but he could be given credit for little else: "the rest was empty smoke, and idle ostentation."[10] As for van Helmont, he was aware that neither the system of Paracelsus nor the disputes of the universities would lead to truth.

But the Remedy which he applied was in effect worse than the Disease, for he founded Physic upon Chemistry, that he would no other certain Way either to its Theory or Practice. After *Helmont, Sylvius de la Böe* first introduced Chemistry in the University of Leyden, and persuaded the Stewards to build a publick Elaboratory for it. Chemistry is certainly a good servant to Physic, but it makes as bad a Master.[11]

In his inaugural lecture for the chair in chemistry Boerhaave railed against the errors of the chemists. Here he spoke of those who interpreted Sacred Scripture by means of the chemical elements and principles. He went on to classify the work of Paracelsus and van Helmont with that of the Rosicrucians. It was a fabulous world they lived in, far removed from that of true science.[12]

6 [Herman Boerhaave] (1742–6), vol. 1, p. 81 (notes on passage continue to p. 85).
7 Boerhaave's *Sermo Academicus de Comparando Certo in Physicis* (1715) is a hymn of praise to the new science. Here see particularly p. 7.
8 Boerhaave (1742–6), vol. 1, p. 48.
9 Ibid., p. 40.
10 Herman Boerhaave (1727), p. 28.
11 Boerhaave (1742–6), vol. 1, p. 40.
12 Hermann Boerhaave (1718). As an example:

But what is the value of chemistry? There is no doubt that medicine has benefitted from the use of chemically prepared medicines. But we also read in Boerhaave's *A New Method of Chemistry* that "Physiology borrows most of its light from chemistry."[13] Here he said, the use of mechanics adds little to our knowledge of matter, but chemistry permits the physician to analyze the fluids of the body. Boerhaave also argued that pathology "is inexplicable by any thing but chemistry,"[14] that urinalysis is properly a chemical investigation, and that we should learn more of the value of foods through chemical analysis.[15]

Boerhaave thus clearly accepted the value of chemistry as long as it was confined to experimental results and was not used as an all-encompassing system of nature and mankind. He felt that the true general science for organic and inorganic matter is physics, to which all others are ancillary. In short,

> Chemistry teaches us the Changes which Bodies suffer of themselves, and when applied to Fire; for Experiments themselves teach us no Falacy; but when we apply the Phaenomena of one Body to account for the Appearances of another, and then draw Conclusions in respect to the human Body, we are frequently deceived. Thus, if any should say, that the fixed Salt of *Tachenius* is proper in the beginning of a Dropsy, his Assertion will be justified by Experience; but if he proceeds to explain the manner in which it operates, it is very possible he may be altogether deceiv'd. . . . if a Chemist takes upon him to account for the Appearances of Bodies, he forgets his own Character, and acts the part of a Philosopher, or too often, of a Rhetorician.[16]

Boerhaave resigned his chair in chemistry and was succeeded in 1729 by Hieronymus David Gaubius (1705–1780). However, his interest in the subject heightened in his final years as he prepared his textbook, the famous *Elementa chemiae* (1732), to replace earlier publications based on notes taken by others in his classroom. This was also a period when he intensified a long-standing interest in transmutational alchemy. The results of his research were published in three parts in the *Philosophical Transactions* of the Royal Society of London in 1734 and 1736 (though he had offered his views on this subject for many years in his lectures). In a

---

O si vesani homines temperassent sibi, nec ipsa Sacra Volumina interpretari voluissent ex Principiis & Elementis Chemicis! Sed pudet, omnia haec de iis dici posse, & refelli non posse! *Paracelsi, Helmontii,* Fratrum *Roseae Crucis,* aliorum, scripta evolvat quis. Stupebit! Nugamentorum pudebit, in quae per veritutum nefas ruit audax omnia fingere Turba Chemicorum. Quae fabulae, superstitio, inscitia!

13 Boerhaave (1727), p. 194.
14 Ibid., p. 195.
15 Ibid., p. 196.
16 Boerhaave (1742–6), vol. 1, pp. 44, 46.

lengthy section on the uses of chemistry in the *New Method of Chemistry* based on those lectures there are pages devoted to the uses of chemistry in alchemy. He concluded that not only could chemical separation techniques isolate gold from other metals, it could also promote the natural growth of gold in a proper matrix through maturation. He commented that "we don't see why this art should be absolutely pronounced false . . ." And as for that branch of alchemy that "teaches how to make gold of other metals, . . . all the world cries out [that it] is impossible, tho' we don't see why . . ."[17]

Boerhaave's experiments on mercury show that he had read the traditional alchemical authors with care. He named many of them and singled out Geber for special praise. Those who read these authors, he said, will see plainly that "the most ancient Alchemists far surpassed the rest in their Accounts of the Nature of Things."[18] Boerhaave was particularly impressed that these authors agreed in so many of their beliefs. He referred to the general acceptance "that Metals are naturally generated in their Veins, are nourished, grow, and multiply like other natural Things, each in their proper Place."[19] He also noted a general agreement that these metallic growth processes required a metallic nutriment, which would be changed by a metallic seed into its own kind. Thus, as the seeds of vegetables and animals change foods into their own nourishment, "so the vivificating Seed of growing Gold, having got a proper Food, in a fit Matrix, by the Help of a suitable and convenient Heat, digests the same into its own particular Nature."[20]

Because the alchemical authors agreed that mercury was the prime ingredient of metals, Boerhaave investigated the possibility of promoting its maturation by lengthy heating, over months and sometimes years. He once heated mercury for fifteen years but found only that it formed a black powder that could be turned into mercury by rubbing. In a similar experiment he heated mercury and obtained a powder that reverted to mercury metal when further subjected to heat. In his description of this process he turned to alchemical terminology, writing that "Thus the Serpent that has bitten itself dies. It arises again more glorious from Death."[21] There is no indication that Boerhaave ever dismissed the real possibility of transmutation.

Boerhaave is seen as a key figure in the development of chemistry in the first half of the eighteenth century not because of specific discoveries but because of his influence and his view of the role of chemistry. To be sure, as professor of both medicine and chemistry he reflects the seventeenth-

---

17 Boerhaave (1727), pt. 2, pp. 215–18.
18 Hermann Boerhaave (1734), p. 6.
19 Ibid., p. 9.
20 Ibid., p. 10.
21 Ibid., p. 40.

century development of both fields; and in his reluctance to reject traditional alchemy he is typical of his time. However, Boerhaave did not consider chemistry a subject primarily of use to the physician, and his chemical textbook was not written for the future pharmacist alone. As for the iatrochemistry of van Helmont and Sylvius, he thought they had clearly gone too far in their interpretations of life processes in terms of chemistry. Their speculations should be supplanted by a new medicine founded on the science of mechanics. In short, Boerhaave favored a chemistry that could be used by physicians for specific purposes, but it should not dominate medicine. It was, then, a chemistry that was losing its close connection with medicine and emerging as a more independent science. His medical and chemical works were translated into numerous languages. The *Elementa Chemiae*, which includes his views on alchemy and the relationship of chemistry to medicine, was published in three French editions: 1748, 1752, and 1754. An abridgment had appeared in French earlier, in 1741.

Like his contemporary Boerhaave, Georg Ernst Stahl (1660–1734) taught both medicine and chemistry.[22] He took his medical degree at Jena in 1684 where he gave the lectures on chemistry that were to become the basis of his *Fundamenta Chymiae*, published nearly forty years later. In 1687 he became a court physician at Weimar, a position he held for seven years. He then accepted a post as the second professor of medicine at the recently founded University of Halle, where he lectured on medical theory and chemistry. In 1715, however, he left the academic world to become a physician at the court of Berlin where he remained to the end of his life.

Stahl's medicine also marked a rejection of the work of the iatrochemists. He believed that the chemical explanations of physiological processes given by van Helmont, Sylvius, and the followers of Tachenius were all wrong and insisted on a sharp differentiation between living and nonliving matter.[23] The latter is particulate and can be studied through the approach of the mechanist. But this is not the case with living matter. At the end of life corruption sets in so there must be something present in a living being that preserves it from corruption and regulates its actions and bodily functions. This is the *anima*, the origin of directive, purposeful motion. Motion in the organic world depends on mechanical causes and can be studied on the basis of the size, shape, and movement of individual particles. In the living orga-

---

[22] Stahl's chemistry is discussed at length by Partington, *History of Chemistry*, vol. 2, pp. 652–90. Still excellent is Hélène Metzger (1930), pp. 91–188. The reader is referred also to David Oldroyd (1973). For Stahl's medical thought, see Lester S. King (1964). King's survey of the work of Stahl is in his biography of Stahl in the *Dictionary of Scientific Biography* (1975), vol. 12, pp. 599–606. Still helpful are Walter Pagel, "Helmont. Leibniz. Stahl." (1931); and Albert Lemoine, *Le vitalisme et l'animisme de Stahl* (1864).

[23] I have largely followed L. S. King's account of the *anima*.

nism, mechanistic explanations are at best only partially useful because it is the anima that directs motion toward a purposeful end. Even in a chemical process it is the *anima* that directs. Stahl differed from the Helmontian tradition, which postulated separate archei in the body organs, each of which carried on their own actions.

For Stahl, Paracelsus and van Helmont had been largely responsible for the invidious influence chemistry had developed in medicine.[24] This must be reversed because, he felt, chemistry is completely useless for any true medical theory. The chemists explain life processes with coagulation and liquefaction, fermentation, volatility, and acrimony. The recent turn to the opposing substances, acid and base, is totally wrong because, he said, it is impossible to find any acid or base in living bodies, or even any neutral body, that produces the effects attributed to it. As Hélène Metzger explained, Stahl felt that it was necessary to rid chemistry and medicine of those ridiculous speculations founded on an imaginary opposition of acid and alkali. Chemists holding to this belief had attempted to account for all natural phenomena, and he felt that these speculations were contrary to good sense and experience.[25]

It is understandable that historians of medicine and historians of chemistry have found so little common ground in their treatments of Stahl. Although he accepted the pharmaceutical value of chemistry, he found the broader iatrochemical speculations on life processes a real danger to the progress of medicine. Even a brief glance at his substantial *Fundamenta Chymiae* shows that this subject for him was largely devoid of medical value. Chemistry is described as the art of resolving compound bodies into principles and recombining them.[26] Chemistry has some medical value, but in his list this would appear to be the least of its uses. The *Fundamenta Chymiae* concentrates on matter and its combinations, descriptions of substances, and chemical processes rather than medicine.

Stahl was strongly influenced by Johann Joachim Becher's (1636–1682) *Physica subterranea* (1669), to which he had prepared an extensive *Specimen Beccherianum* in 1703.[27] Becher had been deeply influenced by contemporary chemical work, but in the *Physica subterranea* he had emphasized a chemistry that was largely inorganic rather than medical. He had postulated three earths necessary for subterranean substances: one for substance, a second for color and combustibility, and a third for form, odor, and weight. These were the *terra vitrescible*, the *terra pinguis*, and the *terra fluida*. The most important of these would prove to be the *terra pinguis*, or fatty earth, a combustible substance, which he also

24 Metzger (1930), pp. 111–13.
25 Ibid., p. 114.
26 G. E. Stahl (1746), p. 1.
27 I have discussed the *Physica subterranea* in *The Chemical Philosophy*, (1977), vol. 2, pp. 458–63.

called sulfur φλογιστὸς. Although the term had roots in ancient philosophical and medical thought, it also had been used by seventeenth-century iatrochemists and, as a concept, bore some similarity to the Paracelsian principle of sulfur. It was a principle that Stahl was to develop at greater length in his *Zymotechnia fundamentalis* (1697). In the course of the eighteenth century, the phlogiston theory was developed into a unified chemical system centered on combustion. It was this nonmedical chemistry that was later to become the target of Lavoisier's chemical studies.

Stahl, as had Boerhaave, concerned himself seriously with questions about transmutation. In the *Specimen Beccherianum* he asked whether a tendency to form metals exists in the subterranean regions, and further, whether metals actually move toward perfection. Stahl favored instant generation to gradual maturation. As he explained in the *Fundamenta Chymiae*,

> . . . it may more easily be conceived, that Metals should be . . . instantaneously generated, than that the imperfect metals should . . . be converted into the perfect . . . by long continued Concoction in the Earth, or by lying therein for some hundreds of years, without the addition of any new matter, or any diminution of the old. . . . [And] if this instantaneous Generation of Metals cou'd once be established, it wou'd give great countenance to the action of the philosophical *Tincture* or *Substance* in the business of Transmutation . . .[28]

Clearly Stahl was sympathetic to the concept of transmutation. In a discussion of philosophical gold he explained that the adepts meant by this

> *Gold* most highly subtilized, and brought to a degree of fermentative mobility; so that being mix'd with pure running Mercury, it may by degrees assimilate the particles thereof to itself, and at length reduce the whole mass to a due degree of spissitude; whence the Mercury also may, in time, become true *Gold*; which, tho' softer than the common, is yet like it, in sustaining all the Proofs whereby the constancy of that is examin'd.[29]

Of special importance for the would-be alchemist was the work of the famed Isaac Hollandus, about whose life little is known. Stahl reprinted Hollandus's treatise on the salts and oils of metals as an appendix to his own thoughts on alchemical transmutation. As with Boerhaave, the study of mercury was of most importance. Stahl wrote in his section on "the Mercuries of Metals" that

> The principal use of these *Mercuries* is their advancement into Gold, by a moderate digestion with highly subtilized or philosophical Gold; whence they are said to be coagulated with it into a fix'd Precipitate; which if

[28] George Ernest Stahl (1730), pp. 249, 251.
[29] Ibid., p. 319.

thrown into Silver or Gold in fusion, there proves and remains good and fix'd Gold[30]

He went on to examine the three basic processes described by the adepts for the making of the philosopher's stone: from vitriol, from niter, and from mercury. Although he discussed these processes in as scientific a fashion as he could, he wrote as any other alchemist when he ascribed success in this endeavor to the Will of God.

> But as the Cautions with regard to all these cases are fundamentally cir-
> cumscribed and defined by the *Divine Will*, which, without all dispute
> governs and directs the thing itself and its success, according to the vari-
> ous Intentions or *moral Circumstances* of the Person; let everyone examine
> himself by this Rule, and accordingly expect success or failure, in his
> attempts.[31]

Stahl's animistic medicine differed greatly from the mechanistic medicine of Boerhaave, but in other areas there are similarities. Both were
reluctant to sever their ties with alchemical tradition, and both sought to
separate chemical speculation from medical theory. Boerhaave was a
mechanist who saw some value in the chemical investigation of living
matter, particularly the body fluids. Stahl was more emphatic in separating the two fields. The *anima* was the director of life processes, and the
speculations of the iatrochemists seemed to him to have gone too far.
Both he and Boerhaave might well have agreed on the usefulness of
chemistry for the preparation of medicines, but Stahl's chemistry was
influenced primarily by Becher's *Physica subterranea*, a work that emphasized the inorganic chemistry of the subterranean world. Thus, with
both authors, the end result was to lessen and nearly eliminate the role
of chemistry as a means of explanation in the understanding of the life
processes. Both Stahl and Boerhaave deemphasized medical chemistry
and sought to establish chemistry as an independent science.

If Stahl's phlogiston chemistry was to become the predominant chemical system in mid-century, his influence on medicine was no less significant. Here again, the French scene is of special importance.[32]
Montpellier had been a center for the introduction of chemical medicines from the mid-sixteenth century, and it continued this tradition in
the eighteenth century with the thirty-year tenure of Antoine Deidier as
its professor of chemistry. Nor had the chemical medicine of the Helmontians been ignored at Montpellier. The use of chemical explanations
for physiological processes had attracted a number of the medical faculty

---

30 Ibid., p. 391.
31 Ibid., p. 424.
32 Of special value is the recent paper by José M. López Piñero, "Eighteenth Century
    Medical Vitalism; The Paracelsian Connection" (1988). Also valuable are the introducto-
    ry chapters to Elizabeth Haigh (1984). A more contemporary account is in M. F. Bérard,
    *Doctrine Médicale de l'École de Montpellier, et Comparison de ses principes avec ceux des autres
    écoles d'Europe* (1819).

there in the late seventeenth century, perhaps most notably Raymond Vieussens. However, with the successes of the new philosophy in the physical sciences there had been a parallel attempt to turn to mechanical explanations in medicine, such as we have seen in the work of Boerhaave. Iatrochemistry may have remained a significant approach in medical circles, but it was generally superseded by the work of the iatrophysicists in the early decades of the eighteenth century. Even Vieussens turned from chemical to mechanical explanations late in life. The teaching of chemistry had been introduced in the seventeenth century primarily for the preparations of chemical remedies. Although the iatrochemists had attempted to broaden chemistry's explanatory value to cover physiological processes, this move was opposed by mechanists; and for the most part, it was pharmaceutical chemistry that retained its importance in the medical education of the late eighteenth century.

As mechanical explanations of life processes became more acceptable in medicine in the early eighteenth century, there remained the problem of explaining what moved the man-machine. Van Helmont had turned to his *Blas* as an answer, but no one suggested a return to this concept. Here Stahl's concept of the *anima* was to prove helpful. François Bossier de Lacroix Sauvages (1706–1767), originally a follower of the iatrophysicist Baglivi, found mechanist answers unsatisfactory for an understanding of the properties and functions of living matter and soon found himself turning to the works of Stahl.[33] He began giving lectures on Stahl's system at Montpellier in 1737, holding to mechanistic explanations as long as possible and turning to the *anima* only when these had been exhausted. His lectures initiated a debate that continued for six or seven years before his views were generally accepted.

To describe the development of vitalistic medicine at Montpellier in any detail would take us beyond our chronological limits. Suffice it to say that the reaction against mechanistic medicine initiated by Sauvages in 1737 continued through the century and beyond. Here we mention only Théophile de Bordeu (1722–1776) and Paul-Joseph Barthez (1734–1806). Bordeu argued in favor of localized vital forces in each organ. In his "Recherches sur les maladies chroniques" (1775) he wrote that "the living body is a collection of several organs which live in their own way, which experience more or less sensation and which move, act and rest in determined times . . . the general life (of the organism) is the sum of all the particular lives."[34] Bordeu read widely, not only the work of Stahl but also that of van Helmont. He believed that "it is impossible to advance even a little into the study of the living body without encountering traces of Van-Helmont." Further, "it is certain that Stahlianism owes its birth to Van-Helmont."[35]

[33] Haigh (1984), pp. 16–31.
[34] Ibid., p. 36.
[35] de Bordeu, "Recherches sur l'Histoire de la Médicine," in *Oeuvres* (1818), vol. 2, p. 671.

Whereas Bordeu thought of many individual vital forces that together formed the total organism, Barthez preferred a single vital principle that made possible all vital phenomena. He was far more critical of van Helmont than Bordeu had been, precisely for this reason. Van Helmont had argued that each organ had its own life force, and this, Barthez countered, was simply unnecessary.[36] It seems evident that the Montpellier vitalists were well aware of their debt to Stahl's animism, and whether or not these physicians agreed with van Helmont, they had some knowledge of his views on the gulf between living and inorganic matter.

Stahl had insisted that chemical explanations were to be eliminated from medical theory. The physicians of Montpellier agreed. Bordeu believed that chemistry was cultivated more at Paris after honored medical figures had started to lecture on Stahl's chemical system, but he also felt that the old chemistry had not been overcome. Some people said they were disciples of Paracelsus, but in truth they did not know even the first principles of the art. Above all they did not properly distinguish chemical from organic processes. The mechanists were surely wrong in their explanations of life processes, and the chemists were no better. For them chemistry

> pursued a thousand flighty questions which amused our fathers too much regarding acid, alkali and their supposed acrimony. Since all this is for the most part imaginary, they did not lead to the true chemical principles of the living body. They are not necessary or useful elements nor are they even possible to maintain.[37]

Bordeu went on to warn his readers that chemistry seeks to take over medicine. With Paracelsus, a man of fire himself, the human body had become a sort of volcano.

> The anatomists have dissected the body down to its infinitely small fibrils and the physicians have transformed man into a machine of levers, pumps, springs, pipes and presses. But the school of Paracelsus would make the body a composite of alembics, ferments, salts, effervescences, distillatory vessels and centers of explosions.[38]

Barthez agreed, stating that the effects of the vital principle are completely different from the phenomena of "dead" nature, and it is the latter phenomena that are determined by the operations of chemistry.[39]

Here then was the result of the reaction against both iatrophysics and

---

36	P. J. Barthez (1858), pp. 24, 93–4.
37	de Bordeu, "Recherches sur l'Histoire de la Médecine" in *Oeuvres* (1818), vol. 2, p. 670.
38	de Bordeu, "Analyse Médicinale du Sang" in *Oeuvres* (1818), vol. 2, p. 930.
39	Barthez (1858), p. 37.
	Les affections du Principe Vital qui produisent et renouvellent, dans un ordre constant, les fonctions nécessaires à la vie, sont absolument différentes des

iatrochemistry in the eighteenth century. Chemistry – other than for pharmaceutical preparations – was divorced from medical theory and physiological explanations. This development had not occurred by 1725, but surely the basic views of Boerhaave and Stahl were already known. The most prominent member of the medical school of Montpellier, Xavier Bichat (1771–1802) was to be in full agreement with his predecessors, Bordeu and Barthez, on this point. In her recent study of Bichat, Elizabeth Haigh has written that "he was one of the last medical theorists of any particular influence to insist uncompromisingly that physics and chemistry were separate sciences from physiology, making specious the application of their principles to the study of living processes."[40] And indeed, this nonchemical and vitalistic medicine was maintained at Montpellier throughout the nineteenth century.

The persistence of alchemy

Perhaps the most surprising aspect of chemistry in the period from the sixteenth through the early eighteenth centuries is the strength of the alchemical tradition. Although the cutting edge of chemical knowledge was centered in Paracelsian medical chemistry in the late sixteenth century, many of these authors continued to believe in the possibility of transmutational alchemy. And with the advent of the chemical physiology of the Helmontians we find little change. Although some scholars simply ignored the subject of alchemy, others turned to van Helmont as one of the legendary alchemists. Nor did the rise of the mechanical philosophy do much to put a stop to this belief in transmutation: Witness Geoffroy's attack on the alchemists in his 1722 paper at the Académie des Sciences. Boerhaave and Stahl were no less interested in traditional alchemy, and we have already noted the flood of early eighteenth-century French publications on this subject. Yet these form but a small proportion of the total alchemical works being published in Germany and the other states of Europe at the time.

The eighteenth century was a period of intense interest in alchemy. The century opened with the publication of J. J. Manget's *Bibliotheca Chemica Curiosa* (1702) in Geneva, while in Germany Friedrich Roth-Scholz published his massive *Deutsches Theatrum Chemicum* (1728, 1730, 1732), a three-volume work comprising some 2,500 pages. In France, a less ambitious but similar collection was compiled, possibly by Jean Maugin de Richebourg, in the four-volume *Bibliotheque des Philosophes*

---

causes productives des mouvements qui ont lieu dans la Nature morte, comme sont ceux que determinent les opérations de la Chimie.
[40] Haigh (1984), p. 15.

Chimiques (1741–54).[41] At the same time many lesser works continued to issue from the French publishing houses.

André Charles Cailleau wrote to instruct Madame Le Febure de la Borle in the secret art (1755), stating that the hidden truths of alchemy made it possible for one

> to cause storms at sea or to appease them, to make a continued calm, to make any of the winds prevail, from the East, the West or the Northwest, to produce clouds or to disperse them, to make the sun appear, to make it rain, thunder snow, hail – and at any time.[42]

Twenty years earlier a Sieur Gosset sought an alchemical union of medicine and the cabala by means of which one might prolong life. The truths of this science had been discovered by none other than Gosset himself.

> I believe, without too great presumption, that I was the first to reveal the Cabalistic science and who demonstrated all its operations and showed what was necessary to do to obtain the great circulé of Paracelsus, this vegetable arcanum, this universal medicine of which the virtues are innumerable for all human illnesses both internal and external.[43]

An otherwise unknown Sieur Raguet (1758) turned to the work of the current medical vitalists and argued that the true universal spirit is phlogiston and that this is the very same spirit "that van Helmont had made so much of and which he presented to us under the name of Archeus. . ."[44]

Even the great French surgeon, Charles Dionis (1710–1776), Doctor Regent in the Parisian Faculty of Medicine, was responsible for a new edition of Sir Kenelm Digby's *Lettre sur la Poudre de Sympathie* (1658). The reason for reprinting this unusual work in 1749 was straightforward. The secret of Digby's powder had been the subject of a dispute among the Abbé de Grély, the Vicar of Embrun, a Parisian apothecary by the name of d'Aliez, and the physician Thieullier.[45] Dionis had prepared the powder, and he printed the Abbé de Grély's recipe for its composition, thinking thereby to present to the medical world an important secret in a volume that had already become very rare.

Perhaps the two most prominent French alchemical scholars of the

---

41 Of Richebourg nothing is known. Ferguson notes that "the compilation was not originally of his making, for there is an edition with the same title that appeared in 1672–8 and bears as the editor's name: le Sieur S. Docteur en Medecine." John Ferguson (1906), vol. 2, p. 273.
42 André Charles Cailleau (1777), p. 74. Cailleau notes that Madame Le Febure de la Borle is the seventh among women philosophers (after Marie, sister of Moses, Pernelle, Cleopatra, Thapuntin, Medeia, and Eutheria). For this quotation, see p. 22.
43 Sieur Gosset (1735), p. 37.
44 Sieur Raguet (1758), p. 19.
45 Charles Dionis (1749), pp. 68–86.

eighteenth century were the Abbé Nicholas Lenglet du Fresnoy[46] (1674–1752/5) and Antoine-Joseph Pernety[47] (1716–1800/1). Du Fresnoy was originally a student of theology, but his interests shifted to chemistry. His three-volume *Histoire de la Philosophie Hermétique* appeared first in 1742 and was reprinted twice in 1744. Lenglet du Fresnoy thought it necessary to write such a history because it had not been done earlier. However, he warned his readers that this did not mean that he believed in the truth of the claims of the alchemists.

> It is necessary to note that there are two kinds of chemistry; the one wise and reasonable, even necessary for the extraction of useful remedies from all things in nature . . . : the other is that foolish and senseless chemistry which is nevertheless the older of the two. . . . The first has been given the name of *Chemistry*, the second that of *Alchemy*.[48]

Accordingly, Lenglet du Fresnoy devoted himself to the composition of a history "of the greatest folly and of the greatest wisdom of which men are capable."[49] The first volume is a history of alchemy, the second contains a group of French translations, and the work closes with a catalog of book titles including a list of chemical papers in the *Mémoires* of the Académie Royale and the *Transactions* of the Royal Society of London.

Although Lenglet du Fresnoy constantly expressed his skepticism of the claims of the alchemists and even reprinted Geoffroy's paper of 1722, there remained in his writings a latent fascination that bordered on belief. This surfaces in his new editions of LeFèvre's *Cours de chymie* (1751) and Alvaro Alonzo Barba's *Metallurgie*, published in the same year. He added two volumes to LeFèvre's work, supplementing it with material from Glaser's *Traité de la Chimie*[50] and adding sections on the powder of sympathy and a dissertation on the nature and analysis of metals and minerals, which are filled with references to astrology and the more mystical chemists of the past including van Helmont, Basil Valentine, and Paracelsus. Even a treatise by Jean-Isaac Hollandus, reputed to be the son of Isaac Hollandus, was translated for this edition.

Du Fresnoy transformed Barba's text on metallurgy even more radically. Writing under the pseudonym Gosford, du Fresnoy noted that for a long time only the Spaniards and the Germans seemed to possess the art of mining and purifying gold and silver. For this reason he had undertaken the task of translating into French the greatest Spanish work of this genre. But in his hands, Barba's severely practical text led to a

---

[46] Jean-Bernard Michauld (1761).

[47] For a survey of Pernety's career and activities (he was among other things the royal librarian of Frederick II at Berlin), see August Viatte (1969), vol. 1, pp. 91–103. Pernety was deeply influenced by Swedenborg whose eighteenth-century followers frequently expressed interest in alchemy.

[48] Nicholas Lenglet du Fresnoy (1742), vol. 1, p. xii.

[49] Ibid., p. 1.

[50] Nicolas Le Fevre (1751), vol. 1, p. xvii.

collection of philosophical and mystical tracts. Indeed, du Fresnoy was convinced that all metals have germs or seeds that grow with the help of the internal heat of the earth and that a knowledge of sympathy and antipathy was essential for our understanding of metallurgy.[51] Among the works included in his edition of Barba was one by Martine de Bertereau, the Baroness of Beau-Soleil, which was written in 1640. Dedicated to Cardinal Richelieu, *La Restitution de Pluton* touched on numerous topics of interest to those concerned with metals and mining.[52] Noting that any person in charge of a mine must be a master of many sciences, she wrote that the first of these is astrology, from which one will learn of the coming of plagues, wars, famines, and floods. If this subject is essential for knowledge of economic conditions and disasters, the stars are no less useful for the miner because they are directly connected with and govern the developing metals and minerals in the earth. This tract, considered to be so important by du Fresnoy, belongs less to metallurgy than to alchemy. The baroness believed that the existence of the universal spirit of life was no less certain than the existence of the Creator, and that this spirit is responsible for the growth and reproduction of all things, inorganic as well as organic in nature.[53] Indeed, she continued, the ancient philosophers prepared from the first matter of the metals their grand elixir, which cures even those illnesses considered to be incurable and also purges the metals of their imperfections.[54] This work by the baroness is typical of du Fresnoy's inclusions in his edition of Barba's practical text on metallurgical procedures.

The mid-century French alchemical adept was able to supplement works such as du Fresnoy's with the publications of Antoine-Joseph Pernety, the royal librarian of Frederick II at Berlin. His *Les Fables egyptiennes et greques dévoilées* (2 vols., 1758; reprinted 1786, 1795) maintained an earlier tradition in its thesis that the whole of ancient mythology was an alchemical allegory. But he felt that an additional work was necessary:

> My treatise on the Egyptian and Greek fables develops part of these mysteries. Obliged as I am to speak the language of the Philosophers, this has resulted in an obscurity that one can only remove by a detailed explanation of the terms that they employ, and of the metaphors which are familiar to them.[55]

A dictionary seemed to Pernety the best way to guide his readers through these texts, and thus he prepared his *Dictionnaire Mytho-Hermetique* (1758; reprinted 1787), which explained the chemical signifi-

---

51 Alvaro Alonzo Barba (1751), vol. 1, p. xxxviii.
52 Martine de Bertereau (1640) in ibid., vol. 2, pp. 56–140.
53 Ibid., p. 76.
54 Ibid., p. 78.
55 Antoine-Joseph Pernety (1758), p. iv.

cance of the allegorical terms used in the art in a volume of nearly six
hundred pages. Nor did he stop with the traditional terminology:

> Many people regard Paracelsian medicine as a branch of the Hermetic
> Science, and that Paracelsus, its author, made use of barbaric terms or took
> them from other languages as did the Disciples of Hermes. I believe that I
> have rendered a service to the public in giving an explanation of these
> terms following the sense in which they are understood by Martin Ruland,
> Johnson, Planiscampy, Becher, Blanchard and many others.[56]

The first edition (1758) of Pernety's extensive alchemical dictionary was
published only eight years prior to the first edition of Pierre Joseph
Macquer's *Dictionnaire de Chymie* (1766), which has been praised as "the
first scientific work of its class." Pernety's second edition (1787) appeared in the same year as Lavoisier's fundamental revision of chemical
nomenclature.

Nor did the *Journal des Sçavans* cease to publish reviews of current
works on alchemy and other mystical subjects. As examples one might
turn to the discussion of Edme Guyot's *Nouveau Systeme de Microcosme*
(1724; reviewed 1727)[57] and Johann Henri Cohausen's *Archeus Febrium
Faber et Medicus* (1731; reviewed 1734).[58] In the former volume the author
sought openly to reestablish the macrocosm–microcosm system based
on the ancient philosophy. He discussed the four elements and insisted
on a universal life spirit, which was no less than the soul of the world
and which contained a celestial seed that entered animals through respiration. The reviewer in the *Journal* was well aware that Guyot's work was
based on ancient alchemical thought, but he felt that Guyot had clarified
the earlier works. For instance, Guyot did not believe that the soul
excites the voluntary movements by means of the animal spirits.[59]
Rather, he argued that excitation is accomplished through a quintessence of the spirit contained within the globules of the blood, which can
expand and contract, thereby affecting the muscular fibers. In short, this
odd work was pictured by the *Journal*'s reviewer as wedding the mystical
world of Renaissance cosmology with that of the mechanist.

Johann Henri Cohausen's *Archeus Febrium Faber et Medicus* was given
an eleven-page review in 1734. Here Cohausen sought to revive van
Helmont's archeus. The reviewer tells us that Cohausen insists that
without the archeus, man would be nothing but a machine and that the
archeus is actually the vital spirit, or the spirit of life, or nature[60]; it is the
principle that gives action to all things in the human body. It is little
wonder that van Helmont is described here as a "Philosophe que notre

56 Ibid.
57 *Journal des Sçavans* (1727), pp. 290–4.
58 Ibid. (1734), pp. 797–808.
59 Ibid. (1727), p. 292.
60 Ibid. (1734), p. 798.

Auteur regarde comme un homme suscité de Dieu pour la reformation & pour l'ornement de la Medecine."[61] The reviewer recommended this book to the reader for further study because even his lengthy review could not suffice to give the reader a complete idea of the book's content.

Even the *Encyclopédie* (1753)[62] is willing to turn from Descartes and Newton in scientific thought. The article "Chymie," though unsigned, had been prepared by Gabriel François Venel (1723–1775), who became professor of chemistry at Montpellier in 1759. Venel deplored the fact that chemistry was so little studied by scientists in his day. "The chemists form a distinct people, small in number, having their own language, laws, mysteries, and living nearly isolated in the midst of a large population little interested in its commerce or its industry."

If there were alchemical charlatans and those who busied themselves only with the preparation of chemical medicines, there also were great systematizers such as Johann Joachim Becher and Georg Ernst Stahl. Indeed, Venel felt that the study of chemistry was essential to all of the sciences. It was necessary, he said, for a new Paracelsus to come forward courageously to point out that many of the errors that have defiled physics have arisen from the works of men who have given themselves the airs of philosophers, but who are ignorant of chemistry. Yet they have sought to explain natural phenomena that only chemistry can explain.[63]

Venel sought to rectify the neglect of the greatest chemists through the history of chemistry that forms an important part of his article. Here he pointed to the achievements of van Helmont, Glauber, Becher, and Stahl. The mechanists were clearly of less interest to him. We note again his fascination with Paracelsus.

> Paracelsus is one of the most singular personnages that literary history presents to us: visionary, superstitious, credulous, dissolute, intoxicated by the chimeras of Astrology, cabala, magic, and all the occult sciences; but bold, presumptious, enthusiastic, fanatic, extraordinary in all things, and determined to give himself to a high degree the luster of a passionate man through the study of his art (he had travelled with this in mind, consulting learned and unlearned men, women, barbers, etc.) and taking for himself the singular title of prince of Medicine and Monarch of Arcana, etc. He has been the author of the greatest revolution that has ever changed the face of Medicine . . . and he has in chemistry the same stature that Aristotle has in Philosophy.[64]

61 Ibid. (1734), p. 799.
62 G. F. Venel (1753), p. 408. Diderot's antimechanistic views have been noted by Charles Coulston Gillispie in his "The *Encyclopédie* and the Jacobin Philosophy of Science" (1962), pp. 255–89, and in his *The Edge of Objectivity* (1960), pp. 184–7.
63 Venel (1753), p. 410.
64 Ibid., p. 431.

Even though his writings are "absolutely unintelligible . . . the real merit of Paracelsus is to be found in the fact that to him is due the propagation and perpetuation of Chemistry."[65]

Conclusion

The study of alchemy and the medicochemical tradition in France presents us with a background to the late eighteenth-century chemical revolution that is very different from what we might expect from the work of Lavoisier and his colleagues, for whom the medical aspects of chemistry were not of major importance. Chemistry became a subject of interest and concern largely because of its relationship with medicine, and it took a century for the Parisian Galenists of the medical faculty to accept the medicines of the chemists. It was only after chemical medicines were approved for internal use in France that chairs of chemistry were finally established, and then in medical faculties. Chemistry was finally accepted, but primarily for the value of its pharmaceutical preparations.

A second chemical influence had also derived from medicine. Attempts to explain disease and physiological phenomena chemically derive ultimately from Paracelsus and his immediate followers, but it was only after the work of van Helmont that this aspect of chemistry became widely influential. Van Helmont described a vitalistic medicine using chemistry and chemical analogies. Willis and Sylvius proposed similar systems, as did Vieussens at Montpellier. These iatrochemists were opposed by the medical mechanists who argued that man and the functions of his organs are best explained in terms of the physics that had proved to be so successful in the study of astronomy and local motion. For these scholars chemical explanations were improper for the study and explanation of living processes. Chemical medicines and the analysis of bodily fluids might be pursued, but these were the limits of chemistry in medicine.

Still, for many people the science of mechanics was unsatisfactory. If a living human was to be understood in terms of physical laws, what was it that gave him life? What was it that gave him motion? These were problems that van Helmont had wrestled with early in the seventeenth century. They were debated again a century later by the doctors at Montpellier, whose answers revived a vitalistic doctrine. However, unlike the work of van Helmont and later iatrochemists, theirs was a medicine devoid of chemistry other than for analyses and for the preparation of medicines. The development of this antimechanistic medicine tended to divorce chemistry and medicine, and the result was a more indepen-

---

[65] Ibid.

dent chemistry that moved farther toward inorganic studies. Had this divorce not occurred, Lavoisier would probably have had to contend more with medical tradition than he did.

In contrast with the constantly changing relationship between chemistry and medicine during the two centuries we have studied, we find a persistent, but rather static, interest in traditional alchemy. The search for the philosopher's stone seems to have been pursued as actively through the eighteenth century as it had been in the sixteenth and the seventeenth, and many people viewed Paracelsus and van Helmont not only as originators of a medical system but also as alchemists of the highest order and discoverers of the true universal medicine. There are tracts as late as the 1780s that accuse Franz Anton Mesmer of plagiarizing the work of Paracelsus and his disciples.[66]

The whole story of French alchemy and the continued interest in the Paracelsian tradition in the mid- and late-eighteenth century would require another book. However, it is my belief that knowledge of the development of chemistry and the vitalistic theories of the Paracelsians from the early sixteenth through the early eighteenth centuries is essential for understanding both the chemical revolution and the Romantic reaction against the mechanical science of the philosophers at the end of the eighteenth century.

[66] See the section on "Joyand's Paracelsian Critique on Mesmer" in Allen G. Debus (1984), pp. 205–8.

Bibliography

This bibliography is arranged alphabetically by primary and secondary sources and then chronologically when an author is represented by more than one work. I have held to original spellings and the use of (or lack of) diacritical marks throughout. The books and papers listed here are those actually cited in the text. Many others have been examined in the course of my research; but even if these had been included, the list would surely be incomplete.

This book is a preliminary attempt to deal with a largely untouched area in the history of science and medicine. Because many of the books listed have lain practically untouched in libraries for hundreds of years, it was a major task to identify the authors and locate the books. These early chemical works seem often to have been dismissed as uninteresting to historians of science or of medicine. The standard bibliographies of alchemy and early chemistry, especially J. Ferguson's *Bibliotheca Chemica* and Denis I. Duveen's *Bibliotheca alchemica et chemica*, were less helpful than I would have wished because neither book covers the Paracelsian tradition. Far better in the search for these titles were J. R. Partington's *A History of Chemistry* and Lynn Thorndike's *A History of Magic and Experimental Science*, both of which cover the Paracelsian debates in considerable detail. Even more specific to this subject were the specialized bibliographies of Karl Sudhoff and Howard Stone, which are listed here. Nevertheless, the original works are for the most part rare, and I cannot claim to have seen all of them. However, I believe that I have examined enough of them to have presented an essentially correct overview of the debate resulting from the introduction of chemistry to medicine in France.

The libraries that proved to be of special value to me were the Wellcome Historical Medical Library and the British Library in London, the National Library of Medicine in Bethesda, Maryland, and the Duveen and Cole Collections at the University of Wisconsin. The Wellcome Library and the National Library of Medicine were particularly helpful in my search because of their chronological card catalogs. Both libraries are rich in the fields of early chemistry and chemical medicine and these catalogs made it possible to follow the literature chronologically at a time in my research when this was particularly helpful. Scarcely less valuable as a "finder" for the Madison Collections is John Neu's *Chemical, Medical, and Pharmaceutical Books Printed before 1800*.

It should be added that biographical information is difficult, sometimes impossible, to find on some of the authors whose works I have discussed. Here Partington is helpful, as is the *Nouvelle Biographie Général universelle*, the

209

Dictionnaire de Biographie Française, and various other standard guides, but many authors outside of the medical establishment were not well known even in their own time. Here the *Dictionary of Scientific Biography* has been of little help, with the exception of some of the shorter biographies prepared by Walter Pagel, Owen Hannaway, myself, and a few other historians who have had an interest in these rather shadowy figures who caused such a stir in their own times.

The secondary sources indicate clearly that although there is increasing interest in the chemistry and Paracelsian medicine of early modern Europe, the number of scholars engaged in such studies, particularly for France, is still relatively small, and there is still much to do. Several important recent dissertations have added to this otherwise sparse material. Bernard Joly's study of Pierre-Jean Fabre is the first serious examination of this prolific figure:

> *Les formes de rationalité à l'oeuvre dans la pensée alchemique au XVIIIeme siècle, Traduction, commentée du Manuscriptum ad Fredericum de Pierre-Jean Fabre.* Thèse de doctorat (nouveau régime) Philosophie sous la direction de Jean-Paul Dumont, 2 vols. (Université de Lille III, 1988).

Although Dr. Joly's thesis reached me in time to refer to it in my text, this was not the case with Hervé Baudry's study of Roch le Bailiff, whose confrontation with the Parisian Medical Faculty was one of the major events in this long story:

> *Contribution à l'Étude du Paracelsisme en France au XVIe Siècle (1560–1580) de la naissance du mouvement aux années de maturité: Le Demosterion de Roch le Baillif (1578).* Étude suivie d'une Edition critique et annotée Thèse doctorat (nouveau régime). (Université de Lille III, 1989).

Although it does not deal specifically with French Paracelsism, note should also be taken of Jole Shackleford's dissertation on Scandinavian Paracelsism, *Paracelsism in Denmark and Norway in the 16th and 17th Century,* which was completed at the University of Wisconsin-Madison in 1989. This, too, has opened new ground in this subject which binds scientific and medical history.

Among other recent Paracelsian studies note should be taken of Bruce T. Moran's investigation of Johannes Hartmann's appointment at Marburg and the role of Moritz of Hessen in introducing medical chemistry there:

> Bruce T. Moran, "Privilege, Communication, and Chemistry: The alchemical circle of Moritz of Hessen-Kassel," *Ambix,* 32 (1985), 110–26.
> "Der alchemistisch-paracelsische Kreis um den Landgrafen Moritz von Hessen-Kassel (1572–1632): Der fürstliche Forschen und die Methode experimenteller Wissenschaft," *Salburger Beitr. Paracelsusforsch.,* 25 (1987), 119–45.
> "Court Authority and Chemical Medicine: Moritz of Hessen, Johannes Hartmann, and the Origin of Academic Chemiatria," *Bulletin of the History of Medicine,* 63 (1989), 225–46.

Among other works that might be added at this point are Nancy Siraisi's *Medical and Early Renaissance Medicine* (Chicago: University of Chicago Press, 1990), Lynn Sumida Joy's *Gassendi the Atomist: Advocate of History in the Age of Science* (Cambridge University Press, 1987), and Peter Dear's *Mersenne and the Learning of the Schools* (Ithaca: Cornell University Press, 1988). Although these works do not deal specifically with the subject of this book, they do attest to the continued interest in reassessing the period of the scientific revolution.

Primary sources

Académie Royale des Sciences (Paris). *Histoire de l'Académie Royale des Sciences . . . Avec les Mémoires de Mathématique & de Physique, . . . Tirées des Registres de cette Académie*, from 1699. I have used the 2nd Amsterdam edition published by Pierre Mortier and others (from 1734).

Agrippa, Henri Cornelius. *La Philosophie Occulte de H.C.A. . . . Divisée en trois Livres, et traduite du Latin.* A la Haye: R. Chr. Alberts, 1727.

Albertus Magnus (pseudo). *Secrets Merveilleux de la Magie Naturelle & Cabalistique du Petit Albert* . . . . Lyon: Heirs of Beringo Fratres, 1743.

Les admirables Secrets d'Albert le Grand Contenant Plusieurs Traités sur la Conception des Femmes, des vertus des Herbes, des Pierres précieuse, & des Animaux . . . . Lyon: Heirs of Beringos Fratres, 1758.

Andreae, Johann Valentin. *Christianopolis. An Ideal State of the Seventeenth Century.* Translated with an historical introduction by Felix Emil Held. New York: Oxford University Press, 1916.

Anon. [Gui Patin (?), Jean Riolan Jr. (?)]. *Advertissement a Théophraste Renaudot Contenant Les Mémoires pour justifier les Anciens droicts & privileges de la Faculté de Medecine de Paris.* Paris: no publisher noted, 1641.

Le Parnasse assiegé où La guerre declarée entre les Philosophes Anciens & Modernes. Lyon: Antoine Boudet, 1697.

Explication de quelques Doutes touchant la Medecine. (s. 1, s.p., ca. 1700).

Lettre a un ami, touchant La Dissolution Radicale & Philosophicale de l'Or, & de l'Argent, sans corrosifs. Avec des Remarques Sur l'opiniòn général, qu'il ne faut point chercher de Reméde à la Goutte. London: Pierre Dunoyer, 1719.

Arnaud, E. R. Docteur en Medecine. *Introdvction a la Chymie, ov á la Vraye Physique. ov le Lecteur trevvera la definition de toutes les Operations de la Chymie; La façon de les faire, & des Exemples en suite tres-rares sur chaque Operation; & le tout dans vn tres-bel ordre.* Lyon: Claude Prost, 1650.

D'Atremont. *Le Tombeau de la Pauvreté. Dan lequel il est traité clairement de la transmutation des Metaux, & du moyen qu'on doit tenir pour y parvenir. Par un Philosophe inconnu. Reveuë & augmentée de la Clef, ou Explication des mots obscurs. Avec un Songe Philosophique sur le sujet de l'Art.* Paris: L. D'Houry, 1681.

Aubertus Vindonis, Iacobus. *De metallorum ortu & causis contra chemistas brevis & dilucida explicatio.* Lyon: I. Berion, 1575.

Duae apologeticae responsiones ad Iosephus Quercetanum. Lyon: I. Ausulti, 1576.

d'Aubry, L'Abbé Jean. *Apologie . . . Contre Certains Docteurs en Medecine: Les persecuteurs de son emprisonnement, Respondant à leurs calomnies, que l'Autheur a guery par Art Magique beaucoup de maladies incurables & abandonnées.* Paris: Chez l'Autheur, ca. 1638.

Le Triomphe de l'Archée et la Merveille du Monde, ov La Medecine Vniverselle, et Veritable Povr toutes sortes de Maladies les plus desesperées . . . Traisléme Edition.

Augumentée de l'Apologie de l'Autheur, Contre certains Docteurs en Medicine. No place, publisher or date [ca. 1660].

Auda, Dominico. *Les Admirables Secrets de la Medecine Chimique Du Sr. Joseph Quinti, Docteur Venetien. Qu'il a Recueillis avec beaucoup de soin & de travail: lesquels ont été plus d'une fois experimentez par lui même en plusieurs infirmitez, & maladies dangereuses* [a new translation from the Italian]. Venice: A. Liege, Chez J. F. Broucart, 1711.

Barba, Alvaro Alonzo. *Metallurgie, ou l'art de Tirer et de Purifier les Métaux, Traduite de l'Espagnol d'Alphonse Barba; avec Les Dissertations les plus rares sur les Mines & les Opérations Métalliques. Dédiée a M. Grassin. Directeur Général des Monnoyes de France*. Translated by Abbé Nicolas Lenglet Du Fresnoy. 2 vols. Paris: Didot, 1751.

Barin, Théodore. *Le Monde Naissant ou La Création du Monde, Démonstrée par des principes tres simples & tres conformes à l'Histoire de Moyse*. Utrecht: Pour la Compagnie les Libraires, 1686.

Barlet, Annibal. *Le Vray et Methodiqve Covrs de la Physiqve Resolvtive, Vvlgairement dite Chymie. Representé par Figures generales & particulieres. Povr Connoistre la Theotechnie Ergocosmiqve, C'est à dire L'Art de Dieu, en L'Ovvrage de l'Vnivers*. 2nd ed. Paris: N. Charles, 1657.

Barthez, P. J. *Nouveau Éléments de la Science de L'Homme*. 3rd ed. 2 vols. Paris: Germer Baillière, 1858; 1st ed., 1778; 2nd ed., 1806.

Beguinus, John. *Tyrocinium Chymicum: or, Chymical Essays, Acquired from the Fountain of Nature, and Manual Experience*. Translated by Richard Russell. London: Thomas Passenger, 1669.

[Belin, Jean Albert]. *Les Avantvres dv Philosophe Inconnu, en la recherche & en l'inuention de la Pierre Philosophale. Divisees en Qvatre Liures. Av Dernier Desqvels il est parlé si clairement de la façon de la faire, que jamais on n'en a parlé auec tant de candeur*. 2nd ed. Paris: Iacqves de Laize-de-Bresche, 1674.

de Bertereau, Martine. Dame & Barones de Beau-Soleil. "La Restitution de Pluton" (1640). See Barba, *Metallurgie* (1751) vol. 2, pp. 56–140.

Besson, Daulphinois, Jacques. Professeur és Sciences Mathematiques. *Art en Moyen Parfaict de Tirer Hvyles et Eaux, de tovs Medicaments simples & Oleogineaux. Premierement Receu d'un certain Empirique qu'on estimoit Alleman, & depuis confirmé par raisons & experiences* (newly corrected and augmented with a second book). Paris: Galiot du Pré, 1573.

Boerhaave, Hermann. *Sermo Academicus de Comparando Certo in Physicis*. Leiden: Petrum vander Aa, 1715.

Sermo Academicus de Chemia Suos Errores Expurgante, Quem habuit, Quum Chemiae professionem in Academiâ Lugduno-Batavâ auspicaretur xxi. Septembris 1718. Lugduni Batavorum: Sumptibus Petri Vander Aa, 1718.

A New Method of Chemistry; Including the Theory and practice of that Art: Laid down on Mechanical Principles and accommodated to the Uses of Life. The whole making a Clear and Rational System of Chemical Philosophy. To Which is prefix'd a Critical History of Chemistry and Chemists, From the Origin of the Art to the Present Time. Translated by P. Shaw and E. Chambers. London: J. Osborn and T. Longman, 1727.

Some Experiments Concerning Mercury. . . . Translated from the Latin, communicated by the Author to the Royal Society. London: J. Roberts, 1734.

Academical Lectures on the Theory of Physics. Being A Genuine Translation of his Institutes and Explanatory Comment . . . . 6 vols. London: W. Innys, 1742–46.

Bordelon, Laurent. *A History of the Ridiculous Extravagancies of Monsieur Oufle; Occasion'd by his reading Books treating of Magick, the Black-Art, Daemoniacks, Conjurers, Witches, Hobgoblins* . . . , *and other Superstitious Practices. With Notes containing a multitude of Quotations out of those Books, which have either Caused such Extravagant Imaginations, or may seeme to Cure them.* London: J. Morphew, 1711.

de Bordeu, Théophile. *Oeuvres complètes de Bordeu, Précédées d'une Notice sur sa vie et sur ses Ouvrages par le Chevalier Richerand.* 2 vols. Paris: Caille et Ravier Libraires, 1818.

B. (Bostocke), R. *The difference betwene the auncient Phisicke, first taught by the godly forefathers, consisting in vnitie peace and concord: and the latter Phisicke proceeding from Idolaters, Ethnikes, and Heathen: As Gallen, and such others consisting in dualities, discorde, and contrarietie.* . . . London: Robert Walley, 1585.

Boyle, Robert. *The Works of the Honourable Robert Boyle.* 6 vols. London: J. and F. Rivington et al., 1772.

Brunschwig, Hieronymus. *Book of Distillation.* Introduction by Harold J. Abrahams. Sources of Science, No. 79. New York: Johnson Reprint, 1971.

Cailleau, André Charles. *Clef du Grand Oeuvre, ou Lettres du Sancelrien Tourangeau a Madam L. D. L. B^{xxx}. T.D.F.A.T.* A Corinte et se trouve a Paris: Cailleau, 1777.

Cardan, Jerome. *De varietate libri XVII.* Basel: Henricus Petrus, 1557.

De subtilitate Libri XXI. Lugduni: Stephan Michael, 1580.

The First Book of Jerome Cardan's De subtilitate. Latin text, commentary, and translation by Myrtle Marguerite Cass. Williamsport, Pa.: Bayard Press, 1934.

de Castaigne, Gabriel. *Ausmosnier du Roy. Tant Medicinales que Chymiques, diuisées en quatre principaux traitez: I Le Paradis Terrestre, II Le grand miracle de la nature metallique, III L'Or Potable, IV Le Thresor Philosophique de la Medicine Metallique.* 2nd ed. Paris: Iean Dhoury, 1661.

Cattier, Isaac. *Seconde Apologie de l'Vniversité en Medecine de Montpellier.* . . . Paris: Jean Piot, 1653.

Joseph Chambon. *Principes de Physique, Rapportes à la Medicine Pratique, & autres Traitez sur cet Art.* Nouvelle ed. Paris: dans la boutique de Claude Barbin, chez la Veuve Jombert, 1711.

Traité des Metaux, Et des Mineraux, Et des Remedes qu'on en peut tirer; avec des Dissertations sur le Sel & le Soulphre des Philosophes, & sur la Goute, la Gravelle, la petite Vérole, la Rougeole & autres Maladies: avec un grand nombre de Remédes choisis. Paris: Claude Jombert, 1714.

Principes de Physique, Rapportés à Médecine-Pratique Nouvelle Edition. Paris: Charles-Antoine Jombert, 1750.

Charas, Moyse. *Apoticaire Artiste du Roy en son Jardin Royale des Plantes. Pharmacopée Royale Galenique et Chymique.* Paris: Chez l'Auteur, 1676.

Chartier, Jean. *La Science dv Plomb Sacre des Sages, ov de l'Antimoine, ov sont D'crites ses rares & particulieres Vertus, Puissances & Qualitez.* Paris: I de Senlecque & François Le Cointe, 1651.

Chevalier, Claude and Sabine Stuart. *L'Existence de la Pierre merveilleuse des Philo-*

sophes. Prouvée par des faits incontestables. Dédié aux Adeptes par un Amateur de la Sagesse. En France, 1765.

de Clave, Estienne. *Nouvelle Lumiere Philosophique des Vrais Principes et Elemens de Nature, & qualité d'iceaux. Contre l'opinion commune.* Paris: Olivier de Varennes, 1641.

Collesson, Jean. Doyen de Maigné. *L'Idée Parfaicte de la Philosophie Hermetiqve, Ou L'Abbregé de la Theorie & Practique de la Pierre des Philosophes.* 2nd ed. Paris: Herué du Mesnil, 1631. First edition, 1630.

L'Idée Parfaite de la Philosophie Hermetique. Ou L'Abregé de la Théorie & Pratique de la Pierre des Philosophes, Troisième edition. Paris: Laurent d'Houry, 1719.

Colonne, François Marie Pompée [here as Crosset de la Haumerie]. *Les Secrets les plus cachés de la Philosophie des anciens découverts et expliqués a la suite d'une Histoire des plus curieuses.* Paris: d'Houry, 1722.

Abregé de la Doctrine de la Paracelse, et ses Archidoxes. Avec une explication de la nature des principes de Chymie. Pour servir d'éclairissement aux Traitez de cet Auteur & des autres Philosophes. Suivi d'un Traité-Pratique de differentes manieres d'operer, soit par la voye Séche, ou par la voye Humide. Paris: d'Houry fils, 1724.

Les Principes de la Nature, ou de la Generation de Choses. Paris: André Cailleau, 1731.

"The Seed of the Chemical Philosophers." Wellcome Historical Medical Library MS 1737 (92 pp. with additional 42 pp. of notes, ca. 1850). Extracts from Paracelsus, the *Cabbala Denudata,* etc.

de Comitibus, Ludovicus. Philosophe & Medecin, *Discovrs philosophiqves Traitans des devx merveilles de l'Art & de la Nature: C'est à dire: De la liqueur de l'Alchaest, & de la Medecine vniverselle. De la matiere de l'une & de l'autre. Du moyen d'operer. Et de la voye qu'il faut tenir pour faire le Sel de Tartre volatil.* Translated by Robert Prevdhomme. Paris: Aux dépens de l'Auteur, 1669.

Cotta, John. *A Short Discoverie of the Unobserved Dangers of severall sorts of ignorant and unconsiderate Practisers of Physicke in England.* London: [R. Field] for W. Jones and R. Boyle, 1612.

Courtin, Germain. *Adversus Paracelsi de tribus principiis, auro potabile totáque pyrotechniâ, portentosas opiniones, disputatio.* Paris: Ex Officina Petri L'Huillier, 1579.

Crasellame, Fra Marc-Antonio. *La Lumiere sortant par soy me'me des Tenebres ou Veritable Theorie de la Pierre des Philosophes écrite en vers Italiens, & amplifiée en Latin par un Auteur Anonyme, en forme de Commentaire; le tout traduit en François par B. D. L.* Paris: Laurent D'Houry, 1687.

Crollius, Oswald. *Basilica chymica.* Frankfurt: Godfrid Tampach, [1623].

La Royalle Chymie. Translated into French by J. Marcel de Boulene. Rouen: Charles Osmont, 1634.

Discovering the Great and Deep Mysteries of Nature. In *Philosophy Reformed and Improved.* Translated by H. Pinnell. London: M. S. for Lodowick Lloyd, 1657.

D. J. B. D. F. Y. C. *La Messager de la Verité Traité. Contenant la Composition & Proprieté d'un Remède Spécifique pour toutes sortes de Maux; La maniére de s'en servir avec le régime de vivre, nourritures & boissons; . . . L'explication de la Figure Philosophique & du Globe Céleste. . . .* Paris: Theodore le Gris, 1722.

D. L. B. *Traité de la Poudre de Projection, Divisé en deux Lettres. Analyse tirée de l'Ecriture Sainte. Moiens pour parvenu à la Poudre de Projection Par l'humide substantial premier principe.* Bruxelles: n.p., 1707.

Dariot, Claude. *La Grand Chirvrgie de Philippe Aoreole Theophraste Paracelse grand Medecin & Philosophe Allemand, Tradvite en François, de la version Latine de Iosquin d'Alhem . . . par M. Claude Dariot . . . Plus vn discours de la goutte & causes d'icelle, auec sa guerison. Item III. Traittez de la preparation des medicamens, auec vne table pour l'intelligence da temps propre au recueil, composition & garde des herbes, fruits & semences.* 3rd ed. Montbeliart: Iacques Foillet, 1608.

Davisson, William. *Philosophia Pyrotechnia, . . . sev cvrricvlvs Chymiatricvs nobillissima illa & exoptatissima Medicinae parte pyrotechnica instructus.* 4 parts. Paris: Ioannem Bessin, 1633, 1635.

Les Elemens de la Philosophie de l'Art du Feu ou Chemie. Contenans les plus belles obseruations qui se rencontrent dans la resolution, preparation, & exhibition des Vegetaux, Animaux, & Mineraux, & les remedes contre toutes les maladies du corps humain, comme aussi la Metallique, appliquée à la Theorie, par vne verité fondée sur vne necessité Geometrique, demonstrée à la maniere d'Euclide . . . . Translated by Iean Hellot. Paris: F. Piot, 1651.

Commentariorum in . . . Petri Severini Dani Ideam Medicinae Philosophicae propediem proditurorum Prodromus. The Hague: Adrian Vlacq, 1660.

Deidier, Antoine. *Institutiones Medicinae Theoricae Phisiologiam & Pathologiam complectentes.* Montpellier: Honore Pech, 1711.

Chimie raisonnée. Où l'on tâche de découvrir la nature & la maniere d'agir des Remedes Chimiques les plus en usage en Medecine & en Chirurgie. Lyon: Marcellin Duplain, 1715.

Descartes, René. *Discourse on Method.* Translated by F. E. Sutcliffe. Baltimore: Penguin Books, 1968.

Didier, J. Docteur en Medecin. *Refvtation de la Doctrine Novvelle dv Sievr Helmont touchant les Fievres.* Sedan: François Chayer, 1653.

Dionis, Charles. Docteur Régent de la Faculté de Médecine en l'Université de Paris. *Dissertation sur le Taenia ou Ver-Plat, Dans laquelle on prouve que ce Ver n'est pas Solitaire; Avec Une Lettre sur la Poudre de Sympathie, propre contre le Rhumatisme simple ou gouteux. On y a joint la manière de del'apprêter & de s'en servir, & le Discours prononcé par M. le Chevalier Digby sur l'efficacité de cette Poudre.* Paris: P. G. Le Mercier, 1749.

Dorn, Gerard. *La Monarchie dv Ternaire en Vnion, Contre la Monomachie dv Binaire en Confvsion.* Paris: Gutenberg Reprints, ca. 1985. First ed. (s.l.), 1577.

Du Breil, André. Angeuin, Docteur regent en la faculté de Medecine à Paris: & ordonné pour la ville de Rouen. *La Police de l'Art et Science de Medecine, contenant la Refvtation des erreurs, & insigner abus, qui s'y commetent pour le iourdhuy: tres-utile & necessaire à toutes personnes, qui ont leur santé & vie en recommendation.* 1st ed., 1580. Paris: Leon Cavellat, 1586.

Duchesne, Joseph (Quercetanus). *Ad Iacobi Avberti Vindonis de ortv et cavsis metallorum contra chymicos explicationem . . . eivsdem de exqvisita mineralium, animalium, & vegitibilium medicamentorum spagyrica praeparatione & vsu, perspecua tractatio.* Lyon: Apud Ioannem Lertotium, 1575.

The Sclopotarie of Iosephus Quercetanus, Phisition, or His booke containinge the cure of wounds receiued by shot of Gunne or such like Engines of warre. Wherevnto is added his Spagericke antidotary of medicines against the aforesayd wounds. Translated by John Hester. London: Roger Ward for John Sheldrake, 1590.

A Breefe Aunswere . . . to the exposition of Iacobus Aubertus Vindonis, concerning the original, and causes of Mettalles. Set foorth against Chimistes. Another exquisite and plaine Treatise of the same Josephus, concerning the Spagericall preparations, and use of minerall, animall, and vegitable secretes, not heeretofore knowne of many. Translated by John Hester, practitioner in the Spagericall Arte. London: 1591, n.p.

Le Grand Miroir dv Monde. 2nd ed. Lyon: Pour les Heretiers d'Eustache Vignon, 1593.

Ad Veritatem Hermeticae medicinae ex Hippocratis veterumque decretis ac Therapeusi, nec non viuae rerum anatomiae exegesi, ipsiusque naturae luce stabiliendam, adversus cuiusdam Anonymi phantasmata Respondio. Frankfurt: Ex Officina Typographica Wolffgangi Richteri, Impensâ Conradi Nabenii, 1605.

The Practise of Chymicall, and Hermeticall Physicke, for the preseruation of health. Translated by Thomas Tymme. London: Thomas Creede, 1605.

Liber De Priscorum Philosophorum verae medicinae materia, praeparationis modo, atque in curandis morbis, praestantia. Déque simplicium, & rerum signaturis, tum externis, tum internis, seu specificis, à priscis & Hermeticis Philosophis multa cura, singularíque industria comparatis, atque introductis, duo tractatus. His accesserunt ejusdem Ios. Quercetani de dogmaticorum medicorum legitima, & restituta, medicamentorum praeparatione, libri duo. Leipzig: Thom. Schürer and Barthol. Voight, 1613.

Le Povrtraict de la Santé. Où est au vif representée la regle vniuerselle & particuliere, de bien sainement, & longuement viure. Enrichy de plusieurs preceptes, raisons, & beaux exemples, tirez des Medecines, Philosophes & Historiens, tant Grecs que Latins, les plus celebres. S. Omer: Charles Boscart, 1618.

Traicté de la matiere, preparation et excellente vertu de la Medecine balsamique des Anciens Philosophes. Auquel sont adioustez deux traictez, l'un des Signatures externes des choses, l'autre des internes & specifiques conformément à la doctrine & pratique des Hermetiques. Paris: C. Morel, 1626.

Du Clos, Sr. Conseiller & Medecin ordinarie du Roy & l'un des Physiciens de l'Academie Royale des Sciences. *Dissertation sur les Principes des Mixtes Naturels. Faite en l'An 1677.* Amsterdam: Daniel Elsevier, 1680.

Ducret, Toussaint. *De Arthritide vera assertio, eivsqve cvrandae methodvs, adversvs Paracelsistas.* Lyon: Bartholomaeus Vincentius, 1575.

du Fresnoy, Nicholas Lenglet. *Histoire de la Philosophie Hermetique. Accompagnée d'un catalogue raisonné des écrivains de cette science. Avec le véritable Philalethe, revû sur les originaux.* 3 vols. Paris: Coustelier, 1742.

Du Gault, Antoine de Fregeville. *Palinodie Chimique ov les Erreurs de cest Art sont moins plaisamment, que serieusement refutez par le Sieur du Gault.* Paris: Pierre Sevestre, 1588.

Du Hamel, Ioan. Bapt. *De consensv Veteris et Novae Philosophiae Libri Dvo. In Priori Libro Platonis, Aristotelis, Epicuri, Cartesii, & aliorum de Principiis rerum naturalium placita excutiuntur, ac Physica generalis penè tota pertractatur. In Posteriori agitur de Elementis, & Chymicorum Principiis, necnon de mixtione, & dissolutione corporum, ubi Chymia ferè universa explicatur.* Paris: Carolum Savreux, 1663.

Duncan, Daniel. *La Chymie Naturelle ou l'Explication Chimique et Mechanique de la Nourriture de l'Animal.* Paris: Laurent d'Houry, 1683. Although I have not seen an earlier edition, the first part of *La Chymie Naturelle* seems to have been printed in 1681 since there is a review of that date in the *Journal des Sçavans.*

Seconde et Troisieme Partie de la Chymie Naturelle ou L'Explication Chimique et

Mechanique De l'Evacuation particuliere aux Femmes, & de la Generation. Paris (printed at Montaubon): Laurent d'Houry & Daniel Horthemels, 1687.

Du Soucy, François. *Sommaire de la Medecine Chymique: Où l'on void clairement beaucoup de choses que les autheurs ont tenues iusques icy dans l'obscurite.* Paris: Pierre Billaine, 1632.

Erastus, Thomas. *Disputationum de medicina nova P. Paracelsi. Pars prima, in qua quae de remediis superstitiosus et magicis curationibus prodidit praecipue examinantur.* [Basel]: 1572.

Disputationum de nova P. Paracelsi medicina. Pars altera: In qua philosophiae Paracelsicae principia et elementa explorantur. [Basel]: 1572.

D'Espagnet, Jean. *La Philosophie Natvrelle Restablie en sa Pvreté. Où l'on void à découuert toute l'oeconomie de la Nature & ou se manifestent quantité d'erreurs de la Philosophie Ancienne, estant redigée par Canons & demonstrations certains. Auec le Traicté de la Ouurage Secret de la Philosophie d'Hermez, qui enseigne la matiere, & la façon de faire la Pierre Philosophale. Spes mea est in Agno.* Paris: Edme Pepingvé, 1651.

Enchyridion Physicae Restitutae: or The Summary of Physics Recovered. Wherein the true Harmony of Nature is explained, and many Errours of the Ancient Philosophers, by Canons and certain Demonstrations, are clearly evidenced and evinced. London: W. Bentley for W. Sheares and Robert Tutchein, 1651.

Fabre, Pierre-Jean. *Alchymista Christianus. In quo Deus rerum Author omnium, & quamplurima Fidei Christianae mysteria, per analogias Chymicas & Figuras explicantur, Christianorumque Orthodoxa, doctrina, vita & probitas non oscitantur ex chymica arte demonstrantur.* Tolososae Tectosagum: Petrum Bosc, 1632.

L'Abregé des Secrets Chymiques, ov l'on void la Nature des animaux vegetaux & mineraux entierement découuert: Avec les vertus et Proprietez des principes qui composent & conservent leur estre; & vn Traitté de la Medecine generale. Paris: Anthoine de Sommaville, 1636.

Traité de la Peste selon la doctrine des médecins spagyriques. Toulouse: Castres, 1653.

Fenotus, Jeannes Antonius. *Alexipharmacum, sive antidotus Apologetica, ad virulantias Josephi cuiusdam Quercetani Armeniaci, euomitas in libellum Jacobi Auberti, de ortu & causis Metallorum contra Chymistas . . . In quo . . . omnia argumēta refelluntur, quibus Chymistae probare conantur, aurum argentumq; arte fieri posse. . . .* Basel: s.d. [1575].

Fernel, Jean. *Universa Medicina, Primum quidem studio & diligentia Guiljelmi Plantii, Cennomanni elimata, Nunc autem notis, observationibus, & remediis Ioann. & Othonis Heurni, Untraject. et Aliorum Praestantissimorum Medicorum Scholiis illustrata. Cui accedunt Casus & observationes rariores, Quas Cl. D.D. Heurnius . . . in diario practico annotavit.* Traiecti ad Rhenum (Utrecht): typis Gilberti à Zyll & Theod. ab Ackersdijck, 1656.

Figulus, Georgius. *Dilingani Philosophi & Chymiatri. Novum & Inauditum Medicinae Universalis Speculum Cabalisto-Chymicum.* Brussels: Joannis Mommarti, 1660.

Fontani, D. Gabrielis. *Iacobi Filii. Artivm et Medicinae Doctoris, Medicorvm Massiliensium Collegio aggregati. De Veritate Hippocraticae Medicinae Firmissimis rationum & experimentorum momentis stabilita, & demonstrata; sev Medicina Antihermetica, In qua Dogmata Medica physiologica, pathologica, & therapeutica, contra Paracelsi, & Hermeticorum placita clarissimé promulgantur: non reiectis penitus Chymicorum inuentis, ad Hippocraticam artem conferentibus. Adiectus est ad calcem generalis index rerum in hoc opere contentarum: necnon introductio ad methodum medendi; atque Apologeticon aduersus Van-helmont. vbi firmissimè demonstratur, quatuor humores Galenistarum non esse fictitios: caetera octauo abhinc folio recensentur.* Lyon: Philip Borde, Lavr Arnavd, & Cl. Rigavd, 1657.

Geoffroy, E. F. "Probleme de Chimie. Trouver des Cendres qui ne contiennent aucunes parcelles de fer." *Mémoires de l'Academie Royale des Sciences* (1705), 478–80. 2nd ed. Amsterdam: Pierre Mortier, 1746.

"Des Supercheriés concernant la Pierre Philosophale." *Mémoires de l'Academie Royale des Sciences* (1722). Paris: de l'Imprimerie Royale, 1722, 61–70; Amsterdam: Pierre de Coup, 1727, 81–93.

Germain, Claude. Dr. Regent en la Faculté de Medecine à Paris. *Orthodoxe ov de l'abvs de l'Antimoine, Dialogue tres-necessaire povr detromper ceux qui donnent ou prennent le Vin & Pouldre Emetique.* . . . Paris: Thomas Blaise, 1652.

Gesner, Conrad. *The Treasure of Euonymus: Conteyninge the wonderfull hid secrets of nature.* . . . Translated by P. Morwyng. London: John Daie, 1559.

The New Jewell of Health. London: H. Denham, 1576.

Glaser, Christophle. *Traite de la Chymie Enseignant par une brieue et facile methode toutes ses plus necessaires preparations.* Paris: Chez l'Autheur, 1663.

Glauber, Johann Rudolph. *La Description des Novveaux Fovrneavx Philosophiques ov Art Distillatoire, Par le moyen duqel sont tirez les Esprits, Huiles, Fleurs, & autres Medicaments: Par vne voye aisée & auec grand profit, des Vegetaux, Animaux, & Mineraux. Auec leur usage, tant dans la Chymie, que dans la Medecine.* Translated by Le Sieur Bernard Dv Teil. Paris: Thomas Iolly, 1659.

The Works of the Highly Experienced and Famous Chymist, John Rudolph Glauber: Containing, Great Variety of Choice Secrets in Medicine and Alchymy. . . . Translated by Christoper Packe. London: Thomas Milbourn, 1689.

Gohory, Jacques. *De Vsu & Mysteriis Notarum Liber. In quo vetusta literarum & numerorum ac divinorum ex Sibylla nominum ratio explicatur.* Paris: Vincent Serternas, 1550.

I. G. P. (translator) [Jacques Gohory, Parisien]. *Le Dixiesme Livre d'Amadis de Gaule, auquel . . . est traité de la furieuse guerre qui fut entre les Princes Gaulois & Grecz pour le recourirement de la belle Helene d'Apolonie. Et des auentures estranges que suruindrent durant ce temps.* Paris: Vincent Sertenas, 1555.

(translator). *Hypnerotomachie ov Discours du Songe de Poliphile, Deduisant comme Amour le combat à l'occasion de Polia, Soubz la fiction de quoy de aucteur monstrant que toutes choses terrestres ne sont que vanité traicté de plusieurs matieres profitables, & dignes de memoire.* Paris: Jacques Keruer, 1561.

(as Leo Suavius). *Theophrasti Paracelsi philosophiae et medicinae utriusque universae, compendium, ex optimi quibusque eius libris: Cum scholijs in libros IIII eiusdem De vita longa, plenos mysteriorum, parabolorum, aenigmatum.* Basel: Per Petrum Pernam, 1568.

Gosset, Sieur. Dr. aggregé au College de Medecins de la Ville d'Amiens. *Revelations Cabalistiques d'une Medecine Universelle Tirée du Vin: Avec une Maniere d'extraire le Sel de rosée: Et une Dissertation sur les Lampes sepulchres.* Amiens: Loüis Godart, 1735.

Grévin, Jacques. *Discovrs . . . sur les vertus & facultez de l'Antimoine. Contre Ce qu'en a escrit maistre Loys de Launay . . . .* Paris: André Wechel, 1566.

Le Second Discovrs de Iacques Grévin, Docteur en Medecin a Paris, sur les vertus & facultez de l'Antimoine, Avqvel Il est sommairement traicté de la nature des Mineraux, venins, pestes, & de plusieurs autres questiōs naturelles & medicinales, pour la confirmation de l'aduis des Medecins de Paris, & Pour seruir d'Apologie contre ce qu'a escrit M. Loïs de Launay, Empirique. Paris: Iacques du Puys, 1567.

De Venenis Libri duo. Antwerp: Christopher Plantin, 1571.

Guinter (Guintherius) von Andernach, Johannes. *De medicina veteri et noua tum cognoscenda, tum faciunda commentarij duo.* 2 vols. Basel: Henricpetrina, 1571.

Harvet, Israel. Medici Aurelianensis. *Defensio Chymiae Adversus Apologiam, & Censuram Scholę Medicorum Parisiensium. Et in easdem Gvlielmi Bavcyneti Medici item Aurelianensis Notationes.* Paris: Apud Guillelmum Auuray, 1604.

Hecquet, Philippe. *De Digestion, et des Maladies de L'Estomac suivant de Systême de la Trituration & du Broyement, sans l'aide de Levains ou de la Fermentation, dont on fait voir l'impossibilité en santé & en maladie.* 2 vols. Paris: Guillaume Cavalier, 1730; 1st ed. 1712.

van Heer, Henricus. *Spadacrene, hoc est fons Spadanus; ejus singularia, bibendi modus, medicamina bibentibus necessaria.* Liége: Arn. de Corswaremia, 1614.

van Helmont, Jean Baptiste. *Ortus medicinae. Id est, initia physicae inaudita. Progressus medicinae novus, in morborum ultionem, ad vitam longam.* Amsterdam: Ludovicus Elsevir, 1648. Reprinted Brussels: Culture et Civilisation, 1966. This is the standard – and first edition of the complete works of van Helmont.

Deliramenta catarrhi: or the Incongruities, Impossibilities and Absurdities couched under the Vulgar Opinion of Defluxions . . . . Translated by Walter Charleton. London: E. G. for William Lee, 1650.

Doctrine Novvelle de Iean Baptiste de Helmont, Seigneur de Royenborch, Pellines, &c natif de Bruxelles: Tovchant les Fievres. Tradvite par Abraham Bavda. Sedan: Iean Iannon, n.d.; dedication dated 8 October 1652.

Oriatrike or Physick Refined. The Common Errors therein Refuted, And the whole Art Reformed & Rectified. Being a New Rise and Progress of Philosophy and Medicine, for the destruction of Diseases and Prolongation of Life. Translated by J(ohn) C(handler). London: Lodowick Loyd, 1662. A useful translation of the complete *Ortus medicinae.*

Les Oevvres . . . Traittant des Principes de Medecine et Physique, pour la guerison assurée des Maladies. Translated by Jean le Conte, Docteur Medecin. Lyon: Jean Antoine Hvgvetan & Gvillavme Barbier, 1671.

Herman, Philip. *An Excellent Treatise.* Translated by John Hester. London: J. Charlwood, 1590.

Homberg, Guillaume. "Essais de Chemie." *Mémoires de la Académie Royale des Sciences* (1702–1709). Amsterdam edition (1702), 44–70; (1705), 117–28; (1706), 336–51; (1709), 133–47.

Hovel (or Hoüel), Nicholas. *Traité de la Peste avqvel est Amplement Discovrv de l'Origen, cause, signes, preseruation & curation d'icelle. Avec Les vertus & facultez de l'electuaire de l'oeuf: duquel iadis soulait vser ce grand Empereur Maximilien.* Paris: Galiot du Pré, 1573.

Journal des Sçavans. From 1666, in various editions. Paris and Amsterdam.

L. S. S. (S.L.S. in the British Library catalog). *Discours Responsif à celuy d'Alexādre de la Tourete, sur les secrets de l'art Chymique & confection d l'Or potable, faict en la defense de la Philosophie & Medicine antique, contre la nouuelle Paracelsique.* Paris: Ian de l'Astre, 1575.

de la Brosse, Guy. *De la Nature, Vertue, et Vtilité des Plantes diuisé en cinq liures.* Paris: Rollin Baragnes, 1628.

De La Chastre, René. Gentil-homme Berroyen. *Le Prototype ov Tres Parfait et Analogiqve Exemplaire de l'Art Chimicq; a la Phisiqve ov Philosophie de la science Naturelle. Contenant les Cavses principes & demonstrations scientifiq; de la certitude dudit Art.* Paris: Jean Anthoine Ioallin, 1620.

La Faveur, Sebastian Matte. Distillateur & Demonstrateur ordinaire de la Chymie en la faculté de Medecine de Montpellier. *Pratique de Chymie . . . Avec un avis sur les eaux minerales.* Montpellier: Daniel Pech, 1671.

de la Martinière, Pierre Martin. Medecin & Operateur ordinaire du Roy. *Tombeau de la Folie. Dans lequel se Void les plus fortes raisons que l'on puisse apporter pour faire connoître la réalité & la possibilité de la Pierre Philosophale, & d'autres raisons & experiences qui en font voir l'abus & impossibilité.* Paris: Chez l'Auteur (after 1669).

de la Tourette, Alexandre. *Bref Discours des Admirables vertus de l'Or-Potable. Auquel sont traictez les principaux fondemens de la medecine, l'origine & cause de toutes maladies, & quels sont les medicamens plus propres à leur guerison, & à la conservation de la santé humaine: Composé par le sieur de la Tourette, n'aguires President des generaux maistres des monnoyes de France . . . Avec une Apologie de la tres vtile science d'Alchimie.* Lyon: Pierre Roussin, 1575.

de Launay, Loys. Medecin ordinaire de la Rochelle. *De la Facvlté & vertu admirable de l'Antimoine, auec responce à certaines calomnies.* La Rochelle: Barthelmi Berton, 1564.

Responce av Discovrs de Maistre Iacqves Grevin, Docteur de Paris, qv'il à Escript contre le livre de Maistre Loys de l'Aunay, Medecin en la Rochelle, touchant la faculté de la Antimoine. La Rochelle: Barthelmi Berton, 1566.

le Baillif, Roch. Edelphe Medecin Spagiric. *Le Demosterion . . . Auquel sont contenuz Trois cens Aphorismes Latins & François. Sommaire veritable de la Medicine Paracelsique, extraicte de luy en la plus part, par le dict Baillif.* Renne: Pierre le Bret, 1578.

Sommaire Defence . . . aux demandes des docteurs, & faculté de Medecine de Paris. Paris: n.p., 1579.

Dv Remede de la Peste, Charbon et Plevrisie, et dv moyen cognoistre quel Element les excite, &.les hommes qui pour le temps y sont assubiettez, fait en faueur du Public. Paris: Abel l'Angelier, 1580.

Premier Traicte de l'Homme, et son essentielle, Anatomie, auec les Elemens, & ce qui est en eux: De ses Maladies, Medecine & absoluts remedes és Tainctures d'Or, Corail, & Antimoine: & Magistere des Perles: & de leur extraction. Paris: Abel l'Angelier, 1580.

Le Breton, Charles. *Remèdes Choises et Éprouvés Tant de Medecine, que de Chyrurgie, pour les maladies du Corps humain, dont un grand nombre n'ont pas encore esté imprimés.* Paris: Claude Jombert, 1716.

Les Clefs de la Philosophie Spagyrique, Qui donnent la connoissance des Principes & des véritables Operations de cet Art dans les Mixtes des trois genres. Paris: Claude Jombert, 1722.

le Doux, Gaston. Dit de Claves. *Traité Philosophique de la Triple Preparation de l'Or de l'Argent.* In *Dictionaire Hermetique, Contenant l'Expliction des Termes, Fables, Enigmes, Emblemes & manieres de parler des vrais Philosophes. Accompagné de deux Traitez singuliers & utiles aux Curieux de l'Art.* Paris: Laurent D'Houry, 1695; reprinted Paris: Gutenberg Reprint, 1979.

Le Fèvre, Nicholas (Nicasius Le Febure). *A Compleat Body of Chemistry.* Translated P.D.C., 2 parts. London: O. Pulleyn, 1670.

Cours de Chymie, pour servir d'Introduction à cette Science. Cinquieme Edition, Revûe corrigée & augmentée d'un grand nombre d'Operations, & enrichie de Figures. Par M. Du Monstrier, Apoticaire de la Marine & des Vaisseaux du Roi: Membre de la Société Royale de Londres & de celle de Berlin. 5 vols. Paris: Jean-Noel Leloup, 1751.

Lemery, L. "Que les Plantes contiennent réelement du fer, & que ce métal entre nécessairement dans leur composition naturelle." *Mémoires de l'Académie Royale des Sciences* (1706). 2nd edition, 2 vols., Amsterdam: Pierre Mortier (1746, 1747), 529–38.

"Reflexions et observations diverses sur une vegetation chimique du Fer, & sur quelques expériences faites à cette occasion avec differentes liqueurs acides & alkalines, & avec differens métaux substituez au Fer, *Mémoires de l'Académie Royale des Sciences* (1707). 2nd edition, 2 vols., Amsterdam (1746, 1747), 388–425.

"Nouvel éclairicissement sur la prétendue production artificielle du Fer, publiée par Becher & soutenne par Mr. Geoffroy." *Mémoires de l'Académie Royale des Sciences* (1708). 2nd edition, 2 vols., Amsterdam: Pierre Mortier (1750), 482–515.

Lemery, Nicholas. *A Course of Chymistry. Containing An easie Method of Preparing those Chymical Medicins which are used in Physick with Curious Remarks and Useful Discourses upon each Preparation, for the benefit of such who desire to be instructed in the Knowledge of this Art.* Translated Walter Harris, M.D. 2nd English ed. from the 5th French ed. London: R. N. for Walter Kettilby, 1686.

de Longeville, Harcouet. *Histoire des Personnes qui ont vecu plusieurs siècles et qui ont Rajeuni avec le Secret du Rajeunissement, Tiré d'Arnauld de Villeneuve.* Paris: la Veuve Charpentier and Laurent le Comte, 1715.

Le Lorrain, Pierre. Abbé de Vallemont. *Curiosities of Nature and Art in Husbandry and Gardening.* London: D. Brown, A. Roper and Fran. Cogan, 1707.

Curiositez de la Nature et de l'Art sur la Vegetation: ou l'Agriculture et le Jardinage dans leur Perfection . . . . Paris: Par la Societe's, 1711. First French edition, 1705.

Le Pelletier, Jean. *L'Alkaest ou le Dissolvant universel de Van-Helmont, Revelé dans plusieurs Traitez qui en découvrent le Secret.* Rouen: Guillaume Behourt, 1704.

Libavius, Andreas. *Alchymia, recognita, emendata, et aucta, tum dogmatibus & experimentis nonullis . . . .* Frankfurt: Excudebat Joannes Saurius, impensis Petri Kopffii, 1606. Printed with Andreas Libavius, *Commentariorvm Alchymiae . . .* [Separate title page (1616)].

[de Limojon de Saint Didier, Alexandre Toussaint]. *Le Triomphe Hermetique ou La Pierre Philosophale Victorieuse. Traitté Plus complet & plus intelligible, qu'il y en ait eû jusques ici, touchant le Magistere Hermetique.* Amsterdam: Henry Walstein, 1699.

Der Hermetische Triumph Oder der Siegende Philosophische Stein. Ein Tract . . . von der Hermetischen Meisterschaft. Leipzig: J. G. Laurentio, 1707.

Le Triomphe Hermétique: Introduction et notes d'Eugène Canseliet. Ouvrage precédé du Mutus Liber avec une hypotypose de Magophon. Paris: E. P. Denoël, 1971.

de Locques, Nicholas. *Les Vertvs Magnetiqves dv Sang, De son vsage interne & externe. Pour la guarison des maladies.* Paris: Iacques le Gentil, 1664.

Les Rvdimens de la Philosophie Natvrelle Tovchant le Systeme dv Corps Mixte. Covrs

Theorique, Où clairement expliquez les Precepts & les Principes de la Chymie, qui ont esté jusques icy cachez des anciens Philosophes. Paris: Geoffroy Marcher, 1665.

Lvssavld, Sieur. Conseiller & Medecine ordinarie du Roy. *Apologie povr les Medecins, Contre ceux qui les accusent de deferer trop à la Nature, & de n'avoir point de Religion.* Paris: En la Boutique de P. Rocolet chez Damien Foucault, 1663.

Massard, Iacqves. Docteur en Medecine, aggregé au College des Medecins de Grenoble. *Panacée, ov Discovrs svr les Effets singuliers d'un Remede experimenté, & commode pour la geurison de la pluspart des longues maladies; même de celles qui semblent incurables . . . Avec un Traité d'Hypocrate de la cause des maladies, & de l'ancienne Medecine, traduit en François par l'Auteur.* Grenoble: Chez l'Auteur; 1679; 2nd part, Grenoble: P. Fremon, 1680.

Mattioli, M. Pierre Andre. Medecin Senoys. *Les Commentaires . . . sur les six liures des Simples de Pedacius Dioscoride Anazarbeen.* Lyon: A L'Escu de Milan par Gabriel Cotier, 1561.

Mercure Française. Le dixiesme Tome. Paris: Iean & Estienne Richer, 1625.

Mersenne, Marin. *La verite des sciences. Contre les septiques ou Pyrhonniens.* Paris: Toussainct Du Bray, 1625. Reprint Stuttgart/Bad Cannstaat: Friedrich Fromann Verlag [Gunther Holzboog], 1969.

Correspondance du P. Marin Mersenne. Religieux Minime. Pub. Mme Paul Tannery. Edited by Cornelis de Waard with the collaboration of René Pintard, 10 vols. (1617–41). Paris: P.U.F. Centre National de la Recherche Scientifique, 1921–67.

Meurdrac, Marie. *La Chymie Charitable et Facile, En faveur des Dames.* Paris: Se vend ruë des Billettes & ruë de Plastre proche la ruë S. Avoye, 1666.

Michauld, Jean-Bernard. *Mémoires pour servir à l'histoire de la vie et des ouvrages de Monsieur l'abbé Lenglet Du Fresnoy.* Londres et se trouvent à Paris: Duchesne, 1761.

Mongin, Mons. J. *Le Chimiste Physicien. Ou l'on montre que les Principes naturels de tous les Corps sont veritablement ceux que l'on découvre par la Chimie. Et où par des Experiences & des Raisons fondée sur les Loix des Mechaniques, aprés avoir donné des moyens faciles pour les separer des mixtes; on explique leurs proprietez, leurs usages & les Principaux Phenomenes qu'on observe es travaillant en Chimie.* Paris: Laurent d'Houry, 1704.

de Montaigne, Michel. *Essais: Reproduction Photographique de l'Édition Originale de 1580 avec une introduction de l'édition originale de 1580 . . . publiee par Daniel Martin.* 2 vols. Genève: Librairie Slakine/Paris: Librairie Champion, 1976.

An Apology for Raymond Sebond. Translated and edited with an Introduction and Notes by M. A. Screech. London and Harmondsworth: Penguin Books, 1987.

Montesquieu, Charles Louis de Secondat. *The Persian Letters . . . now first Completely translated into English with Notes and Memoirs by John Davidson . . . .* 2 vols. Philadelphia: George Barrie, n.d.

[Mr. Moreau, Doct. en Med.] *La Defense de la Faculté de Medecine de Paris, Contre son Calomniateur. Dediée a Monseigneur l'Eminentissime Cardinal Dvc de Richelieu.* Paris: n.p., 1641.

Morin, Jean Baptiste. *Refvtation des Theses Erronees de Anthoine Villon dit le soldat Philosophe, & Estienne de Claues Medecin Chymiste, par eux affichées publiquement*

à Paris, contre la Doctrine d'Aristote le 23. Aoust. 1624 à l'encontre desquelles y a
  eû censure de la Sorbonne, & Arrest de la Cour de Parlement. Ou sont doctement
  traictez les vrays principes des corps & plusieurs autres beaux poincts de la Nature;
  & prouuee la solidité de la Doctrine d'Aristote. Paris: Et se vendent chez l'Au-
  theur, dans l'Isle du Palais, en la Place Dauphine, à l'Escu de France, 1624.
Naudé, Gabriel. *Instrvction a la France svr la Verité de l'Histoire des Freres de la Roze-
  Croix.* Paris: François Ivlliot, 1623.
*The History of Magick By Way of Apology For All the Wise Men who have unjustly
  been reputed Magicians, from the Creation to the present age.* Translated by J.
  Davies. London: John Streater, 1657.
Apologie pour tous les grands hommes, qui ont este accusez de Magie. Paris Iacqves
  Cotin, 1659.
Nicholas Cusanus. *The Idiot in Four Books. The first and second of Wisdome. The third
  of the Minde. The fourth of staticke Experiments, or Experiments of the Ballance.*
  London: William Leake, 1650.
Unity and Reform. Selected Writings of Nicholas de Cusa. Edited by John P. Dolan.
  South Bend: University of Notre Dame Press, 1962.
de Nuisement, Jacques. Receueur General au Comté de Ligny en Barrois. *Traittez
  De L'Harmonie Et Constitution Generalle du Vray Sel, Secret des Philosophes, et de
  l'Esprit universel du Monde . . . .* Paris: Ieremie Perier & Abdias Buizard,
  1621.
Palissy, Bernard. *The Admirable Discourses of Bernard Palissy.* Translated by Aurèle
  La Rocque. Urbana: University of Illinois Press, 1957.
*Oeuvres Complètes . . . Édition conforme aux Textes Originaux imprimés du vivant
  de l'Auteur; avec des notes et une notice historique par Paul-Antoine Cap.* Nouveau
  Tirage augmenté d'Avant-Propos de M. Jean Orcel. Paris: Albert Blanchard,
  1961. In this edition the "Traité des Metavx et Alchimie" (pp. 188–223) and
  the "Traité de l'Or Potable" (pp. 224–31) are to be found as part of the
  Discours Admirables.
Recepte Veritable. Edition critique par Keith Cameron. Geneva: Librairie Droz,
  1988.
Paracelsus. *La grande, vraye et parfaicte chirurgie.* Translated by M. Pierre Hassard
  d'Armentieres, medecin et chirurgien. Anvers: Guillaume Silvius, 1568.
*De la Peste, et ses Cavses et Accidents, comprins en cincq liures, nouuellemēt traduits
  en François par M. Pierre Hassard d'Armentieres Medecin.* Anvers: Christopher
  Plantin, 1570.
De restituta vtriusque Medicinae vera Praxi. Edited by Gerard Dorn. Lyon: Jacobo
  Dv Pvys, 1578.
*A hundred and fourteene Experiments and Cures of the famous Physitian Philippus
  Aureolus Theophrastus Paracelsus: Translated out of the Germane tongue into the
  Latin. Whereunto is added certaine excellent and profitable workes by B. G. a Portu
  Aquitano. Also certaine Secrets of Isacke Hollandus concerning the Vegetall and
  Animall worke. Also the Spagericke Antidotarie for Gunne-Shot of Iosephus Quir-
  sitanus.* Collected by Iohn Hester. London: Vallentine Sims, 1596.
Opera Bücher und Schrifften. 2 vols. Edited by Johann Huser. Strasbourg: L.
  Zetzner, 1616.
Chirurgische Bücher und Schrifften. Edited by Johann Huser. Strasbourg: L.
  Zetzner, 1618.
Les XIV Livres des Paragraphes de Ph. Theoph. Paracelse . . . Où sont contenus en

Epitome ses secrets admirables, tant Physiques que Chirurgiques . . . Plus vn abregé des preparations Chimiques . . . Vn autre Discours excellent de l'Alchimie . . . Translated by C. De Sarcilly. Paris: Jean Guillemot, 1631.

Of the Supreme Mysteries of Nature. Translated by R. Turner. London: J. C. for N. Brook and J. Harison, 1656.

Sämtliche Werke. 15 vols. Edited by Karl Sudhoff and Wilhelm Matthiessen. Munich/Berlin: R. Oldenbourg (Vols. vi–ix: O.W. Barth), 1922–1933.

Volumen medicinae paramirum. Translated and preface by Kurt L. Leidecker. Supplement to Bulletin of the History of Medicine, No. 11. Baltimore: Johns Hopkins Press, 1949.

(Paré) Parey, Ambroise. *The Works . . .* Translated out of Latin and compared with the French by Th. Johnson. London: Th. Cotes and R. Young, 1634.

Oeuvres complètes d'Ambroise Paré. Notes and introduction by J. F. Malgaine. 3 vols. Paris: J. B. Baillière, 1840–1.

Pascal, Jacques. Maistre Apothecaire de Beziers. *Discours Contenant la Conference de la Pharmacie Chymique, ou Spagirique, auec la Galenique, ou Ordinaire. Ensemble La Demonstration des abus qui se commettent sur les principaux medicamens officinaux de l'Apothecaire ordinaire.* Beziers: Iean Martel, 1616.

[Patin, Gui]. *Le nez povrry de Theophraste Renavdot, Grand Gazettier de France, et Espion de Mazarin.* [S.l. n.d. (ca. 1644)].

Lettres . . . Nouvelle Édition augmentée de lettres inédites, précédée d'une notice Biographique . . . par J. -H. Reveillé-Parise. 3 vols. Paris: J. -B. Baillière, 1846.

de Peiresc, Nicolas-Claude Fabri. *Lettres de Peiresc publiées par Philippe Tamizey de Larroque . . . Tome quatrième. Lettres de Peiresc à Borilly, à Bouchard et à Gassendi. Lettres de Gassendi à Peiresc 1626–1637.* Paris: Imprimerie national, 1893.

Pernety, Antoine-Joseph. *Dictionnaire Mytho-Hérmetique, dans lequel on trouve les Allégories Fabuleuses des Poetes, les Métaphores, les Enigmes et les Termes barbares des Philosophes Hermétiques expliqués.* Paris: Bauche, 1758.

Perreau, Jacques. *Rabbat-Ioye de L'Antimoine Triomphant, ov Examen de l'Antimoine Iustifié de M. Evsèbe Renaudot.* Paris: Gaspar Metvras, 1655 (over 1654).

de Planis Campy, David. *L'hydre morbifique exterminee par L'hercvle ov Les sept Maladies tenuës pour incurable iusques à present rendues guerissables par l'Art Chymique Medical . . .* Paris: Herué du Mesnil, 1628.

Les Oevvres . . . Contenant Les plus beaux traictez de la Medecine Chymique que les Anciens Autheurs ont enseigné. . . . Paris: Denys Moreau, 1646.

Poleman, Joachim. *Nouvelle Lumière de Medecine, du Mistere ou Souffre des Philosophes.* Rouen: Guillaume Behourt, 1721.

Poli, Martino. Spargirico in Roma, aggregato alla Reale Accademia delle Scienze in Parigi. *Il Trionfo degli Acidi vendicati dalle calunnie di molti Moderni: Opera Filosofica e Medica Fondata sopra de Principij Chemici & adornata di varij esperimenti; Contro Il Sistema, e Prattica delli Moderni Democritici & Epicurei Reformati . . .* Rome: Giorgio Placho, 1706.

[Pousse, François]. *Examen des Principes des Alchymistes sur la Pierre Philosophale.* Paris: Daniel Jollet Chez Berthelmy Girin, 1711.

Raguet, Sieur. *Dissertation sur Diverses Maladies et sur l'Usage de l'Esprit Philosophique; Avec un Recueil des principales quérisons opérées par ce Reméde.* Paris: Aux depéns du Sieur Raguet, Auteur de l'Esprit Philosophique, 1758.

Renaudot, Eusèbe. Conseiller Medecin du Roy, Docteur Regent en la Faculté de Medecin à Paris. *L'Antimoine Ivstifie et L'Antimoine Triomphant ov Discours*

Apologetique faisant voir que la Poudre; & la Vin Emetique & les autres remedes tirés de l'Antimoine ne sont point veneneux, mais souuerains pour guerir la pluspart des maladies, qui y sont exactement expliquées. Auec leurs preparations les plus curieuses tant de la Pharmacie, que de la Chymie. Paris: Iean Henault, [1653].

Editor. *A General Collection of Discourses of the virtuosi of France, upon Questions of all sorts of philosophy, and other natural knowledge.* Translated by G. Havers. London: Thomas Dring and John Starkey, 1664.

Another Collection of Philosophical Conferences of the French Virtuosi upon Questions of all Sorts; For the Improving of Natural Knowledge. Made in the Assembly of the Beaux Esprits at Paris, by the most Ingenious Persons of that Nation. Translated by G. Havers and J. Davies. London: Thomas Dring and John Starkey, 1665.

Editor. *Recveil General des Qvestions traitées és Conferences du Bureau d'Adresse, sur toutes sortes de Matieres. Par les plus beaux Esprits de ce Temps.* 6 vols. Lyon: Antoine Valançol, 1666.

Del Rio, Martin Antoine. *Disquisitionum magicarum.* Lugduni: Apud Horativm Cardon, 1612. First edition, 1599.

Riolan, Jean (the Elder). *Ad Libavi Maniam . . . Responsio pro Censura Scholae Parisiensis contra Alchymiam lata.* Paris: In Officina Plantiniana, apud Adrianum Perier, 1606.

[Riolan, Jean (the Younger)]. *Ioannis Antarveti Medicinae Candidati. Apologia pro iudicio Scholę de Alchimia. Ad Harueti & Baucyneti recoctam crambem.* Paris: Hadrian Perier, 1604.

Riolan, Jean (the Younger). *Cvrievses Recherches svr les Escholes en Medecine, De Paris et de Montpelier, Necessaires d'estre sçeuës, pour la conseruation de la vie.* Paris: Gaspar Metvras, 1651.

de Rochas, Henry. *Sieur d'Ayglun, Medecin ordinaire du Roy. La Vray Anatomie Spagyrique, des Eaux Mineralles, et de Toutes les Choses qui les composent, auec leurs qualitez & vertus, curieusement obseruées.* Paris: Pierre Billaine, 1637.

La physique Reformee, contenant la Refvtation des Erreurs populaires, et le Triomphe des veritez philosophique, La Genealogie des Elemens, & des Principes, l'origine, & les operations de la Nature, en la generation & production des Animaux, Vegetaux, & Mineraux. Paris: Pierre Lamy, 1638.

[Rosicrucians]. *The Fame and Confession of the Fraternity of R:C: Commonly of the Rosie Cross. With a Praeface annexed thereto, and a short Declaration of their Physicall Work.* By Eugenius Philalethes (Thomas Vaughan). London: J. M. for Giles Calvert, 1652.

S. D. E. M. Sieur. *Bibliotheque des Philosophes [Chymiques] ou Recueil des Oeuvres des Auteurs les Plus approuvez qui ont écrit de la Pierre Philosophale. Tome Premier Contenant sept Traitez qui sont énoncez dans la page suivant. Avec un Discours, servant de Preface, sur la verité de la Science, & touchant les Auteurs qui sont dans ce Volume. Et une Liste des Termes de l'Art, & des Mots anciens qui se trouvent dans ces Traitez, avec leur explication.* Paris: Charles Angot, 1672. A second volume appeared in 1678.

de Saint André, François. *Docteur en Medecine de la Faculté de Caen. Entretiens sur l'Acide et sur l'Alkali, Où sont examineés les objections de Mr. Boyle contre ces principes. Avec une replique à la Lettre de Mr. S . . . Docteur en Medecine aggregé au College de^{xxx} touchant la nature de ces deux sels.* Paris: Lambert Roulland, 1677. 1st ed., 1672; 3rd ed., 1680.

Sanctorius, Sanctorius. *La Medecine Statique de Sanctorius, ou l'Art de se conserver la santé par la transpiration.* Translated by Charles Le Breton. Paris: Claude Jombert, 1722.

Scot, Reginald. *The Discoverie of Witchcraft* [1584], with an introduction by the Rev. Montague Summers. New York: Dover, 1972.

[Sendivogius, Michael]. *Cosmopolite ou Nouvelle Lumière Chymique, Pour servir d'éclairissement aux trois Principes de la Nature, exactement décrits dans les trois Traitez suivans. Le Ier. De la Nature en générale, où il est parlé du Mercure. Le II. Du Soufre. Le III. Du vray Sel des Philosophes. Derneire Edition, Revûë & Augmentée De la Lettre Philosophique d'Antoine Duval. Et de l'Estrait d'une autre Lettre assez curieuse.* Paris: Laurent d'Houry, 1723.

Servetus, Michael. *A Complete Account of Syrups Carefully Refined According to the Judgment of Galen.* . . . In Michael Servetus, *A Translation of his Geographical, Medical and Astrological Writings with Introductions and Notes.* Translated by Charles Donald O'Malley. Philadelphia: American Philosophical Society, 1953.

Severinus, Peter. *Idea medicinae philosophicae. Continens Fundamenta totius doctrinae Paracelsicae Hippocraticae & Galenicae.* 3rd ed. Hagae-Comitis, 1660.

Sonnet, Thomas. *Sieur de Courval, Docteur en Medecine, Gentilhomme Virois. Satyre. Contre les Charlatans et Pseudomedecins Empiriques. En laquelle sont amplement descouuertes les ruses & tromperies de tous Theriacleurs, Alchemistes, Chimistes, Paracelsistes, Distillateurs, Extracteurs, & de Qvintescences, Fondeurs d'or Potable, Maistres de l'Elixir, & telle pernicieuse engeance d'imposteurs.* . . . Paris: Iean Milot, 1610.

Stahl, George Ernest. *Philosophical Principles of Universal Chemistry: Or, The Foundation of a scientific Manner of Inquiring into and Preparing the Natural and Artificial Bodies for the Uses of Life* . . . *Design'd as a General Introduction to the Knowledge and Practice of Artificial Philosophy; Or, Genuine Chemistry in all of its Branches. Drawn from the Collegium Jenense of Dr. George Ernest Stahl. By Peter Shaw M.D.* London: Printed for John Osborn and Thomas Longman, 1730.

——— *Fundamenta Chymiae Dogmaticae et Experimentalis, et quidem tum communioris physicae mechanicae pharmaceuticae ac medicae tum sublimioris sic dictae Hermeticae atque alchymicae. Olim in privatos auditorum usus posita, jam vero indultu autoris publicae luci exposita. Annexus est ad coronidis confirmationem tractatus Isaaci Hollandi de salibus et oleis metallorum.* 2nd ed., Nuremburg: Imbensis B. Guolfg. Maur. Endteri, 1746.

Suau, Jean. *Traitez contenans la pvre et vraye Doctrine de la Peste & de la Coqueluche, Les Impostures Spagyriques, & plusieurs abus de la Medecine, Chirurgie, & Pharmacie, tres doctes, & tres-vtiles.* Paris: Didier Millot, 1586.

Suavius, Leo. See Jacques Gohory.

Sylvius, Franciscus de la Boë. *Opera Medica.* Amsterdam: Daniel Elsevier and Abraham Wolfgang, 1680.

Theatrum chemicum. Edited by Lazarus Zetzner. 2nd ed., 4 vols., Strasbourg: Zetzner, 1613; 5th vol., 1622. 3rd ed., 6 vols., Strasbourg: Zetzner, 1659–61.

[Thévart, Jacques]. *La Defense De la Faculté de Medecine de Paris. Contre Me Françoise Blondel Docteur Regent en ladite Faculté.* British Library copy missing title page, ca. 1666. A second defense by Thévart appeared in 1668.

Tollius, Jacobus. *La chemin du ciel chymique.* Paris: Laurent d'Houry, 1688.

Tymme, Thomas. *A Dialogue Philosophicall.* London: T. S[nodham] for C. Knight, 1612.

Venel, Gabriel François. "Chymie." In *Encyclopédie, ou Dictionnaire Raissonné des Sciences, des Arts et des Métiers.* Edited by M. Diderot and M. D'Alembert. Vol. 3. Paris: Briasson, David, Le Breton and Durand, 1753.

Vieussens, Raymond. Medecin de la Faculté de Montpelier. *Deux dissertations . . . Le Premiere Touchant l'extraction du Sel acide du Sang, La Second Sur la proportion de quantité de ses principes sensibles.* Montpelier: Honoré Pech, 1698.

Medecin ordinaire du Roi, de l'Académie des Sciences de Paris, & de la Societé Royale de Londres. *Traité Nouveau de la Structure et des Causes du Mouvement Natural du Coeur.* 2 vols. Toulouse: Jean Guillemette, 1715.

de Vigenère, Blaise. *Traicte dv Fev et dv Sel.* Rouen: Iacqves Caillové, 1642.

A Discovrse of Fire and Salt, Discovering many Secret Mysteries, as well Philosophical as Theologicall. Translated by Edward Stephens. London: Richard Cotes, 1649.

Villars, Nicholas Pierre Henri de Montfaucon. *Le Comte de Gabalis, ou Entretiens sur les sciences secrets. Nouvelle edition, augmentés des Genies assistans & des Gnomes irreconciliables.* Londres: Chez les Freres Vaillant, 1742.

Violet, Fabius. *La Parfaicte et Entiere Cognoissance de tovtes les Maladies du corps humain, causées par obstruction.* Paris: Pierre Billaine, 1635.

Wier, Jean. *Cinq Livres de l'impostvre et tromperie des diables: des enchantements & sorcelleries. . . .* Translated by Jacques Grévin. Paris: Iacques du Puys, 1567.

Histoires Dispvtes et Discovrs des Illvsions et Impostvres des Diables, des Magiciens infames, sorcieres et Empoisonnevrs: des Ensorcelez et Demoniaques. . . . 2 vols. Paris: Aux bureaux du Progrès Médical and A. Delahaye et Lescrosnier, 1885. This is a reprint of the 1579 edition which includes two dialogues on sorcerers and their punishment by Thomas Erastus.

Willis, Thomas. *Practice of Physick. . . .* Translated by S. Pordage. London: T. Dring, C. Harper and J. Leigh, 1681.

Wimpenaeus, Johannes Albertus. *De concordia Hippocraticorum et Paracelsistarum libri magni excursiones defensiuae, cum appendice, quid medico sit faciundum.* Munich: Adamus Berg, 1569.

Woodall, John. *The Surgions Mate.* London: E. Griffen for L. Lisle, 1617.

Secondary sources

Appleby, John H. "Arthur Dee's Associations Before Visiting Russia Clarified, Including Two Letters from Sir Theodore Mayerne." *Ambix*, 26 (1979), 1–15.

Astruc, Jean. *Mémoires pour servir a l'Histoire de la Faculté de Medecine de Montpellier . . . .* Revus & publiés par M. Lorry. Paris: P. C. Calalier, 1767.

Baader, G. "Jacques Dubois as a Practitioner." In A. Wear, R. K. French, and I. M. Lonie, Editors. *The Medical Renaissance of the Sixteenth Century,* pp. 146–54. Cambridge University Press, 1985.

Badel, Pierre-Yves. "De quelques lectures alchimiques du *Roman de la Rose.*" Paper presented at the Renaissance Conference of the Newberry Library. Spring, 1987.

Baumann, E. D. *François de la Boë Sylvius (1614–1672).* Leiden: E. J. Brill, 1949.

Bérard, M. F. *Doctrine Médicale de l'Ecole de Montpellier, et Comparison de ses principes avec ceux des autres écoles d'Europe.* Montpellier et a Paris: Librairie au Rabais, 1819.

Bila, Constantin. *La croyance a la magie au XVIIIe siécle en France dans les contes, roman & traités*. Paris: J. Gambier, 1925.

Boas, Marie. "Acid and Alkali in Seventeenth-Century Chemistry." *Archives Internationales d'Histoire des Sciences, 9* (1956), 13–28.

Brockliss, L. W. B. "Medical Teaching at the University of Paris 1600–1720." *Annals of Science, 35* (1978), 221–51.

"Aristotle, Descartes and the New Science: Natural Philosophy at the University of Paris 1600–1750." *Annals of Science, 38* (1981), 33–69.

French Higher Education in the 17th and 18th Centuries: A Cultural History. Oxford: Clarendon Press, 1987.

"The Medico-Religious Universe of an Early 18th Century Parisian Doctor: The Case of Philippe Hecquet." In *The Medical Revolution of the 17th Century.* Edited by Roger French and Andrew Wear. Cambridge University Press, 1989, pp. 191–221.

Broeckx, C. *Commentaire de J. B. van Helmont sur le premier livre du Régime d'Hippocrate: Peri diaites.* Antwerp: 1849.

Interrogatoires de J. B. van Helmont sur le magnétisme animal. Anvers: Buschmann, 1856.

Buck, A. "La contribution humaniste à la formation de l'esprit scientifique." In *Sciences de la Renaissance* (VIIIe Congrès International de Tours), pp. 41–8. Edited by Jacques Roger. Paris: J. Vrin, 1973.

"La polémique humaniste contre les sciences." In *Sciences de la Renaissance* (VIIIe Congrès International de Tours), pp. 33–40. Edited by Jacques Roger. Paris: J. Vrin, 1973.

Cafiero, Lisa. "Robert Fludd e la polemica con Gassendi." *Revista Critica di Storia della Filosofia, 19* (1964), 367–410; *20* (1965), 3–15.

Chevalier, A. G. "The 'Antimony-War' – A Dispute Between Montpellier and Paris." *Ciba Symposia, 2* (1940), 418–23.

Clarke, Jack A. *Gabriel Naudé, 1600–1653.* Hamden, Conn.: Archon Books, 1970.

Copeman, W. S. C. *Doctors and Disease in Tudor Times.* London: William Dawson and Sons, 1960.

Corleiu, Dr. August. *L'ancienne Faculté de Médecine de Paris.* Paris: V. Adrien Delahaye et C^c, Libraires-Éditeurs, 1877.

Couliano, Ioan P. *Eros and Magic in the Renaissance.* Translated by Margaret Cook with a foreword by Mircea Eliade. Chicago: University of Chicago Press, 1987.

Crombie, A. C. *Augustine to Galileo: The History of Science A.D. 400–1650.* Cambridge, Mass: Harvard University Press, 1953.

Daems, Willem F. *Stimmi Stibium Antimon: Eine substanzhistorische Betrachtung.* Arlesheim, Switzerland: Weleda AG, 1976.

Debus, Allen G. "Robert Fludd and the Circulation of the Blood." *Journal of the History of Medicine and Allied Sciences, 16* (1961), 374–93.

"Solution Analyses Prior to Robert Boyle." *Chymia, 8* (1962), 41–61.

"An Elizabethan History of Medical Chemistry." *Annals of Science, 18* (1962, published 1964), 1–29.

"Robert Fludd and the Use of Gilbert's *De magnete* in the Weapon-Salve Controversy." *Journal of the History of Medicine and Allied Sciences, 19,* (1964), 389–417.

"The Paracelsian Aerial Niter," *Isis, 55* (1964), 43–61.

"The Significance of the History of Early Chemistry." *Cahiers d'Histoire Mondiale*, 9 (1965), 39–58.

"The Sun in the Universe of Robert Fludd." *Le Soleil à la Renaissance – Sciences et Mythes*, Travaux de l'Institut pour l'étude de la Renaissance et de l'Humanisme, 2, pp. 257–78. Brussels: P.U.B./P.U.F, 1965.

The English Paracelsians. London: Oldbourne Press, 1965; New York: Franklin Watts, 1966.

"Fire Analysis and the Elements in the Sixteenth and the Seventeenth Centuries." *Annals of Science*, 23 (1967), 127–47.

"Mathematics and Nature in the Chemical Texts of the Renaissance." *Ambix*, 15 (1968), 1–28; 211.

"Palissy, Plat and English Agricultural Chemistry in the 16th and 17th Centuries." *Archives Internationales d'Histoire des Sciences*, 21 (1968), 67–88.

The Chemical Dream of the Renaissance. Churchill College, Cambridge. Overseas Lecture Series, No. 3. Cambridge: Heffer, 1968.

Science and Education in the Seventeenth Century. The Webster Ward Debate. London: Macdonald and Co.; New York: American Elsevier, 1970.

"Joseph Duchesne." In *Dictionary of Scientific Biography*, vol. 4, pp. 208–10. New York: Scribner's, 1971.

"Guintherius-Libavius-Sennert: The Chemical Compromise in Early Modern Medicine." In *Science, Medicine and Society in the Renaissance*, vol. 1, pp. 151–65. 2 vols. Edited by Allen G. Debus. New York: Science History Publications, 1972.

"The Paracelsians and the Chemists: The Chemical Dilemma in Renaissance Medicine." *Clio Medica*, 7 (1972), 185–99.

"Motion in the Chemical Texts of the Renaissance." *Isis*, 64 (1973), 4–17.

"A Further Note on Palingenesis: The Account of Ebenezer Sibly, in *The Illustration of Astrology* (1792)." *Isis*, 64 (1973), 226–30.

"La philosophie chimique de la Renaissance et ces Relations avec la chimie de la fin du XVIIᵉ siècle." *Sciences de la Renaissance. VIIIᵉ Congrès Internationalde Tours* (1965), pp. 273–283. Edited by Jacques Roger. Paris: J. Vrin, 1973.

"Alchemy." *Dictionary of the History of Ideas*, 1, pp. 27–34. 5 vols. Executive Editor, Philip P. Wiener. New York: Charles Scribner's Sons, 1973–4.

"Petrus Severinus." In *Dictionary of Scientific Biography*, vol. 12, pp. 334–6. New York: Scribner's, 1975.

The Chemical Philosophy: Paracelsian Science and Medicine in the Sixteenth and Seventeenth Centuries. 2 vols. New York: Science History Publications, 1977.

Man and Nature in the Renaissance. Cambridge University Press, 1978.

"Chemistry, Pharmacy and Cosmology: A Renaissance Union." *Pharmacy in History*, 20 (1978), 125–37.

Robert Fludd and His Philosophical Key: Being a Transcription of the manuscript at Trinity College, Cambridge, with an Introduction by Allen G. Debus. New York: Science History Publications, 1979.

"The Paracelsians in Eighteenth Century France: A Renaissance Tradition in the Age of the Enlightenment." *Ambix*, 28 (1981), 36–54.

"The Paracelsians in Eighteenth Century France: A Renaissance Tradition in the Age of the Enlightenment." In *Transformation and Tradition in the Sciences: Essays in Honor of I. Bernard Cohen*, pp. 193–214. Edited by Everett Mendelsohn. Cambridge University Press, 1984.

"History with a Purpose: The Fate of Paracelsus." *Pharmacy in History, 26* (1984), 83–96.

"Chemistry and the Quest for a Material Spirit of Life in the Seventeenth Century." In *Spiritus: IV° Colloquio Internazionale del Lessico Intellettuale Europeo, Roma, 7–9 gennaio 1983,* pp. 245–63. Edited by M. Fattori and M. Bianchi. Rome: Edizioni dell'Ateneo, 1984.

"The Role of Chemistry in the Scientific Revolution." *Lias: Sources and Documents Relating to the Early Modern History of Ideas,* 13 (1986), 139–50.

"Chemistry and Iatrochemistry in Early Eighteenth-Century Portugal: A Spanish Connection." In *Historia e Desenvolvimento da Ciência em Portugal: I Colóquio – até ao Século XX. Lisboa, 15 a 19 Abril de 1985.* 2 vols., pp. 1245–62. Secretary-General of the colloquium, Prof. Doutor António Vasconcellos Marques. Lisboa: Academia das Ciências de Lisboa, 1986.

"Chemistry and the Universities in the Seventeenth Century." *Academiae Analecta: Klasse der Wetenschappen, 48* (1986), 13–33.

Chemistry, Alchemy and the New Philosophy, 1550–1700. London: Variorum Reprints, 1987.

"Myth, Allegory, and the Scientific Truth: An Alchemical Tradition in the Period of the Scientific Revolution." *Nouvelles de la Republique des Lettres,* 1987. Part 1, 13–35.

"The Chemical Philosophy and the Scientific Revolution." In *Revolutions in Science: Their Meaning and Relevance,* pp. 27–48. Edited by William R. Shea. Canton, Mass: Science History Publications, 1988.

"Alchemy in an Age of Reason: The Chemical Philosophers in Early Eighteenth Century France." In *Hermeticism and the Renaissance: Intellectual History and the Occult in Early Modern Europe,* pp. 231–50. Edited by Ingrid Merkel and Allen G. Debus. Washington: Folger Books; The Folger Shakespeare Library/London and Toronto, Associated University Presses, 1989.

"Quantification and Medical Motivation: Factors in the Interpretation of Early Modern Chemistry." *Pharmacy in History* 31 (1989), 3–11.

"Iatrochemistry and the Chemical Revolution." In *Alchemy Revisited: Proceedings of the International Conference on the History of Alchemy at the University of Groningen 17–19 April 1989,* pp. 51–66. Edited by Z. R. W. M. von Martels. Leiden, New York, Copenhagen, Köln, 1990.

Dictionary of Scientific Biography. Charles C. Gillespie, Ed. in Chief. 16 vols. New York: Scribner's, 1970–80.

Dictionnaire des Biographies. Publié sous la Direction de Pierre Grimal. 2 vols. Paris: Presses Universitaires de France, 1958.

Dulieu, Louis. *La pharmacie à Montpellier.* Avignon: Les Presses Universelles, 1973.

La Medecine à Montpellier. 3 vols. [I. Le Môyen Age, 1975; II. La Renaissance, 1979; III. L'Époch classique, 1983.] Avignon: Les Presses Universelles.

Duveen, Denis I. *Bibliotheca alchemica et chemica.* London: Dawsons, 1949.

Felix, Annette. "Les débuts et les titulaires de la chaire de chimie à la Faculté de Medecine de l'ancienne Université de Louvain." *RBPH: Revue Belge de Philologie et d'Histoire,* 64 (1986), 234–55.

Ferguson, John. *Bibliotheca Chemica: A Bibliography of Books on Alchemy, Chemistry and Pharmaceutics.* 2 vols. London: Derek Verschoyle Academic and Bibliographical Publications Ltd., 1954. 1st ed. 1906.

Forbes, R. J. *Studies in Ancient Technology.* Vol. 7. Leiden: E. J. Brill, 1963.

Fourés, Auguste. *Les Hommes de l'Aude*. 2 vols. Narbonne: impr. F. Caillard, 1889, 1891.

Galluzzi, Paolo. "Motivi Paracelsiani nella Toscana di Cosmio II e di Don Antonio Dei Medici: alchemia, medicina 'chimica' e riforma del sapere." In *Scienza credenze occulte livelli di cultura*, pp. 31–62. Florence: Olschki, 1982.

Gardner, F. Leigh. *A Catalogue Raissonné of Works on the Occult Sciences. Vol. 1. Rosicrucian Books*. Introduction by Dr. William Wynn Westcott. 2nd ed., privately printed, 1923.

Gibbs, F. W. "Boerhaave's Chemical Writings." *Ambix*, 6 (1958), 117–35.

Gibson, Thomas. "A Sketch of the Career of Theodore Turquet de Mayerne." *Annals of Medical History*, N.S., 5 (1933), 315–26.

Giese, Ernest and Benno Von Hagen. *Geschichte der medizinische Fakultat der Friedrich-Schiller-Universitat Jena*. Jena: VEB Gustav Fischer Verlag, 1958.

Gillispie, Charles C. *The Edge of Objectivity*. Princeton: Princeton University Press, 1960.

"The *Encyclopédie* and the Jacobin Philosophy of Science." In *Critical Problems in the History of Science*, pp. 255–89. Edited by Marshall Clagett. Madison: University of Wisconsin Press, 1962.

Goltz, Dietlinde. "Die Paracelsisten und die Sprache." *Sudhoffs Archiv für Geschichte der Medizin und der Naturwissenschaften*, 56 (1972), 337–52.

Guerlac, Henry. "Guy de La Brosse and the French Paracelsians." In *Science, Medicine and Society in the Renaissance: Essays to Honor Walter Pagel*. Vol. 1, pp. 177–99. Edited by Allen G. Debus. 2 vols. New York: Science History Publications, 1972.

Gunther, R. T. *Early Science in Oxford*. 15 vols. Oxford: Printed for the Subscribers, 1922–67.

Early Science in Cambridge. Oxford: Printed for the Author at the Press, 1937.

Haigh, Elizabeth. *Xavier Bichat and the Medical Theory of the Eighteenth Century. Medical History*, Supplement 4. London: Wellcome Institute for the History of Medicine, 1984.

Halleux, Robert. "Un alchimiste liégeois au XVIIe siècle?" *Bull. de l'Institut Archélogique Liégeois*, 87 (1975), 21–30.

"Gnose et expérience dans la philosophie chimique de Jean-Baptiste Van Helmont." *Bulletin de l'Académie royale de Belgique* (Classe des Sciences), 5th série, 65 (1979), 217–29.

"Helmontiana." *Academiae Analecta*, 45 (1983), 33–63.

"Le Mythe de Nicolas Flamel ou les Mécanismes de la Pseudépigraphie alchimique." *Archives internationales d'Histoire des Sciences*, 33 (1983), 234–55.

Hamy, E. T. "Quelques notes sur la mort et la succession de Guy de La Brosse." *Bulletin du Muséum d'Histoire Naturelle*, 2 (1897), 152–4.

"Un précurseur de Guy de la Brosse. Jacques Gohory et le Lycium Philosophal de Saint-Marceau-les-Paris (1571–1576)." *Nouvelles Archives du Museum d'Histoire naturelle*. 4th Ser., 1 (1899), 1–26.

"La famille de Guy de La Brosse." *Bulletin du Muséum d'Histoire Naturelle*, 6 (1900), 13–16.

Hannaway, Owen. "Jacques Gohory." In *Dictionary of Scientific Biography*, vol. 5, pp. 447–8. New York: Scribner's, 1972.

The Chemists and the Word: The Didactic Origins of Chemistry. Baltimore: The Johns Hopkins Press, 1975.

Howard Rio. "Guy de La Brosse: Botanique et chimie au début de la révolution scientifique." *Revue d'Histoire des Sciences, 31* (1978), 301–26.

"Guy de La Brosse and the Jardin des Plantes in Paris." In *The Analytic Spirit. Essays in the History of Science in Honor of Henry Guerlac,* pp. 195–224. Edited by Harry Woolf. Ithaca: Cornell University Press, 1981.

"Medicine and the royal patronage of science in the early seventeenth century." Unpublished paper presented at the Toronto meeting of the History of Science Society, 1981.

La Bibliothéque et le Laboratorie de Guy de La Brosse au Jardin des Plantes à Paris. Geneva: Libraire Droz, 1983.

Howe, H. A. "A Root of van Helmont's Tree." *Isis, 56* (1965), 408–19.

Hubicki, Wlodzimierz. "The beginnings of chemistry as a university science." *Actes du XIᵉ Congrès Internationale d'Histoire des Sciences. Varsovie-Cracovie 24–31 Août 1965.* Vol. 4, pp. 41–5. Ossolineum: Académie Polonaise des Sciences, 1968.

Isler, Hansruedi. *Thomas Willis 1621–1675. Doctor and Scientist.* London: Hafner, 1968.

Joly, Bernard. *Les formes de rationalité à l'oeuvre dans la pensée alchimique au XVIIᵉᵐᵉ siècle, Traduction commentée du Manuscriptum ad Fredericum de Pierre-Jean Fabre.* Thèse de doctorat (nouveau régime) Philosophie sous la direction de Jean-Paul Dumont. 2 vols. Université de Lille III, 1988.

"La réception de la pensée de Van Helmont dans l'oeuvre de Pierre-Jean Fabre." In *Alchemy Revisited: Proceedings of the International Conference on the History of Alchemy at the University of Groningen 17–19 April 1989,* pp. 206–14. Edited by Z. R. W. M. von Martels. Leiden, New York, Copenhagen, Köln, 1990.

Kent, A. and Owen Hannaway. "Some New Considerations on Beguin and Libavius." *Annals of Science, 16* (1960), 241–50.

King, Lester S. "Stahl and Hoffman: A Study in Eighteenth Century Animism." *Journal of the History of Medicine and Allied Sciences, 19* (1964), 118–30.

The Road to Medical Enlightenment 1650–1695. London: Macdonald; New York: American Elsevier, 1970.

"Georg Ernst Stahl." In *Dictionary of Scientific Biography,* vol. 12, pp. 599–606. New York: Scribner's, 1975.

The Philosophy of Medicine: The Early Eighteenth Century. Cambridge, Mass.: Harvard University Press, 1978.

de la Tourette, Gilles. *Théophraste Renaudot d'Après des documents inédits.* Paris: Plon, 1884.

Lemoine, Albert. *Le vitalisme et l'animisme de Stahl.* Paris: Germer Baillière, 1864.

Lenoble, Robert. *Mersenne ou la naissance de mécanisme.* Paris: Vrin, 1943; reprint 1971.

Lindeboom, G. A. *Herman Boerhaave. The Man and His Work.* London: Methuen & Co., Ltd., 1968.

"Hermann Boerhaave." In *Dictionary of Scientific Biography,* pp. 224–8. Vol. 2. New York: Scribner's, 1970.

Lingo, Alison Klairmont. "Empirics and Charlatans in Early Modern France: The Genesis of the Classification of the 'Other' in Medical Practice." *Journal of Social History, 19* (1985/1986), 583–603.

López Piñero, José Maria. "La iatroquimica de la segunda mitad del siglo XVII."

In *Historia de la Medicina*. Vol. 4, pp. 279–95. Edited by Pedro Lain Engralgo. Barcelona: Salvat Editores, 1973.

"Eighteenth Century Medical Vitalism; The Paracelsian Connection." In *Revolutions in Science: Their Meaning and Relevance*, pp. 117–32. Edited by William R. Shea. Canton, Mass.: Science History Publications, 1988.

Maddison, Francis, Margaret Pelling, and Charles Webster, Editors. *Essays on the Life and Work of Thomas Linacre c. 1460–1524*. Oxford: Clarendon Press, 1977.

Marvick, E. W. "The Character of Louis XIII: The Role of His Physician." *Journal of Interdisciplinary History*, 4 (1974), 347–74.

Marx, Jacques. "Alchimie et Palingénésie." *Isis*, 62 (1971), 274–89.

Meinel, Christoph. "*Artibus Academicus Inserenda*: Chemistry's Place in Eighteenth and Early Nineteenth Century Universities." *History of Universities*, 7 (1988), 89–115.

Merkel, Ingrid, and Allen G. Debus, Editors. *Hermeticism and the Renaissance: Intellectual History and the Occult in Early Modern Europe*. Washington: Folger Books; The Folger Shakespeare Library; London and Toronto: Associated University Presses, 1988.

Metzger, Hélène. *Les doctrines chimiques en France du début du XVIIᵉ à la fin du XVIIIᵉ siècle, prémiere partie*. Paris: P.U.F., 1923.

Newton, Stahl, Boerhaave et la doctrine chimique. Paris: Félix Alcan, 1930.

La méthode philosophique en histoire des sciences: textes 1914–1939. Edited by Gad Freudenthal. Tours: Fayard, 1987.

Mévergnies, Paul Nève de. *Jean-Baptiste van Helmont. Philosophe par le feu*. Paris: Librairie E. Droz, 1935.

"Sur les lettres de J. B. van Helmont au P. Marin Mersenne." *Revue Belge de Philosophie et d'Histoire*, 26 (1948), 61–82.

Montgomery, John Warwick. *Cross and Crucible: Johann Valentin Andreae (1586–1654), Phoenix of the Theologians*. The Hague: M. Nijhoff, 1972.

Multhauf, Robert P. "John of Rupescissa and the Origin of Medical Chemistry." *Isis*, 45 (1954), 359–67.

"Medical Chemistry and 'The Paracelsians'." *Bulletin of the History of Medicine*, 28 (1954), 101–26.

"The Significance of Distillation in Renaissance Medical Chemistry." *Bulletin of the History of Medicine*, 30 (1956), 329–46.

The Origins of Chemistry. London: Oldbourne, 1966.

Murphy, Terence D. "The Transformation of Traditional Medical Culture under the Old Regime." *Historical Reflections/Reflexions Historiques*, 16 (1989), 307–50.

Nelli, René. "Pierre-Jean Fabre médecin spagirique et alchimiste 1588–1658." *La Tour Saint Jacques*, no. 16, July/August 1958, 36–50.

Neu, John, Editor. *Chemical, Medical and Pharmaceutical Books Printed before 1800. In the Collections of the University of Wisconsin Libraries*. Madison and Milwaukee: The University of Wisconsin Press, 1965.

Niebyl, Peter H. "Galen, van Helmont, and Blood Letting." In *Science, Medicine and Society in the Renaissance*, pp. 13–23. Vol. 2. Edited by Allen G. Debus. New York: Science History Publications; London: Heinemann, 1971.

Nouvelle Biographie Général depuis les Temps les plus Reculés jusqu'a 1850–60 avec les Renseignements Bibliographiques et l'indication des sources a consulter. Publiée par MM. Firmin Didot Frères sous la direction de M. Le Dr. Hoefer. 46 vols. in 23 vols. Copenhagen: Rosenkilde et Bagger, 1963–9.

Oldroyd, David. "An examination of G. E. Stahl's *Principles of Universal Chemistry.*" *Ambix*, 20 (1973), 36–52.

O'Malley, C. D. *Andreas Vesalius of Brussels 1514–1564*. Berkeley: University of California Press, 1964.

"Joannes Guinter." In *Dictionary of Scientific Biography*, pp. 585–6. Vol. 5. New York: Scribner's, 1972.

Packard, Francis R. *Guy Patin and the Medical Profession in Paris in the XVIIth Century* (London: Oxford University Press, 1924).

Pagel, Walter. *Jo. Bapt. Van Helmont. Einführung in die philosophische Medizin des Barock*. Berlin: Julius Springer, 1930.

"Helmont. Leibniz. Stahl." *Sudhoffs Archiv für Geschichte der Medizin*, 24 (1931), 19–59.

"The Religious and Philosophical Aspects of van Helmont's Science and Medicine." *Bulletin of the History of Medicine*. Supp. No. 2. Baltimore: Johns Hopkins Press, 1944.

"Harvey and the Purpose of the Circulation." *Isis*, 42 (1951), 22–38.

"The Reaction to Aristotle in Seventeenth-Century Biological Thought." *Science, Medicine and History. Essays in Honour of Charles Singer*, pp. 489–509. Edited by E. A. Underwood. Vol. 1. London: Oxford University Press, 1953.

"J. B. Van Helmont's Reformation of the Galenic Doctrine of Digestion – and Paracelsus." *Bulletin of the History of Medicine*, 29 (1955), 563–8.

"Van Helmont's Ideas on Gastric Digestion and the Gastric Acid." *Bulletin of the History of Medicine*, 30 (1956), 524–36.

"The Position of Harvey and Van Helmont in the History of European Thought." *Journal of the History of Medicine and Allied Sciences*, 13 (1958), 186–98.

Das medizinische Weltbild des Paracelsus: seine Zusämmenhange mit Neuplatonismus und Gnosis. Kosmosophie, Band I. Wiesbaden: Franz Steiner, 1962.

William Harvey's Biological Ideas: Selected Aspects and Historical Background. Basel: S. Karger, 1967.

"Thomas Erastus." In *Dictionary of Scientific Biography*. Vol. 4, pp. 386–8. New York: Scribner's, 1971.

Joan Baptista van Helmont: Reformer of Science and Medicine. Cambridge University Press, 1982.

Paracelsus. An Introduction to Philosophical Medicine in the Era of the Renaissance. Basel: S. Karger, 1958. Reprinted with "Addenda and Errata." Basel: Karger, 1982.

The Smiling Spleen: Paracelsianism in Storm and Stress. Basel: Karger, 1984.

Partington, J. R. *A History of Chemistry*, vol. 2. London: Macmillan, 1961; vol. 3, London: Macmillan, 1962.

Patterson, T. S. "Jean Beguin and his *Tyrocinium Chymicum*." Annals of Science, 2 (1937), 243–98.

Pauli, Wolfgang. "The Influence of Archetypal Ideas on the Scientific Theories of Kepler." In C. G. Jung and W. Pauli, *The Interpretation of Nature and the Psyche*, pp. 147–240. Translated by Priscilla Silz, Bolligen Series, 51. New York: Pantheon Books, 1955.

Pilpoul, Pascal. *La Querelle de l'Antimoine (Essai historique)*. Thèse pour l'Doctorat en Médecine. Paris: Librairie Louis Arnette, 1928.

Pinvert, Lucien. *Jacques Grévin (1538–1570): Étude Biographique et Littéraire*. Paris: A. Fontemoing, 1899.

Rattansi, P. M. "Jean Beguin." In *Dictionary of Scientific Biography*, pp. 571–2. Vol. 1. New York: Scribner's, 1970.

Remington's Pharmaceutical Sciences. Easton Pa.: Mack, 1980.

Roger, Jacques. *Les Sciences de la vie dans la pensée française du XVIIIe siècle: la generation des animaux de Descartes à l'Encyclopédie*. 1963; 2nd ed. Paris: Armand Colin, 1971.

"Chimie et Biologie: des 'molécules organiques' de Buffon à la 'physicochimie' de Lamarck." *History and Philosophy of the Life Sciences*, 1 (1979), 43–64.

Rommelaere, Willem. *Études sur J. -B. Van Helmont*. Brussels: Manceaux, 1868.

Schaff, Georges. "Jean Gontheir d'Andernach (1497–1574) et la médecine de son temps." In *Médecine et Assistance en Alsace XVIe–XXe Siècle: Recherches sur l'histoire de la santé*, pp. 20–40. Edited by Georges Levet and Georges Schaff. Strasbourg: Librairie Isten, 1976.

Secret, François. "Palingenesis, Alchemy and Metempsychosis in Renaissance Medicine." *Ambix*, 26 (1979), 81–99.

Shea, William R. "Descartes and the Rosicrucians." *Annali dell'Istituto e Museo di Storia della Scienza di Firenze*, 4 (1979), 29–47.

Sherrington, C. S. *Endeavour of Jean Fernel*. Cambridge University Press, 1946.

Smeaton, W. A. "Etienne François Geoffroy." In *Dictionary of Scientific Biography*, vol. 5, pp. 352–4. New York: Scribner's, 1972.

"Herman Boerhaave (1668–1738): Physician, Botanist, and Chemist." *Endeavor*, 12 (new series) (1988), 139–42.

Solomon, Howard M. *Public Welfare, Science, and Propaganda in Seventeenth Century France: The Innovations of Théophraste Renaudot*. Princeton, New Jersey: Princeton University Press, 1972.

Van Spronsen, J. W. "The Beginning of Chemistry." In *Leiden University in the 17th Century: An Exchange of Learning*. Edited by Th. H. Lunsingh Scheuleer and G. H. M. Posthumus Meyjes. With the assistance of A. G. H. Bachrach. Leiden: University Press, Brill, 1975.

Stevenson, Lloyd. "'New Diseases' in the Seventeenth Century." In *Bulletin of the History of Medicine*, 39 (1965), 1–21.

Stone, Howard. "The French Language in Renaissance Medicine." *Bibliothèque d'Humanisme et Renaissance*, 15 (1963), 315–46.

Sudhoff, Karl. "Ein Beitrag zur Bibliographie der Paracelsisten im 16. Jahrhundert." *Centralblatt für Bibliothekswesen*, 10 (1893), 316–26.

Bibliographia Paracelsica. Berlin: Verlag Georg Reimer, 1894. Reprinted Graz: Academische Druck- u. Verlagsanstalt, 1958.

Iatromathematiker vor nehmlich im 15. und 16. Jahrhundert. Breslau: J. U. Kern, 1902.

Temkin, Owsei. *Galenism: Rise and Decline of a Medical Philosophy*. Ithaca and London: Cornell University Press, 1973.

Thickett, D. *Estienne Pasquier (1529–1615): The Versatile Barrister of 16th Century France*. London: Regency Press, 1979.

Thorndike, Lynn. *A History of Magic and Experimental Science.* 8 vols. New York: Columbia University Press, 1923–58.

Trevor-Roper, Hugh. "The Sieur de la Rivière, Paracelsian Physician of Henry IV." In *Science, Medicine and Society in the Renaissance. Essays to Honor Walter Pagel,* vol. 2, pp. 227–50. Edited by Allen G. Debus. 2 vols. New York: Science History Publications, 1972.

"The Paracelsian Movement." In *Renaissance Essays.* London: Secker and Warburg, 1985, pp. 149–99.

Vandevelde, A. J. J. "Helmontiana." In *Verslagen en Mededeelingen, K. Vlaamsche Academie voor Taal-en Letterkunde.* 5 parts. Pt. 1 (1929), pp. 453–76; pt. 2 (1929), pp. 715–37; pt. 3 (1929), pp. 857–79; pt. 4 (1932), pp. 109–22; pt. 5 (1936), pp. 339–87.

Viatte, August. *Les sources occultes du Romanticisme – Illuminisme – Théosophie 1770–1820.* 2 vols. Paris: Champion, 1927; reprinted Paris: Champion, 1969.

Walker, D. P. *Spiritual and Demonic Magic from Ficino to Campanella.* London: The Warburg Institute, 1958.

Walzer, R. *Galen on Jews and Christians.* London: Oxford University Press, 1949.

Wear, A. R., K. French, and I. M. Lonie, Editors. *The Medical Renaissance of the Sixteenth Century.* Cambridge University Press, 1985.

Wightman, W. P. D. *Science and the Renaissance: An Introduction to the Study of the Emergence of the Sciences in the Sixteenth Century.* 2 vols. Edinburgh: Oliver and Boyd, 1962.

Yates, Frances A. *The French Academies of the Sixteenth Century.* London: Warburg Institute, University of London, 1947.

Giordano Bruno and the Hermetic Tradition. Chicago: University of Chicago Press, 1964.

"The Hermetic Tradition in Renaissance Science." *Art, Science, and History in the Renaissance,* pp. 255–74. Edited by Charles Singleton. Baltimore: Johns Hopkins Press, 1968.

The Rosicrucian Enlightenment. London: Routledge & Kegan Paul, 1972.

Zéphrin, Yolande. "Henry et Henry-Louis Rouvière, apothecaires ordinaires du roi, d'après de nouveaux documents." *Revue d'Histoire de la Pharmacie,* 33 (1986), 219–33.

Index

Printed in the United States
By Bookmasters